The Corporate Transformation of Health Care

Can the Public Interest Still Be Served?

ABOUT THE AUTHOR

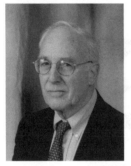

John P. Geyman, MD, is Professor Emeritus of Family Medicine at the University of Washington School of Medicine in Seattle, where he served as department chairman for 14 years. As a board-certified family physician, he has spent 13 years in rural practice and over 25 years in academic medicine.

Dr. Geyman is a member of the Institute of Medicine of the National Academy of Sciences. He was the founding editor of *The Journal of Family Practice* (1973–1990), and served as Editor of *The Journal of the American Board of Family Practice* from 1990 to 2003. He has authored four books of his own, *The Modern Family Doctor and Changing Medical Practice* (1971), *Family Practice: Foundation of Changing Health Care* (1985), *Health Care in America: Can Our Ailing System Be Healed?* (2002), and *Falling Through the Safety Net: Americans Confront the Perils of Health Insurance* (2004). He has co-edited five other books, including *Behavioral Science in Family Practice* (1980), *Family Practice: An International Perspective in Developed Countries* (1983) (translated into Japanese, 1985), *Evidence-Based Clinical Practice: Concepts and Approaches* (2000), and *Textbook of Rural Medicine* (2001). He has also authored or co-authored more than 175 articles and editorials in professional journals concerning various clinical subjects, primary care, medical education, and health policy.

The Corporate Transformation of Health Care

Can the Public Interest Still Be Served?

John P. Geyman, MD

 Springer Publishing Company

Springer Publishing Company, Inc.
11 West 42nd Street
New York, NY 10036

Acquisitions Editor: Ursula Springer
Production Editor: Jeanne W. Libby
Cover design by Joanne Honigman

01 02 03 04 05 / 5 4 3 2 1

Library of Congress Cataloging-in-Publication-Data

Geyman, John P., 1931–
    The corporate transformation of health care : can the public interest be served? / John P. Geyman.
        p. ; cm.
    Includes bibliographical references and index.
    ISBN 0-8261-2466-6
    1. Medical corporations—United States. 2. Medical economics—United States. 3. Multihospital systems—United States. 4. Health mantenance organizations. 5. Public health—United States.
    [DNLM: 1. Delivery of Health Care—economics—United States. 2. Health Facilities, Proprietary—trends—United States. 3. Health Care Reform—organization & administration—United States. 4. Managed Care Programs—economics—United States. 5. Ownership—economics—United States.
    6. Quality of Health Care—United States. W 84 AA.1 G357c 2004] I. Title.

    R728.2.G49 2004
    362.1'0425—dc22   2004019372

Printed in the United States of America by Maple-Vail Book Manufacturing Group.

DEDICATION

To the hundreds of thousands of health professionals laboring under the burdens of our collapsing health care system and the tens of millions of their patients facing its growing unaffordability, may there come a better day.

CONTENTS

LIST OF TABLES AND FIGURES

PREFACE

In 1980 Dr. Arnold Relman, then editor of *The New England Journal of Medicine,* coined the term "medical-industrial complex" and warned of its potentially corrosive effects on health care and health policy. Several years later, study groups within the Institute of Medicine questioned whether investor-owned health care would end up serving the public interest, corporate self-interest, or both. Today we know that a quiet revolution has taken place, although the changes have been too gradual for many to appreciate.

Control of our health care system has shifted over the last 30 years from health professionals and not-for-profit interests to a relatively small number of large health care corporations that are now firmly embedded throughout the health care system. These range from managed care organizations, hospitals, nursing homes, dialysis centers, and medical supply and equipment companies, to a myriad of invisible administrative corporate functions. Many studies which have examined the track records of investor-owned health care corporations are now available. As a result, there are now answers to many concerns raised in the 1980s, such as problems of overuse and fragmentation of services, overemphasis of the business side of health care, and "cream skimming" by commercial interests. As this book will document, the answers are not promising, they call for major reform.

This book has four main goals: (1) to examine the extent of corporate transformation across eight health care industries within the medical-industrial complex; (2) to consider whether this transformation serves the public interest; (3) to assess the impact of these changes on health care costs, on access to and quality of care, and on sustainability of our market-based system; and (4) to consider options for system reform given current political and economic realities. In view of these goals, the focus of this book must necessarily be broad. It cannot be encyclopedic, but will seek out and make sense of credible and up-to-date sources which collectively shed light on questions raised in the 1980s about corporate health care.

My perspective is that of a physician in the broadest of primary care specialties—family practice—with 13 years experience in rural practice, 25 years in academic family medicine (including 14 years as a departmental chairman), and editor of national family practice journals for 30 years. On the basis of my study and research on the health care system, including the publication of *Health Care in America: Can Our Ailing System Be Healed?* and *Falling Through the Safety Net: Americans Confront the Perils of Health Insurance,* I have come to the conclusion that incremental reforms of today's market-based system will continue to be ineffective without conversion to some kind of health insurance based on social goals. I will endeavor to make the case for single-payer health insurance on the basis of evidence, not ideology, but at the same time I will give voice to the arguments by others for reform alternatives.

The intended audience for this book includes physicians (including residents and medical students in training); other health professionals; policy makers; legislators; business and labor groups; citizens' reform groups, and others involved in planning, financing, delivery, or evaluation of health care services. The book should also be of interest to many consumers and lay readers concerned about the growing unaffordability of, decreasing access to, and inconsistent quality of our present health care system.

The book is organized in three parts. After an introductory chapter highlighting the growth of investor-owned corporate health care over the last 30 to 40 years, Part I describes eight corporate health care industries and their impact on the health care system. Part II examines four major ways in which health care corporations protect their interests. Part III compares the advantages and disadvantages of privatized and public utility models of health care, as well as possible approaches to reform.

The economic boom of the 1990s, though it served many health care corporations and their investors well, has not been kind to U.S. health care. With more than 43 million uninsured Americans and, tens of millions *under*insured, the health care system is collapsing around us. Inflation of health care costs continues unabated, rendering health care increasingly unaffordable to a large and growing part of the population, currently estimated at about 50%. Yet we are being told by corporate interests and many politicians in both parties that incremental reforms of our market-based system will be effective if we just give them more time. This book provides an up-to-date analysis of the failing medical marketplace and suggests an approach to urgently needed structural reform.

John P. Geyman, MD
May 2004

ACKNOWLEDGMENTS

Feedback and encouragement from many colleagues have helped to make this book possible. Selected chapters were reviewed and commented upon by Drs. Richard Deyo (Professor of Medicine and Co-Director of the Center for Cost and Outcome Research at the University of Washington), Don McCanne (past President of Physicians for a National Health Program), Fitzhugh Mullan (Contributing Editor to *Health Affairs*), John Saultz (Professor and Chairman of Family Medicine at Oregon Health Sciences University), and Eric Wall (regional medical director of Lifewise, a Premera Health Plan based in Portland). Discussions with other colleagues also contributed to the genesis of this book: William Burnett (former head of the California Health Manpower Policy Commission), Dr. Richard Clover (Dean, School of Public Health at the University of Louisville), Dr. William Fowkes (former head of the Division of Family and Community Medicine at Stanford University), Dr. Harold Holman (Professor of Medicine at Stanford University), Dr. Donald Light (Professor of Comparative Health Systems at the University of Medicine and Dentistry of New Jersey), Dr. John Midtling (Department of Family Medicine at the University of Tennessee in Memphis), Dr. Charles North (PHS Indian Hospital in Albuquerque, New Mexico), and Dr. Michael Prislin (Department of Family Medicine at the University of California, Irvine).

I am in debt to Dr. Ida Hellander (executive Director of Physicians for a National Health Program), for sharing data updates and teaching slides developed by PNHP over the years, as well as reports of the Kaiser Family Foundation, Commonwealth Fund, Robert Wood Johnson Foundation, Public Citizen, and the Institute of Medicine. Thanks are due to the journals and publishers who granted permission to reprint or adapt material originally published by them, as cited throughout the book.

Virginia Gessner, my administrative assistant for 28 years, typed the entire manuscript meticulously, converting handwritten drafts to finished text. Graphics were skillfully prepared by Pat McGifford at Uwired Health Sciences at the University of Washington and Bruce Conway at Lightwatcher, Friday Harbor, Washington.

Finally, I thank Dr. Ursula Springer (President of Springer Publishing Company in New York), Jeanne Libby, and their colleagues who provided editorial help and encouragement along the way to transform manuscript into published book. And, as is always the case with any of my projects, the ongoing support of Gene, my wife of 48 years, has made this book possible from start to finish.

Chapter 1

GROWTH OF INVESTOR-OWNED CORPORATE HEALTH CARE

As we know only too well, the mere mention of Enron has come to symbolize all the worst of investor-owned corporations in this country. It would be one thing if the Enron story were just an exception, but unfortunately there are many other similar cases throughout corporate America in this current deregulatory era. WorldCom, Tyco International, and Imclone are just some of the examples of firms infected by similar scandals, with each example bringing to light previously hidden conflicts of interest in other industries as well, ranging from accounting firms, investment banks, and Wall Street analysts. Public opinion is now shifting, as evidenced by a *Business Week*/Harris poll in 2000 in which about 80% of respondents voiced concerns about the increasing corporate power over too many aspects of American life. (Hartmann, 2002, p. 131).

A new period of deregulation and corporate-friendly policies began in 1980 as the country reasserted free market principles in pursuit of a dominant role in a global economy. Taxes on the rich were reduced, and corporations were given more freedom to merge and downsize their workforces (Korten, 2001). Appointments to the Supreme Court were once again more conservative and another "gilded age," reminiscent of the late 1800s, was launched. Income gaps within the society grew to unprecedented levels. Corporate CEO compensation grew from 40 times that of a median U.S. worker in 1978, to 500 times as much by 2000, while the average family in the middle quintile of income saw its income barely increase during that period from $31,700 to $33,200 (Phillips, 2002).

In contrast to the history of most U.S. corporations, most health care corporations are a more recent phenomenon. With only a few exceptions such as General Electric, the rise of investor-owned corporate health care in America dates back only to the 1960s, and most such corporations are younger than that. Since health care is such an essential service within our society, in much the same way as

1

education and fire protection, the question arises as to how health care corporations see their public interest role. Do they engage in the same corporate excesses and abuses being seen in other fields? Are they any more regulated than other kinds of corporations, whether voluntarily or by government? What impact do they have on the health care marketplace? To what extent are those impacts constructive or detrimental? These interrelated questions will be addressed in the following chapters.

This chapter has a three-fold purpose: (1) to briefly review some historical highlights of investor-owned health care corporations; (2) to assess whether their common practices are similar or different from the excesses of corporate self-interest elsewhere in the economy; and (3) to discuss briefly how health care markets differ from other markets and whether health care is just another commodity for sale or a basic human right.

INVESTOR-OWNED CORPORATE HEALTH CARE: AN HISTORICAL PERSPECTIVE

It was federal legislation that played a large role in the corporatization of American medicine. The creation of Medicare and Medicaid in 1965 opened up new opportunities for corporate investment in many parts of the health care enterprise, including hospitals, nursing homes, home care, and clinical laboratories, and in the insurance industry. In return for their support of Medicare legislation, hospitals were assured that Blue Cross would process the claims and convey a summary to the federal government. As a result, a pro-hospital intermediary stood thereafter between the government and the hospital (Andrews, 1995). Seven years later, in 1972, with the passage of an amendment to the Social Security Act, the treatment of end-stage kidney disease became covered by Medicare. As a result of these new entitlement programs, facilities, providers, and suppliers rushed to fill a large and wide-open market. Reimbursement was on a cost-plus or fee-for-service basis without a uniform rate schedule, regulations were scant, and patients expected either public or private insurers to pay most of their costs of care. In this new environment health care costs rose dramatically, even as the volume of services and the demand for insurance increased (Robinson, 1999).

Today's big corporate hospital chains, together with many other health care corporations, were established within a few years of the passage of Medicare. The largest investor-owned hospital chain,

Hospital Corporation of America (HCA), controlled 23 hospitals in 1970 and 300 in 1980, and as the world's largest hospital company by the mid-1990s had annual revenues of over $10 billion (Andrews, 1995, p. 19). Rapid growth in investor-owned facilities and services likewise took place in health maintenance organizations (HMOs), nursing homes, home care, emergency room services, clinical laboratories, dialysis centers, mental health centers, and health screening programs. Wall Street became enamored of the profits available in health care; the net earnings of publicly-owned health care corporations rose by 30-35% in 1979 (Relman, 1980). Between 1965 and 1990, U.S. corporate profits after taxes increased more than 100-times, and at a pace nearly 20 times greater than profits for all U.S. corporations (U.S. Department of Commerce, 1986). By the mid-1980s, many U.S. hospitals derived more than one-half of their revenue from Medicare, while other programs such as dialysis centers, were almost entirely dependent on Medicare and Medicaid funding (Lindorff, 1992).

In a landmark article in 1980, Arnold Relman, then editor of *The New England Journal of Medicine,* coined the term "medical-industrial complex" to describe the large and growing network of for-profit corporations permeating the health care system. Noting this departure from a long tradition of individual ownership and not-for-profit care, he called for careful study of the corporate trend, warning that the medical-industrial complex "creates the problems of overuse and fragmentation of services, overemphasis on technology, and 'cream-skimming,' and it may also exercise undue influence on national health policy" (Relman, 1980, p. 303).

Three years later, a report by the Institute of Medicine (IOM), *The New Health Care for Profit: Doctors and Hospitals in a Competitive Environment* asked these questions about the emergence of investor-owned corporate health care (Gray, 1983).

> Does the development of for-profit medical care represent a change in the goals pursued by medical professionals and institutions, or is it only a change in the methods by which the traditional goals of service are pursued? Does the growth in for-profit health care represent a decline in the ideals that morally anchored a powerful profession and facilitated necessary patient trust, or does it embody a more honest acknowledgment of realities that have always been present? Or is it a neutral development?

Then again, in 1986, the IOM's Committee on For-Profit Enterprise in Health Care, concerned about the common distinctions between for-

TABLE 1.1. Common Distinctions Between For-Profit and Not-for-Profit Organizations

For-Profit	Not-for-Profit
Corporations owned by investors	Corporations without owners or owned by "members"
Can distribute some proportion of profits (net revenues less expenses) to owners	Cannot distribute surplus (net revenues less expenses) to those who control the organization
Pay property, sales, income taxes	Generally exempt from taxes
Sources of capital include: a. Equity capital from investors b. Debt c. Retained earnings (including depreciation and deferred taxes) d. Return-on-equity payments from third-party payers (e.g., Medicare)	Sources of capital include: a. Charitable contributions b. Debt c. Retained earnings (including depreciation) d. Governmental grants
Management ultimately accountable to stockholders	Management accountable to voluntary, often self-perpetuating boards
Purpose: Has legal obligation to enhance the wealth of shareholders within the boundaries of law; does so by providing services	*Purpose:* Has legal obligation to fulfill a stated mission (provide services, teaching, research, etc.); must maintain economic viability to do so
Revenues derived from sale of services	Revenues derived from sale of services and from charitable contributions
Mission: Usually stated in terms of growth, efficiency, and quality	*Mission:* Often stated in terms of charity, quality, and community service, but may also pursue growth
Mission and structure can result in more streamlined decision making and implementation of major decisions	Mission and diverse constituencies often complicate decision making and implementation

Source: Gray, B. E. (Ed.) (1986). *For-profit enterprise in health care: Supplementary statement on for-profit enterprise in health care.* Washington, D.C: National Academy Press. Reprinted with permission.

profit and not-for-profit organizations (see Table 1.1), warned that a substantial increase in the for-profit sector's share of the health care system could:

1. Put further pressure on hospitals, voluntary organizations, and other facilities that provide needed but less profitable services

2. Create powerful centers of influence to affect public policy
3. Increase the drift of the health care system toward commercialism and away from medicine's service orientation (Gray, 1986).

Two years later, Roger Bulger, then president of the Association of Academic Health Centers, laid down this gauntlet concerning the challenges facing privatized corporate health care:

> Under the deregulated, decentralized systems approach to health care evolving in the United States, the main problem will be how to guarantee a requisite level of care for the poor and underinsured. How we answer that problem will be the true measure of our values, of our national character, and of the quality of our beliefs (Bulger, 1988).

Today, two decades after these warnings, a quiet revolution has taken place. An enormous medical-industrial complex is well entrenched in the U.S., and many of its corporations are active on a worldwide basis through the global economy and the World Trade Organization (WTO). Nine of the 12 largest publicly held health care corporations in the world are American (*The Wall Street Journal* 2002).

Many of the concerns raised during the 1980s about the threat of profit-driven health care have now come to pass, and many of the changes have been too gradual for us to appreciate their true impact. To a considerable degree, Wall Street has already replaced Main Street in the delivery of health care and the formulation of health care policy. Figure 1.1 shows the extent of investor-owned corporate ownership of sectors of the health care industry by 1998 (Himmelstein, Woolhandler, & Hellander, 2001). The figure for general hospitals is misleading on the low side. Investor-owned hospital chains now account for about 15% of U.S. hospitals, but they also own and manage many clinical laboratories, and rehabilitation, long-term care and psychiatric services (VHA Inc., 1998).

DO HEALTH CARE CORPORATIONS BEHAVE DIFFERENTLY FROM OTHER CORPORATIONS?

Although this question may seem naïve, it is worth asking since health care is such a basic human need and an essential part of the social fabric. The concerns raised by Relman, the IOM, and others in the 1980s need to be addressed. To a large extent, the jury is in and the answers are not promising. Part II of this book will provide more

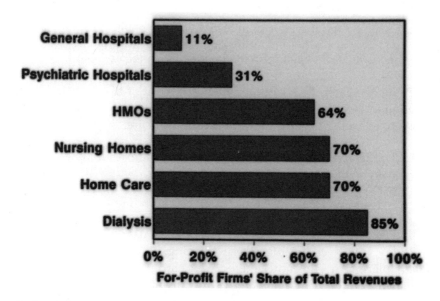

FIGURE 1.1 Extent of for-profit ownership, 1998.
Source: Himmelstein, D., et al. (2001). *Bleeding the patient: The consequences of corporate health care.* Monroe, ME: Common Courage Press. Reprinted with permission.

detailed answers to this question, as I look closely at eight industries within health care. For now, here are some examples which show that the bottom line trumps the social good in the new corporate health care market.

- As an example of the business ethos, Tietelman wrote approvingly, in a 1985 *Forbes Magazine* article on *selective* surgery, of Republic Health's strategies for maximizing profits by identifying surgical procedures that "can be done quickly, often in a few hours, without lots of nurses, tests, meals or general care" and marketing them "just as hotels market cut-rate weekends" (Tietelman, 1985).
- Pfizer manufactured many defective Bjork-Shiley heart valves in its factory in the Caribbean. Although defective valves were known by management to have poor welds, they did not tell the government and ordered the valves to be ground down, weakening the valves further. The defective valves were then marketed worldwide, despite the written protests of their developer Dr. Viking Bjork. These valves are subject to strut rupture, usually accompanied by sudden death. To date there have been 800

valve fractures with 500 deaths. The company paid civil penalties in order to avoid criminal charges and about $200 million in restitution to victims, and later lobbied the Health Industries Manufacturers' Association to ban all lawsuits against manufacturers of body parts. This lobbying effort was almost successful. The Republican Senate leader slipped such a clause into Patients' Rights legislation, but it was later killed when it became public (Palast, 2002).

- After a national study documenting worse outcomes of lumbar fusion in Medicare patients compared with no fusion, special interests initiated a letter-writing campaign to Congress calling for eliminating funding for the Agency for Health Care Policy and Research (AHCPR) and limiting the power of the FDA. One manufacturer of pedical screws, a medical device used in spinal fusion, even lobbied for a court injunction to prevent the AHCPR from producing guidelines for the treatment of low back pain (Deyo, Ciol, Cherkin, Loeser & Bigos, 1993; Psaty, Simon, Wagner, & Omenn, 1997).
- The largest dialysis provider Fresenius, a German firm, took over National Medical Care (NMC) several years ago. Although NMC manufactured dialyzers and labeled them for single use, it regularly reused dialyzers in its own clinics, saving the company about $130 million each year. For-profit dialysis centers are also 55% more likely than not-for-profit centers to use short dialysis periods, which decreases survival while increasing profits (Himmelstein, Woolhandler, & Hellander, 2001, p. 137–138). Fresenius pleaded guilty to charges of conspiracy and fraud, and was forced to pay $486 million in fines and settlements to the government in 2000 (Reuters News Service, 2000; USA Today, 2002; Brown, 2000).
- The pharmaceutical industry is rife with ways to increase profits at the expense of patients, competitors, and payers, including strategies to game patent laws (Los Angeles Times, 2002), contracting with competitors not to produce a cheaper generic drug (Ivins, 2001), fighting against imports of prescription drugs from Canada (Generic Pharmaceutical Association, 2002; Baglole, 2003), promoting "me too" drugs which are no better than older drugs (Relman & Angell, 2002), suppression of unfavorable research results (Deyo, Psaty, Simon, Wagner & Omenn, 1997; CBS 60 Minutes, 1999), devious and misleading direct-to-consumer advertising (Wolfe, 2001) and, because of fears of price controls, lobbying against a prescription drug benefit for Medicare through

a false front organization with the benign-sounding name, Citizens for Better Medicare (Green, 2002).

- Insurance swindles and corporate fraud involving health insurance/HMO/hospital billings are estimated to run between $100 billion and $400 billion each year, about 100 times more than all the combined burglaries in the country (Hartmann, 2002, p. 184).
- After many years of promotion by corporations that make infant formula, a plague of infant deaths occurred around the world when mothers in developing countries mixed the formula with unsanitary water. UNICEF created a global code on infant formula marketing, which included a ban on packaging showing healthy, fat babies. Gerber Foods refused to alter its trademarked logo with its happy, pudgy infant and threatened action under the international trade agreements (GATT). In order to avoid a long and expensive challenge to a WTO tribunal, the Guatemalan government exempted imported baby food products from its labeling restrictions (Wallach & Sforza, 1999).
- Conflict over drug patents has become the most contentious issue facing the WTO as poor nations attempt to obtain essential drugs to deal with public health emergencies. In November 2001, it was agreed that nations could override patents to deal with such crises, such as the AIDS epidemic in Africa. Despite the urgency of such crises, however, pharmaceutical corporations continue to vigorously defend their patents and oppose both unlicensed imports and unlicensed local production of cheaper drugs by other countries (Fisk, 2001).

WHAT'S DIFFERENT ABOUT THE HEALTH CARE MARKETPLACE?

Proponents of the free market in health care have touted for many years the effectiveness of competition in achieving greater efficiencies and cost containment. It is surprising how many economists and health policy analysts still buy into this premise, even as the evidence has proven the opposite. As will be documented in later chapters, the story of investor-owned corporate health care is one of *increased* costs, *reduced* efficiency, *less* value, *lower* quality, resulting from consolidation and profiteering in an increasingly fragmented marketplace

In the largely deregulated health care market since the early 1980s, health care costs have increased far faster than cost of living or purchasing power of much of the population. Over the last five years, for example, while the Consumer Price Index (CPI) increased by an annual average between 2% and 3%, health care costs have increased by double-digit percentages. They soared by an average of 16% in 2003, and are expected to grow by at least that much in 2004. A majority of employers anticipate that similar cost increases will continue through 2007 (Towers Perrin, 2003).

Health care has become unaffordable for lower-income groups as well as for much of the middle class. There is now a "medical divide" in the U.S. at annual incomes of about $50,000. About one-half of the non-elderly U.S. population earn less than $50,000 a year, and have major problems in affording health care (Kaiser Family Foundation, 2002). In their excellent recent book *The Two Income Trap: Why Middle-Class Mothers and Fathers Are Going Broke,* Elizabeth Warren and Amelia Warren Tyagi make the point that the average dual-income middle-class family of four today, despite a combined income 75% more than its one-income counterpart a generation ago, is more strapped by fixed costs and has less discretionary income (Warren & Tyagi, 2003) (Figure 1.2).

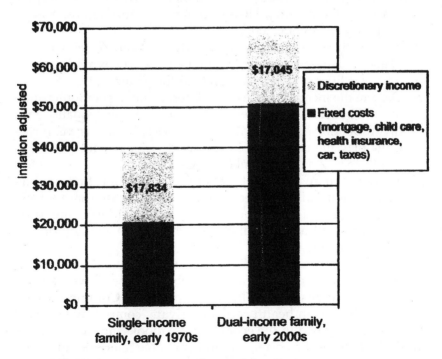

FIGURE 1.2 Fixed costs as a share of family income.

Source: Reprinted with permission from Warren E., & Tyagi, A. W. *The Two-Income Trap: Why Middle-class Mothers and Fathers are Going Broke.* New York: Basic Books, 2003: p. 50–51.

The largely deregulated market over the last 30 years has failed to contain costs through managed competition. The drivers of the market have been costs and profits, not quality and service. Consolidation of the major players within the market has led to oligopoly and often tacit rate setting by large corporate interests.

There are many reasons why markets in health care do not behave the way they do in other areas of the economy, such as automobiles or housing. Here are some of them:

- It is estimated that a metropolitan market of about 400,000 is required to enable any real competition between hospitals or HMOs. Communities of smaller size have a limited number of facilities and providers. More than one-third of Americans live in areas (including 9 entire states) with populations less than 360,000 (Kronick, Goodman, Weinberg, & Wagner, 1993)
- Even in larger metropolitan markets, consolidation among providers often limits choice and competition as monopolies take over; in El Paso, Texas, for example, the two largest hospital chains in the country, HCA and Tenet, control almost 80% of hospital beds (Stein, 2002)
- The health care system is largely driven by care of acute illness; visits for acute or semi-urgent problems are unavoidably limited to facilities and providers within the community.
- Despite the increasing use of the Internet among computer-literate and better educated people, there remains an "equality gap" of information between patients and their physicians; yet physicians play the major role in clinical decisions about the use of health care services (Eisenberg, 1986)
- There are many large subsets of the population that are limited in their ability to seek out, or travel to alternative facilities or providers; these include many elderly, the frail, chronically ill and disabled, and those with literacy or language barriers

In view of these and other factors, Robert Evans, a well-known health care economist at the University of British Columbia, maintains that "there is in health care no 'private, competitive market' of the form described in the economics textbooks, anywhere in the world. There never has been, and inherent characteristics of health and health care make it impossible that there ever could be" (Evans, 1997).

IS HEALTH CARE JUST ANOTHER COMMODITY FOR SALE?

This basic question, important as it is, remains hotly debated and unanswered in the U.S., which stands alone among Western industrial nations in not having some form of social health insurance. In their study of the for-profit enterprise in health care in the early 1980s, the Institute of Medicine framed the issue in these terms:

> Ordinarily, in our predominantly capitalist society, it would be deemed odd to inquire into the implications of making a business of providing services or of making money from such a business. However, the services discussed here help people to keep or regain their health and can affect, at minimum, whether they are able to pursue their life goals, and, at maximum, whether they live or die. Many people see health care as the sort of public good that should be the right of all citizens, but this view has never prevailed in public policy (Gray, 1986, p. xviii).

Whether health care should be a basic human right, and its delivery a public service, generates an ongoing battle of conflicting ideologies. On the conservative side, the argument is made that the right to health care is a "qualified right granted patients but modified by the available resources within the health care system and the rights of physicians to control the practice of their professions." Liberals contend that everyone should have "full and unencumbered access to all available medical services based on the medical needs of the individual" (Kaufman, 1981). The polar ends of the argument are well represented by these two opposing views by Milton Friedman, a leading advocate of free market economics and David Himmelstein, MD and Steffie Woolhandler, MD, general internists and health care activists at Harvard Medical School respectively:

> Few trends could so thoroughly undermine the very foundations of our free society as the acceptance by corporate officials of a social responsibility other than to make as much money for their shareholders as possible (Friedman, 1962).

> In our society, some aspects of life are off-limits to commerce. We prohibit the selling of children and the buying of wives, juries, and kidneys. Tainted blood is an inevitable consequence of paying blood donors; even sophisticated laboratory tests cannot compensate for blood that is sold rather than given as a gift. Like blood, health care is too precious, intimate, and corruptible to entrust to the market (Woolhandler & Himmelstein, 1999).

The U.S. Supreme Court, interestingly enough, on the basis of the Fourteenth Amendment, has recognized "an acknowledged right to health derived from a constitutionally guaranteed right to life and happiness" (Michelman, 1968).

Since resources are limited in any society and some kind of rationing is inevitably required (we already ration care on the basis of class and income), Larry Churchill, an ethicist at the University of Notre Dame, adds this useful perspective:

"There is a moral right to health care, but not of the sort often claimed. It is a right grounded not in purchasing power, merit, or social worth, but in human need. The right to health care finds its rationale in a social concept of the self, in a sense of common humanity, and in a knowledge of common vulnerability to disease and death . . . A right to health care based on need means a right to equitable access based on need alone to all effective care society can reasonably afford . . . A right to health care is not a license to demand care. It is not a right to the very best available or even to all one may need. Some very pressing health needs may have to be neglected because meeting them would be unreasonable in the light of other health needs or social priorities. Health care is unique among needs and should enjoy a high place among our basic requirements for life (Churchill, 1987).

In the real world of politics, policy, and commerce, free market forces still dominate U.S. health care. As a result, our present trends and policies discriminate against lower-income groups, a growing part of the middle class and the elderly. As an example of what this all means for one-half of the nonelderly population in the U.S. earning less than $50,000 a year, Figure 1.3 shows four kinds of access problems which result from the high costs of health care.

CONCLUDING COMMENTS

U.S. health care corporations have made, and continue to make, many of the important technological innovations that have brought today's health care to its advanced state. We have General Electric to thank, for example, for the early development of the X-ray tube, as well as other advances in diagnostic equipment in later years. However, some of these technological advances are adopted before they are shown to be effective, are duplicative or noncurative, or are even found to be more harmful than beneficial. Further, our market-based system increasingly leaves out a growing part of the population which cannot

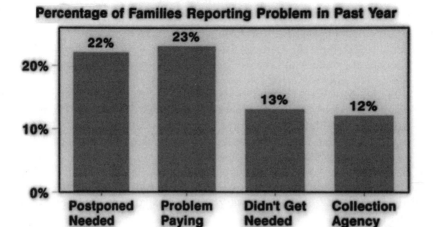

FIGURE 1.3 Access problems for middle class families (income $25,000–$49,999).

Source: Slide Set Show, 2002 edition. Physicians for a National Health Program, Chicago, Illinois. Retrieved from *www.pnhp.org* and reprinted with permission.

afford health care services that are proven to be effective. That is what the rest of this book is about—whether the "social contract" between health care, medicine, and the public interest should be redrawn and, if so, how?

REFERENCES

Andrews, C. (1995). Profit fever: The drive to corporatize health care and how to stop it. Monroe, ME: Common Courage Press.

Baglole, J. (2003, Jan. 22). Glaxo tries new tack on cheap Canadian drugs. *Wall Street Journal*, D2.

Bulger, R. J. (1988). Technology. *Bureaucracy and healing in America: A postmodern paradigm*. Iowa City, IA: University of Iowa Press.

CBS. (1999), Dec. 19). 60 Minutes.

Churchill, L. R. (1987). *Rationing health care in America: Perceptions and principles of justice*. Notre Dame, IN: University of Notre Dame.

Deyo, R. A., Ciol, M. A., Cherkin, D. C., Loeser, J. D., Bigos, S. J. (1993). Lumbar spinal fusion: A cohort study of complications, reoperations, and resource use in the Medicare population. *Spine, 18,* 463.

Deyo, R. A., Psaty,, B. M., Simon, G., Wagner, E. H., Omenn, G. S. (1997). The messenger under attack: Intimidation of researchers by special interest groups. *New England Journal of Medicine, 33,* 1176.

Editorial. (2002, June 10). Gaming the patent drug system. *Los Angeles Times.*

The global giants: Amid market pain, U.S. companies hold greater sway. (2002, Oct. 14). *Wall Street Journal,* R10.

Eisenberg, J. M. (1986). Doctors' decisions and the cost of medical care: The reasons for doctors' practice patterns and ways to change them. Ann Arbor, MI: Health Administration Press Perspectives.

Evans, R. G. (1997). Going for the gold: The redistributive agenda behind market-based health care reform. *Journal of Health Politics, Policy and Law, 22,* 427.

Fisk, M. (2001). Making drugs a public good. *Pharmaceutical News, 8,* 45.

Friedman, M. (1967). *Capitalism and freedom.* Chicago: University of Chicago Press.

Generic Pharmaceutical Association (2002, Nov.) rips PhRMA. *O'Dwyer's PR Services Report,* 15.

Gray, B. H. (Ed) (1983). *The new health care for profit: Doctors and hospitals in a competitive environment.* Washington, DC: Institute of Medicine, National Academy Press.

Gray, B. H. (Ed) (1986). *For-profit enterprise in health care: Supplementary statement on for-profit enterprise in health care.* Washington, DC: Institute of Medicine, National Academy Press.

Green, M. (2002). *Selling out: How big corporate money buys elections, rams through legislation, and betrays our democracy.* New York: Regan Books.

Hartmann, T. (2002). *Unequal protection: The rise of corporate dominance and the theft of human rights.* Emmaus, PA: Rodale Press.

Himmelstein, D. U, Woolhandler, S, & Hellander, I. (2001). *Bleeding the patient: The consequences of corporate health care.* Monroe, ME: Common Courage Press.

Ivins, M. (2001, July). Drug companies can really make you sick. *Public Citizen's Health Research Group Health Letter,* 4.

Kaiser Family Foundation (2002, June 5). Survey.

Kaufman, C. L. (1981). The right to health care: Some cross-national comparisons and U.S. trends in policy. *Social Science in Medicine, 15,* 157.

Kidney dialysis giant guilty of fraud. (2000, Jan. 19). Reuters News Service. USA Today (2002). Medicare fraud. January 20. 3A. Brown, J. G. (2000). Press Release, January 19. Settlement with Fresenius Medical Care. U.S. Department of Health and Human Services, Office of Inspector General, Washington, D.C.

Korten, D. C. (2001). *When corporations rule the world.* San Francisco: Berrett-Koehler Publishers, Inc.

Kronick, R., Goodman, D. C., Weinberg, J., & Wagner, E. (1993). The marketplace in health care reform. The demographic limitations of managed competition. *New England Journal of Medicine, 328,* 148.

Lindorff, D. (1992). *Marketplace medicine: The rise of the for-profit hospital chains.* New York: Bantam Books.

Michelman, F. (1968). Forward: On protecting the poor through the Fourteenth Amendment. *Harvard Law Review, 83,* 7.

Palast, G. (2002). *The best democracy money can buy.* Sterling, VA: Pluto Press.

Phillips, K. (2002, Nov./Dec.). Wealth and Democracy: Rich-poor gap, corruption are harbingers of economic decline. *Public Citizen News, 22* (6), 7.

Relman, A. S. (1980). The new medical-industrial complex. *New England Journal of Medicine, 303,* 963.

Relman, A. S., & Angell, M. (2002, Dec. 16). America's other drug problem. *The New Republic,* 47.

Robinson, J. C. (1999). *The corporate practice of medicine: Competition and innovation in health care.* Berkeley, CA: University of California Press.

Stein, L. (2002, Sept. 20). Pulling the plug. *Metro.* Silicon's Valley's weekly newspaper, *September 20.*

Towers Perrin (2003). Health Care Cost Survey. Available at *www.towersperrin.com*

Tietelman, R. (1985, Apr. 22).Selective surgery. *Forbes Magazine,* 75–76.

U.S. Dept. of Commerce (1986). The National Income and Product Accounts of the United States, 1929–82: Statistical Tables, Table 6.21B.

U. S. Department of Commerce (1993). *Survey of Current Business,* Table 6.19C.

VHA Inc. (1998). *Environment assessment: Setting foundations for the millennium.* Irving, TX: Author.

Wallach, L., & Sforza, M. (1999). Whose trade organizations? Corporate globalization and the erosion of democracy. *Public Citizen,* 1.

Warren, E. & Tyagi, A. W. (2003). *The Two-Income Trap: Why Middle-Class Mothers and Fathers are Going Broke* (pp. 50–51). New York: Basic Books.

Wolfe, S. M. (2001, Sept.) Direct-to-consumer (DTC) ads: Illegal, unethical or both? *Public Citizen's Health Research Group Health Letter,* 3.

Woolhandler, S. & Himmelstein, D. U. (1999). When money is the mission: The high costs of investor-owned care. *New England Journal of Medicine, 341,* 444–446.

Part I

CORPORATE CONTRIBUTIONS TO THE SOARING COSTS OF HEALTH CARE

Chapter 2

HOSPITALS AND NURSING HOME CHAINS

The industrialization of episodic medicine was not the original intent of the market idealists of the early 1970s who favored health maintenance organizations. Many of them regard chain hospitals and emergicenters as the antithesis of what they had in mind. They wanted corporate involvement to change the nature of health care; it seems likely, in the foreseeable future, to reproduce the defects of the traditional system on a grander scale.

—*Paul Starr*
Professor of Sociology, Princeton University

In a way, we're kind of like a utility.

—*Thomas Frist, Jr.*
Chairman, Hospital Corporation of America

The above comments cited in Starr (1982) and Lindorff (1992) provide a useful backdrop to this chapter. The first reveals the concerns of Paul Starr, a professor of Sociology at Princeton, more than 20 years ago after his comprehensive study of health care in the United States. The second reflects the perceptions and beliefs of a corporate insider, the CEO of Hospital Corporation of America (HCA), now the largest investor-owned hospital chain, during its formative years. We will return to these two different views of the health care world at the end of this chapter to see whether they can be reconciled.

Investor-owned chains of hospitals and nursing homes cannot be pigeonholed as such—they often extend into other areas of the health care system, such as surgicenters, urgent care clinics and even ownership of insurance companies. The purpose of this chapter is threefold: (1) to provide a brief historical overview of trends involving for-profit investor-owned hospital and nursing home chains; (2) to present five case examples of large chains of general, rehabilitation, and psychiatric hospitals, and nursing homes; and (3) to briefly discuss

19

three ongoing policy issues resulting from the impact of these corporate chains on U.S. health care.

HISTORICAL OVERVIEW AND TRENDS

Ironically, public programs (e.g., Medicare and Medicaid in the 1960s) and their later reimbursement policies have been the major stimuli of what has become an enormous corporate empire of diverse, intertwined investor-owned chains of hospitals and other health care facilities and service providers. In earlier years, most hospitals and nursing homes were small, individually owned and operated companies. These companies became the launching pads for investor-owned corporations to enter into the delivery of medical care, as they bought them and organized them into chains. As these corporate enterprises grew, they typically diversified into related phases of health care, each new acquisition adding to their overall market share. Here are two examples of corporate integration, which had developed during the early 1980s:

- In 1984, the 8 largest investor-owned corporations together owned and operated 426 acute care hospitals, 102 psychiatric hospitals, 272 long-term care units, 62 dialysis centers, 89 ambulatory care centers, and a variety of other ambulatory and home health services (Gray, 1986)
- By 1980, National Medical Care (NMC) owned 120 dialysis centers; in addition, one of its subsidiaries made dialysis supplies and equipment and another performed laboratory tests for dialysis patients while NMC was also diversifying into psychiatric care and respiratory therapy (Starr, 1982, p. 443)

Today, investor-owned hospital chains have often set up their own financing mechanisms as an alternative to negotiating with third-party insurers. Early examples were the insurance plans established by Humana and HCA in the mid-1980s. In one of these plans Humana Care Plus offered free choice of physicians, but penalized subscribers for using hospitals that were not owned by Humana (Kirchner, 1985). Other strategies used by investor-owned hospital chains to increase their market share within an area are the development of urgent-care clinics, freestanding "emergicenters," and other "patient feeder" systems (Lindorff, 1992, p. 26).

Claiming cost containment and greater efficiencies through market discipline in a free health care market, investor-owned chains of hospitals invariably cut costs, especially by cutting nursing staff and other clinical personnel (Woolhandler & Himmelstein, 1997). Quality of care is thereby compromised as cost savings achieved through these "efficiencies" are passed along as profits and dividends to shareholders rather than being used for institutional investment and improvement in patient care services. The chains seek out profitable markets and avoid "poor-pay" patients, whose care then falls to public and not-for-profit hospitals. Unprofitable services are often shut down regardless of community need (Coye, 1997; (Martinez, 2002; (White, 2002). Most chain hospitals are 100 to 200 beds in size, typically without residency training programs. Their administrative and general service costs are invariably higher than their not-for-profit counterparts. These higher costs are usually claimed to be due to higher interest expenses and financial services after acquisitions and mergers, but they also tend to add to the bottom line through complex billing procedures to payers (Himmelstein, Woolhandler, Hellander, 2001; Kuttner, 1996). Perhaps most important, ownership, policy and decision making are usually transferred from the community to distant corporate headquarters elsewhere in the country. This obviously interferes with the ability of public and not-for-profit facilities to develop coordinated health care systems that are responsive to the needs of the local community and surrounding region (Starkweather, 1981; (Starr, 1982).

Mergers and consolidation became common during the 1990s as hospitals struggled to survive in a time of declining patient census and reduced reimbursement by payers. Some not-for-profit hospitals were forced to close; many converted to for-profit status, often being acquired by investor-owned chains.

As a result of these changes over the last 30 or more years, there has been an enormous shift in relationships and influence between physicians, hospitals, HMOs and insurers.

Table 2.1 provides an historical overview of these changes. (Bodenheimer & Grumbach, 2002). In past years, hospitals were dependent on the loyalty of physicians for admission of patients and maintaining their daily census and revenue. More recently, hospitals have had to negotiate contracts with HMOs for sources of patients, while physicians in the community may have contracts with multiple HMOs, thus dividing their loyalty to any given hospital (Freudenheim & Abelson, 2003). Within this increasingly competitive marketplace, managed care has made it more difficult for many physicians to provide charity care. The higher the HMO penetration in a region, the lower the amount of charity care, and some for-profit HMOs even forbid physicians from seeing non-paying patients. (Himmelstein, Woolhandler & Hellander, 2001, p. 77).

TABLE 2.1. Historical Overview of U.S. Health Care

1945–1970: Provider-insurer pact
Independent hospitals and small private practices
Many private insurers
Providers tended to dominate the insurers, especially in Blue Cross and
   Blue Shield
Purchasers (individuals, businesses, and, after 1965, government) had
   relatively little power
Reimbursements for providers were generous

The 1970s: Tensions develop
Purchasers (especially government) become concerned about costs of
   health care
Under pressure from purchasers, insurers begin to question generous
   reimbursements of providers

The 1980s: Revolt of the purchasers
Purchasers (business joining government) become very concerned with
   rising health care costs
Attempts are made to reduce health cost inflation through Medicare
   DRGs, fee schedules, capitated HMOs, and selective contracting

The 1990s: Breakup of the provider-insurer pact
Spurred by the purchasers, selective contracting spreads widely as a
   mechanism to reduce costs
Price competition is introduced
Large integrated health networks are formed
Large physician groups emerge
Insurance companies dominate many managed care markets
For-profit institutions increase in importance
Insurers gain increasing power over providers, creating conflict and
   ending the provider-insurer pact

Source: Bodenheimer, T. S., & Grumbach, K. (2002). *Understanding health policy:
A clinical approach.* New York: Lange Medical Books/McGraw-Hill. Reprinted
with permission.

CASE EXAMPLES OF INVESTOR-OWNED CHAINS

Acute Care Hospitals
The two investor-owned hospital chains that I am about to describe
are representative of the industry. They are both the largest chains in
the country and have demonstrated their success in the open marketplace in economic terms. But they have strayed far from the stan-

dards and values of traditional not-for-profit community hospitals, which maintain local ownership and governance.

HCA

Today's largest investor-owned hospital chain, HCA took root in Nashville, Tennessee in the mid-1960s. Thomas Frist, a cardiologist there, having established his own new 50-bed acute care facility, sought funding from local investors to expand his hospital. Unable to raise local funding, he decided to team up with his surgeon son, Thomas Frist, Jr., and Jack Massey, the developer of the Kentucky Fried Chicken chain, to start a chain of hospitals. Their idea was to model after Holiday Inn, creating opportunities to buy supplies in bulk, and to raise money from Wall Street investors as a national corporation. Their timing could not have been better. The Medicare and Medicaid programs, established in 1965, brought new access to care for many millions of Americans and a reimbursement stream for expanded hospital services. By 1987, HCA had become the nation's largest for-profit hospital chain, owning almost 200 acute-care facilities in 28 states as well as 45 in 8 foreign countries (Lindorff, 1992, pp. 39–41). By 1995, HCA was the 53rd largest corporation in the U.S., with a market value approximating Boeing, Chrysler, and Time Warner (Derber, 1998).

In 1994, HCA was acquired by Columbia Healthcare Corporation, a large Texas-based chain founded in 1987 by Richard Scott, previously a successful surgical supply wholesaler. The resulting corporate giant, Columbia/HCA, soon entered upon hard times. Its prodigious growth was fueled by aggressive, even predatory, business practices that created widespread public backlash and attracted the scrutiny of regulators. Its attempt to purchase Blue Cross and Blue Shield (BCBS) of Ohio, for example, was met by public outcry and a lawsuit by the state's Attorney General to block the proposed acquisition, which would have provided over $15 million in severance payments to the three top BCBS executives as "consulting fees and noncompete agreements" (Kuttner, 1996). In 1996, federal agents first raided Columbia/HCA all over the country, soon including laboratory and home care services as well as hospitals, and extensive investigations of alleged fraud were begun. Scott was soon forced out, Thomas Frist, Jr. took the reins, and the company (renamed simply HCA) started damage control against widespread allegations of fraud. In December of 2002, HCA announced a settlement with the Justice Department of more than $880 million, raising its total amount of civil fines and criminal penalties in recent years to $1.7 billion (Associated Press, 2002). These fraudulent practices included falsification of patient records, billing for services that were not ordered by treating physicians and/or not provided, devious accounting procedures intended to increase reimbursements, and kickbacks to physicians for patient referrals to their hospitals (Sparrow, 2000). .

In its pursuit of profits from hospital services as a chain business, its philosophy was expressed in these terms by Richard Scott soon after becoming president and CEO of Columbia/HCA:

> Do we have an obligation to provide health care for everybody? Where do we draw the line? Is any fast-food restaurant obligated to feed everyone who shows up? (Ginsberg, 1996)

Scott disparaged his not-for-profit competitors as "social parasites," (referring to their tax-exempt status) and rejected the arguments of critics that his hospitals should take more responsibility for care of the poor and the needs of the community.

Here are examples of typical practices of HCA and/or Columbia over the years, at various stages in their evolution:

- aggressive acquisition practices, typically involving secret negotiations, avoiding competitive bids, intensive lobbying efforts, and payoffs to helpful participants
- buying up underperforming hospitals, cutting staff and services, and then either making them profitable or closing them down
- taking over a Florida hospital and closing its emergency room, leaving the residents of the community with a 45-minute drive during rush hour traffic to the nearest emergency room
- gross overcharging for services (e.g., a Columbia-owned hospital in Georgia charged $14,584 for an average hospital stay for a stroke patient compared with $6,735 in a similar public hospital)
- after HCA's purchase of Good Samaritan Health System in San Jose, California, nurses' contracts were unilaterally terminated, many nurses were fired, quality of care deteriorated under a chronic staffing shortage, and charity care was cut by 89% (Ginsberg, 1996; (Kuttner, 1996; (Stein, 2002)

Tenet Healthcare Corporation (Tenet)
Tenet Healthcare Corporation is the second largest investor-owned hospital chain in the U.S. With headquarters in Santa Barbara, Cali-

fornia, the company by 2002 owned 114 acute-care hospitals in 16 states. Through many of the same practices as HCA, its national marketing plan focuses on highly reimbursed services in cardiology, orthopedics, and neurology. Its hospitals are located in large communities across Southern California, Texas, Louisiana, and South Florida, where a growing population of aging baby boomers need these services (White, 2002).

Tenet, until 1995 known as National Medical Enterprises (NME), has been the target of recurrent federal investigations for many years. Recently, the U.S. Justice Department sued the company for up to $323 million in damages, alleging that the company falsified patient diagnoses on Medicare claims from 1992 through 1998 to inflate its revenue (White, 2003). The company is now under investigation for exorbitant Medicare claims involving "outlier payments," which are designed to reimburse hospitals for extra care given to the sickest patients. Tenet was found by a state agency to have the highest average charges of any private hospital system in California, with charges 60% to 90% higher than statewide averages for 7 common diagnoses (Rapaport, 2002). Tenet hospitals in California were also found to charge an average of 10 times the cost of drugs, with one hospital charging 18 times their cost (Abelson, 2002).

In 1995, after contending with ongoing investigations, settlements and fines for fraudulent practices, NME sought to remove the cloud of scandal by changing its name to Tenet Healthcare, chosen because it was thought to represent integrity and "shared values" (Gentile, 2003). In 2004, Tenet is in the process of selling more than one-quarter of its hospitals after recurrent government investigations. (Rundle, 2004).

Rehabilitation Hospitals
HealthSouth is the largest investor-owned chain of for-profit rehabilitation hospitals in the country. It is now besieged by federal investigations for longstanding accounting and tax fraud. HealthSouth, with about 1,800 facilities in all 50 states and abroad, bills itself in its marketing materials as committed to providing high-quality, cost-effective care. Yet its claims are belied by a persistent story of predatory greed since its founding. Health South is a classic example of the dichotomy in ethics of corporate business and health care services.

Founded in 1984 by Richard Scrushy in Birmingham, Alabama, the company went public two years later. Scrushy, a former physical therapist, was the driving force in building a large chain of health care and rehabilitation facilities, including inpatient, outpatient, surgical, diagnostic, occupational, and other medical centers (Freudenheim & Abelson, 2003). HealthSouth became the largest employer in Birmingham (3,500 employees), and Scrushy became well known as a flamboyant executive. He was one of the University of Alabama's main donors, and his contributions helped to finance a school for health-related professions that bears his name (Romero, 2003). Stock in the company climbed to over $30 a share in 1998, but then plummeted to less than $4 a share when its fraudulent practices became public (Freudenheim, 2003). HealthSouth and Scrushy were accused of adding at least $1.4 billion to earnings between 1999 and 2003 and inflating assets by $800 million in an effort to boost its attractiveness to investors. The Securities and Exchange Commission (SEC) believes that reported earnings for 1999 to 2001 were 100 times the correct amount (Norris, 2003). Scrushy has been charged with insider trading for selling about $100 million in HealthSouth shares in the weeks before the company disclosed concerns about a change in Medicare reimbursement rates that was certain to reduce earnings. The company is also being sued by the Justice Department for billing Medicare for "one-on-one therapy by licensed physical therapists when the patients were actually treated in groups, often by unlicensed HealthSouth employees" (Freudenheim, 2003).

While the government continues its investigations, HealthSouth has had to scramble to arrange financing to avoid bankruptcy. It is being closely monitored by suppliers and insurers, and some believe that it will rival WorldCom and Enron for its brazen fraud (Atlas, 2003). After five months of widening investigations by the Justice Department, 14 former HealthSouth executives agreed to plead guilty to fraud (Weil & Mollencamp, 2003). The case is also expected to carry over into investigations of auditors and investment bankers who have advised the company over the years (Romero & Freudenheim, 2003).

Psychiatric Hospitals

Investor-owned for-profit psychiatric hospitals have been a growth industry since the 1970s. Between 1978 and 1983, they were increasing by more than 30% per year. (Gray, 1986, p. 476) Their record for quality of care and service has been disturbing, however, as reflected in these two examples during the 1990s (Sparrow, 2000, pp. 25–26):

- As one of the country's largest investor-owned psychiatric chains, National Medical Enterprises (NME, now Tenet, as already discussed) agreed to a settlement with the federal government of $362 million, then the largest settlement between the government and any health care provider (Myerson, 1994). NME had already paid out over $230 million to settle suits by 16 private insurers and more than 130 patients. The allegations included holding patients against their will, and paying kickbacks and bribes to community and church workers for patient referrals (Freudenheim, 1993).

- After cutbacks in mental health coverage by private insurers in the 1980s, psychiatric hospitals became more dependent on Medicare and Medicaid revenues. In Massachusetts, these two programs accounted for 72% of psychiatric admissions in 1997, up from 40% in 1990. Over those seven years, locked wards had increased markedly, with psychiatric admissions to these beds increasing by more than 50%. An exposé by reporters of the *Boston Sunday Globe* found a number of patients, after voluntary admissions, being admitted to locked wards not for medical reasons, but as one staff member admitted "because the census is down" (Kong & O'Neill, 1997).

Nursing Homes

Although nursing homes have been for-profit for many years, until 1970 most of them were small, individually owned facilities tied to their communities. By 1970 that was changing, since many of these facilities could no longer meet new building and safety standards, and were either closed or acquired by investor-owned chains. By 1984, the three largest chains (Beverly Enterprises, Hillhaven (a subsidiary of NME), and ARA Living Centers) together operated about 1,500 nursing homes across the country, controlling six times as many beds as not-for-profit nursing homes. These investor-owned nursing homes thrived on Medicare and Medicaid reimbursement policies, which covered operating costs as well as some profit factor. As we saw for other investor-owned hospital chains, administrative and other costs immediately went up as the proportions of spending on patient care services went down (Gray, 1986, pp. 32–33, 505, 524). Today about 70% of nursing home beds are in investor-owned facilities.

Although some investor-owned nursing home chains were the darlings of Wall Street during the early and mid-1990s, the industry has fallen on hard times as a result of federal cutbacks in reimbursements, especially from Medicaid. The majority of nursing home patients are on Medicaid, and the 17,000 nursing homes in the U.S. are now experiencing a $3.7 billion shortfall each year in meeting costs of care for these patients. Medicare reimbursement has been more liberal, and actually subsidizes some of this shortfall, but only 10-15% of nursing home patients are on Medicare. As a result, as states face deficits and have to make cuts in Medicaid spending, the financial health of the industry today has become precarious (Sherrid, 2002).

About 1.6 million Americans live in nursing homes This population has a high degree of disability and chronic illness, and presents a particular challenge to around-the-clock care. Many are unable to walk without assistance, one-half are incontinent, one-quarter have joint contractures, and many have dementia (Harrington & Carrillo, 2001).

Quality of care in U.S. nursing homes has varied widely for many years. Federal legislation that was passed in 1987 set standards for nursing home care and mandated periodic surveys. However, in 1997 only 29% of nursing homes surveyed could meet federal standards. One-quarter of nursing homes in the country had deficiencies that had either caused actual harm to patients or put them at risk for death or serious injury (Harrington & Carrillo, 2001). Persistent problems included low staffing levels with underpaid and inadequately trained staff, not enough nurses, and high staff turnover rates (Harrington, 1996).

Compared with not-for-profit nursing homes, for-profit nursing homes have been shown to have lower staffing levels and worse quality of care. (Harrington, Woolhandler, Mullen, Carillo & Himmelstein, 2001) Investor-owned nursing home chains avoid unionized staff, and often treat their staff badly. According to records of the National Labor Relations Board, the largest for-profit nursing home chain, Beverly Enterprises, accumulated 1,000 violations of workers' rights in 1987 (Lindorff, 1992, p. 271). In addition, fraud has been a pervasive problem throughout much of the for-profit nursing home industry. As Louis Freeh, director of the F.B.I. testified before Congress in 1995:

> Nursing home and hospice operators exploit the elderly and Alzheimer's patients by fraudulently billing for services, incontinence supplies and medications; tragically choosing patients who have difficulty understanding or remembering what was and what was not done, much less complaining to their insurer or alerting law enforcement. (Freeh, 1995).

CONTENTIOUS POLICY ISSUES

Three policy issues stand out for their continuing controversy and importance to the health care system.

Is the corporate business ethic consistent with quality of care?

Although investor-owned chains tout their commitment to quality of care, increased efficiency and value, there is growing evidence that their emphasis on cost-cutting and bottom-line profits ends up compromising the quality of care provided. Since the late 1980s, the evidence consistently shows that corporate shareholder interests trump values of service and quality of care.

- a 1989 study found death rates 6% lower at private, not-for-profit hospitals than at for-profit hospitals (Hartz et al., 1989)
- a large 1999 study found death rates 7% lower at not-for-profit nonteaching hospitals and 25% lower at major teaching hospitals (almost all not-for-profit) than at for-profit nonteaching hospitals (Taylor, Whellan, & Sloan, 1999)
- other studies in the late 1990s showed higher rates of postoperative complications (Kovner & Gergen, 1998) and preventable adverse events (Thomas, et al., 1998) at for-profit hospitals than at private, not-for-profit hospitals
- investor-owned HMOs score worse on all 14 quality of care measures than not-for-profit HMOs (Himmelstein, Woolhandler, Hellander & Wolfe, 1999)
- a 2002 systematic review and meta-analysis of all studies comparing mortality rates at for-profit private hospitals with rates at their not-for-profit counterparts found consistently higher mortality rates at for-profit hospitals; this study represented more than 26,000 hospitals and 38 million patients (Devereaux, Choi, Lacketti, Weaver & Schunemann et al., 2002); it is estimated that this difference would result in 14,312 additional deaths each year if all U.S. hospitals were converted to for-profit status (Woolhandler, 2002)
- a 2001 study found quality of care deficiencies more than 40% higher in investor-owned nursing homes compared with either not-for-profit or public facilities (Harrington, Woolhandler, Mullen, Carillo, & Himmelstein, 2001)

A major underlying reason for consistently worse quality of care in investor-owned for-profit facilities is their aggressive cost-cutting of staff, especially nurses, as they seek to achieve at least 10-15% profits for their stockholders (Devereaux et al., 2002; Woolhandler & Himmelstein, 1997).

Should Not-for-Profit, Charitable Hospitals be Sold to Investor-Owned Chains?

This might seem at first glance a naïve and irrelevant question, since many not-for-profits have already been sold to for-profit chains. The question, however, is a complex one, and there are both ethical and legal reasons to question these conversions. As Robert Kuttner points out, the not-for-profit hospital often has had land deeded to it under a charter to provide charity care, while the worth of the hospital represents many years of philanthropy, exempted taxes, other public investments, and the contributions of many in the community. A not-for-profit hospital struggling to compete and survive may see the funding and size of a chain buyer as attractive. The acquiring chain has a stable of analysts, accountants, attorneys, and consultants ready to put together a low-ball proposal, often in secret without competing bids, and with financial inducements to trustees or executives. The chain generally assures the hospital that its mission will be honored and preserved through a charitable foundation to be set up when the purchase is concluded. There are, however, many ways in which the chain can backtrack on such a commitment. One way is not to fund the foundation, which happened after Columbia/HCA bought HealthONE, a six-hospital system in Denver (Kuttner, 1996; Meyer, 1995).

State laws and regulatory policies with respect to hospital conversions to for-profit status vary widely from one state to another. Many states have little or no oversight of these transactions, while others take an active role in oversight and control through their state attorneys general. In Massachusetts, for example, the attorney general intervened in the purchase of two community hospitals by Columbia/HCA, retained an independent accounting firm to determine fair market value, obtained a commitment to keep both emergency rooms open for at least 3 years, and improved other community benefits, including the terms of the foundation (Office of the Attorney General, 1996). Other states have strengthened their oversight of these conversions. Nebraska, for example, enacted a law empowering its attorney general to block the conversion of a not-for-profit hospital on the basis of any of nine criteria, including conflicts of interest of board members, too low a purchase price, and "whether the purchaser has made a commitment to provide care to the disadvantaged, the uninsured, and the underinsured, and to provide benefits to the affected community to promote improved health care" (Nebraska State Legislature, 1996).

Whose Interests Do Specialty Hospitals Serve?

A new battleground has opened up in recent years between specialty hospitals and acute care hospitals. As of 2003, there were about 100 operational specialty hospitals across the country with 20 to 30 more under construction. They are for-profit, investor-owned (often by local physicians), and usually have under 100 beds. They emphasize lucrative procedures, especially cardiac care and orthopedic surgery, and claim to be more efficient due to shorter turnaround times between surgeries, less bureaucracy, and the motivation of their physician investors (McGinley, 2003; Page, 2003). Full-service, acute care hospitals, however, see them as skimming away profitable parts of their operations, leaving them with poorly reimbursed essential services (e.g., emergency and trauma services, burn units) and less ability to make ends meet. They also point out that specialty hospitals take less responsibility for the care of lower income patients and generally care for patients with less severe illnesses than those in general hospitals, as was shown by a 2003 study by the General Accounting Office (Voelker, 2003; General Accounting Office, 2003). In view of concerns raised by critics of specialty hospitals, the 2003 Medicare reform law imposed an 18-month moratorium on reimbursing physicians who self-refer to a specialty hospital built after November, 2003, and also called for studies on the financial impact and referral patterns of specialty hospitals (Silverman, 2004).

In their backlash to the threat of specialty hospitals, acute care hospitals have several strategies at their disposal, including blocking specialty hospitals through the "certificate of need" process (still operational in one-half of the states) and termination of privileges for physicians working at a competing specialty hospital. Specialty hospitals are now gathering data on their outcomes of care, but there is little reason to believe that they will be less costly and their impact on acute care hospitals is likely to be detrimental.

CONCLUDING COMMENTS

Returning to the opposing views quoted at the beginning of this chapter, it is clear that Paul Starr's predictions were on target. The defects of the health care system have indeed been magnified over the last 21 years by the corporatization of health care. Despite the claims by investor-owned chains of greater efficiency and value, their costs are higher, value has declined, and quality of care is worse than at their not-for-profit counterparts. The five investor-owned chains profiled here cannot be dismissed as anecdotal or unrepresentative of the industry since these are the largest chains of their types. The suggestion by Thomas Frist, Jr., chairman of HCA, that hospitals are "kind of like a utility" seems disingenuous since HCA and other investor-owned, for-profit chains go to great lengths to avoid public control. Having monitored corporatization of U.S. health care for years from his seat on the House Ways and Means Health Subcommittee, California Representative Pete Stark has this to say:

> Making fat profits on hospitals at the expense of the poor and the sick may not be a prison offense in this country. What is a crime is the galloping privatization of the nation's health resources and the rise of a competitive health care system that has less and less to do with health and access to care, and everything to do with money. (Lindorff, 1992, p. 22).

REFERENCES

Abelson, R. (2002, Nov. 24). Nurses' Association says in study that big hospital chain overcharges patients for drugs. *The New York Times.*

Associated Press (2002). Hospital chain ends fraud case. *The New York Times,* December 19, C9.

Atlas, R. D. (2003, Mar. 22). HealthSouth is scrambling to arrange financing to avert bankruptcy. *The New York Times,* C1.

Bodenheimer, T. S., & Grumbach, K. (2002). *Understanding health policy: A clinical approach.* New York: Lange Medical Books/McGraw-Hill.

Coye, M. J. (1997). The sale of Good Samaritan: A view from the trenches. *Health Affairs (Millwood), 16*(2), 107.

Derber, C. (1998). *Corporation nation: How corporations are taking over our lives and what we can do about it* (p. 246). Griffin, NY: St. Martin's Press.

Devereaux, P. J., Choi, P. T., Lacketti, C., Weaver, B., Schumenann, H.J., Haines, T. (2002). A systematic review and meta-analysis of studies comparing mortality rates of private for-profit and private not-for-profit.hospitals. *Canadian Medical Association Journal, 166,* 1399.

Freeh, L. (1995, Mar. 21). Federal Bureau of Investigation statement before the Special Committee on Aging, U.S. Senate, Washington, D.C., p 4.

Freudenheim, M. (1993, Dec. 14). National Medical resolves last of insurance disputes. *The New York Times,* C5.

Freudenheim, M. (2002, Feb. 7). F.B.I. is investigating HealthSouth trades. *The New York Times,* B1.

Freudenheim, M. (2003, Mar. 20) Hospital chain accused of accounting fraud. *The New York Times,* A1.

Freudenheim, M., & Abelson R. (2003, Mar. 21). HealthSouth regroups in effort to avoid bankruptcy. *The New York Times,* March 21.

General Accounting Office. (2003, Apr. 18). Specialty hospitals: Information on national market share, physician ownership and patients served. GAO-03–683R.

Gentile, R. (2003, Jan. 19). Tenet Healthcare woes mirror past scandals. *Contra Costa Times.*

Ginsburg, C. (1996, Nov. 18). The patient as profit center: Hospital Inc. comes to town. *The Nation,* November 18, 18.

Gray, B. H., (Ed.) (1986). For-profit enterprise in health care. Washington, DC: Institute of Medicine, National Academy Press.

Harrington, C. (1996). The nursing home industry: Public policy in the 1990s. In: P. Brown (Ed.), *Perspectives in Medical Sociology.* Prospect Heights, IL: Waveland Press. Harrington, C., & Carrillo, H. (2001). The regulation and enforcement of federal nursing home standards, 1991–1997. In C. Harrington & C. L. Estes (Eds.), *Health Policy,* Sudbury, MA: Jones & Bartlett.

Harrington, C., Woolhandler, S., Mullen, J., Carilló, H., & Himmelstein, D. U. (2001). Does investor-ownership of nursing homes compromise the quality of care? *American Journal of Public Health, 91,* 1.

Hartz, A. J., Krakauer, H., Kuhn, E. M., Young, M., Jacobsen, S. I., Gay, G. (1989). Hospital characteristics and mortality rates. *The New England Journal Medicine, 321,* 1720.

Himmelstein, D. U., Woolhandler, S., Hellander, I., & Wolfe, S. M. (1999). Quality of care in investor-owned vs not-for-profit HMOs. *Journal of the American Medical Association, 282.*

Himmelstein, D. U., Woolhandler, S., Hellander, I. (2001). *Bleeding the patient: The consequences of corporate health care.* Monroe, ME: Common Courage Press.

Kirchner, M. (1985, Nov. 25). Will you have to join a hospital chain to survive? *Medical Economics,* November 25, 164–172.

Kong, D., & O'Neill, G. (1997, May 11). Locked wards open door to booming business. *Boston Sunday Globe,* May 11, A1. Kovner, C., & Gergen, P. J. (1998). Nurse staffing levels and adverse events following surgery in U.S. hospitals. *Image Journal Nursing Schools, 30,* 315.

Kuttner, R. (1996). Columbia/HCA and the resurgence of the for-profit hospital business. *The New England Journal of Medicine 335,* 446.

Lindorff, D. (1992). *Marketplace medicine: The rise of the for-profit hospital chains (p. 276).* New York: Bantam Books. Martinez, B. (2002, Apr. 12). After an era of dominant HMOs, hospitals are turning the tables. *The Wall Street Journal Online.*

McGinley, L. (2003, May 16). Niche hospitals draw criticism from lawmakers. *The Wall Street Journal.*

Meyer, H. (1995, June 5). The deal. *Hospitals & Health Networks,* June 5, 22, 24, 26, 28.

Myerson, A. R. (1994). Hospital chain sets guilty plea: Kickbacks, bribes paid for referrals. *The New York Times,* C1.

Nebraska State Legislature (1996). Legislative Bill 1188, the Nonprofit Hospital Sale Act, Sections 7 and 8. Lincoln, NE: Author.

Norris, F. (2003, March 20). In U.S. eyes, a fraud particularly bold. *The New York Times,* C1.

Office of the Attorney General. (1996, Apr. 1). Harshbarger reaches agreement with MetroWest and Columbia/HCA on hospital deal. News release, Boston, Massachusetts.

Page, L. (2003, March). Battle lines: Acute care and specialty hospitals square off in turf wars over lucrative medical procedures. *Medical Economics,* March, 14–17.

Rapaport, L. (2002, Nov. 27). Tenet's fees for Medicare tops in state. *Sacramento Bee.* Retrieved from sacbee.com.

Romero, S. (2003, Mar. 21). The rise and fall of Richard Scrushy, entrepreneur. *The New York Times,* C4.

Romero, S., & Freudenheim, M. (2003, Mar. 26) HealthSouth advisors said to be under scrutiny. *The New York Times,* C1.

Rundle, R. L. (2004, Jan. 27). Tenet remains on tenuous ground. *The Wall Street Journal,* C5.

Sherrid, P. (2002, May 27). Money and business. Long-term blues: Nursing homes to Congress: We really need Medicare. Retrieved from *U.S.news.com.*

Silverman, J. (2004, Feb. 1). Fewer Medicaid patients seen at specialty hospitals. *Family Practice News,* p. 120.

Sparrow, M. K. (2000). *License to steal: How fraud bleeds America's health care system.* Boulder, CO: Westview Press.

Starkweather, D. B. (1981, Apr. 22). U. S. Hospitals: Corporate Concentration vs. Local Community Control. Public Affairs Report, Bulletin of the Institute of Governmental Studies, University of California, Berkeley.

Starr, P. (1982). *The social transformation of American medicine.* New York: Basic Books.

Stein, L. (2002, Sept. 20). Pulling the plug. *Metro, Silicon Valley's Weekly Newspaper.*

Taylor, D. H. Jr., Whellan, D. E., Sloan, F. A. (1999). Effects of admission to a teaching hospital on the cost and quality of care for Medicare beneficiaries. *The New England Journal of Medicine, 340,* 293.

Thomas, E. J., et al. (1998, Nov. 8–10). Hospital ownership is associated with preventable adverse events. Proceedings of Enhancing Patient Safety and Reducing Errors in Health Care, Rancho Mirage, California, November 8–10.

Voelker, S. (2003). Specialty hospitals generate revenue and controversy. *Journal of the American Medical Association, 289,* 409.

Weil, J., & Mollencamp, C. (2003, Aug. 6). HealthSouth options award is off the charts. *The Wall Street Journal,* August 6, C1.

White, R. D. (2002, Jan. 5). Tenet continuing resurgence. *Los Angeles Times*.

White, R. D. (2003, Jan. 10). U. S. files suit against Tenet over billings. Retrieved from Latimes.com.

Woolhandler, S., & Himmelstein, D. U. (1997). Costs of care and administration at for-profit and other hospitals in the United States. *The New England Journal of Medicine, 336,* 769.

Woolhandler, S. (2002, May 28). Physicians for a National Health Program, press release, Chicago, Illinois.

Chapter 3

HEALTH MAINTENANCE
ORGANIZATIONS (HMOs)

There is a broad spectrum of HMOs in terms of motivation, practices, and values. Not-for-profit HMOs such as Kaiser Permanente and Group Health Cooperative of Puget Sound tend to be more socially oriented and emphasize prevention, patient education, and evidence-based, cost-effective care. At the other end of the spectrum are investor-owned, for-profit HMOs, driven strongly by the mission to make money for their shareholders. Although the distinction between the two types of HMOs can at times be blurred, many studies over the years have demonstrated major differences between these polar opposites in terms of costs, access, and quality of care.

About two-thirds of the nation's HMOs are now for-profit and fall at the investor-owned end of the spectrum. This chapter will focus on the impact of corporate investor-owned HMOs on health care costs, access, and quality of care, including a discussion of (1) their history and present status; (2) common practices not in the public interest; and (3) some major controversial and unresolved issues.

HISTORICAL PERSPECTIVE

The federal government promoted expansion of the concept of the HMO in the early 1970s in the hope that costs could be contained based on the promise of not-for-profit HMOs, which had already emphasized prevention and service for many years. The Health Maintenance Organization Act of 1973 was passed by Congress as part of President Richard Nixon's health care reform strategy. The Act overrode previous state bans on prepaid group practice that had been lobbied for earlier by organized medicine, and provided some start-up funds for new HMOs. The basic principle of prepaid group practice was that "an organized system of care accepts the responsibility to provide or otherwise assure comprehensive care to a defined population for a fixed periodic payment per person or per family." (Somers & Somers, 1977). The Independent Practice Association (IPA) model joined group and staff models as a legitimate HMO. Under the IPA model, the fiscal intermediary contracts with a loose group of physicians, working in independent practices or multispecialty group practices, to provide care to HMO enrollees. (Kovner & Jones, 1999). The regulation required large and medium-sized business that offered health insurance to their employees to also offer at least one federally qualified HMO, if available in the area, as an alternative to fee-for-service coverage. In order to qualify for employer mandate startup funding, new plans had to meet federal requirements for benefits coverage and guarantee coverage, at uniform community-rated prices, to all enrollees regardless of health status. An HMO was required to offer, as basic services, a comprehensive range of services, including physicians' care, emergency care, laboratory and diagnostic services, hospitalization, mental health care, home health services, family planning and alcohol and drug abuse services (Starr, 1982).

The movement to HMOs was slow during the 1970s, but picked up steam in the 1980s as employees gravitated to what was initially a comprehensive benefits package with lower out-of-pocket costs compared with traditional indemnity insurers, which typically reimbursed beneficiaries specified amounts, usually as partial payments, toward the cost of services (Somers & Somers, 1977, p. 112). HMO growth was further fueled by investor ownership as commercial insurers started new HMOs and as many not-for-profit plans converted to for-profit status. Although the HMO Act of 1973 banned explicit underwriting, insurers found many subtle ways to attract a favorable patient risk mix, and a longstanding debate was started over the extent to which for-profit HMOs "cherry pick" the market (Robinson, 1999).

In their early years, IPA model HMOs acted mainly as brokers between participating physicians and HMOs. In that model, individual physicians could contract with one or several HMOs while practicing in a loosely organized IPA. In later years, IPA type HMOs took a more active role in authorizing services, deciding on selection and retention of physicians, and assessing quality of care. A more tightly organized HMO model is the integrated medical group, whereby physicians are employees of a larger organization that owns and manages their practices. Still another HMO model involves a network of contractual relationships which can link the HMO with hospitals, physician groups, pharmacies, home health agencies, and other provider groups. These virtually integrated network HMOs may not provide direct health care services at all, instead serving as middle-men for negotiating contracts between the participants (Bodenheimer & Grumbach, 2002).

Capitation became the major method of payment to providers by HMOs. This was a system in which providers were paid a contracted amount each month for each enrollee ("covered life"). Financial risk was thereby shifted from insurers to providers. Later modifications of risk-sharing were made under different contractual agreements, including various systems for risk adjustment, "carve-outs" for special types of services, stop-loss provisions, and withholds/bonuses distributed at the end of each year. Capitation placed physicians in positions of potential conflict of interest whereby the physician earned more income by delivering less care. While capitation reimbursement of providers has been successful in many other Western industrialized countries for years, as well as in staff-model not-for-profit HMOs in the U.S., it has not been successful in the for-profit HMO industry in terms of cost containment or quality of care. In IPA model HMOs, many physicians belong to several IPAs and may contract with multiple HMOs. These are not circumstances which nurture the development of an efficient, quality-focused group practice culture (Bodenheimer & Grumbach, 2002, pp. 44–51).

The 1980s were years when business and government became very concerned about rising health care costs, and capitated HMOs and selective contracting were among their strategies to address the problem. The 1990s saw consolidation of larger insurers, more aggressive selective contracting, and more frequent conversion to for-profit status. By the mid-1990s, there were more for-profit HMOs than not-for-profits.

For-profit HMOs increasingly assumed the role of deciding how, where, and by whom the enrollees' health care was to be provided. Clinical decision making was infringed upon by business-oriented managers, leading to a growing chasm between providers and insurers, as well as tension between providers and their patients. With denial of services widespread and accountability of HMOs almost nonexistent, a widespread public backlash to HMOs emerged during the 1990s. A 1998 Wall Street Journal/NBC News poll found that 86% of respondents felt that HMOs were more concerned with cost control than providing good care. HMOs were blamed for limiting access to specialists and intruding upon the physician-patient relationship (Duff, 1998). They were suddenly being forced to the defensive under a flurry of lawsuits and the threat of government regulation. Consequently, the era of managed competition gave way to unmanaged competition as HMOs began charging more for premiums, offering less in capitation payments to providers, easing the gatekeeper roles whereby primary care physicians could limit access to specialists and other services, and enabling point-of-service access to specialists whereby patients could pay more out-of-pocket to see a provider who is not part of the HMO's regular provider panel. In effect, of course, as HMOs loosened their grip on the delivery system, costs again skyrocketed and HMOs merely passed these costs on to consumers (Robinson, 1999, p. 62).

As for-profit HMOs became discredited as a strategy for cost containment and delivery of care, one of the founders of the HMO concept, Dr. Paul Elwood, had to conclude "For those of us who devoted our lives to reshaping the health system trying to make it better for patients, the thing (managed care) has been a profound disappointment" (Phillips, 1998).

Ralph Nader went further in this overview of the for-profit HMO industry:

> As costs annually far exceeded the general inflation rate and health care absorbed ever greater percentages of the GNP, the alternative of "managed care" emerged as a way to control costs. A dominant format also emerged—the giant, for-profit HMOs and their entrepreneurial billionaire bosses securing large clusters of customers and seeking more and more mergers. A series of perverse economic incentives were insinuated from top to bottom so as to seriously compromise the independent clinical judgments of physicians and other health professionals and often turn the pocket- book allegiance of the health care servers against the interests of their patients, as with gag rules, bonuses for not referring and the like. The HMO and its deepening swamp of commercialism over service, of profiteering over professionalism, of denial or rationing of care where such care is critically needed, of depersonalization of intensely personal kinds of relationships, are all occurring and spreading without sufficient disclosure, accountability and structural responsibility before the damage to life and health is done. (Nader, 1999).

Today, after a period of intense competition, mergers and consolidation of HMOs during the 1990s, a smaller number of large, mostly-for-profit HMOs still cover about 80 million people in the U.S. Public suspicion continues about their conflict of interest between making money for their CEOs and shareholders and their responsibility to assure good medical care. As a result of changing policies of for-profit HMOs to allow more direct access to specialists, some physicians are starting to feel less encumbered by HMO restrictions. A 2001 survey by the Center for Studying Health System Change found, for example, that almost 86% of responding specialists felt they had enough clinical autonomy, up from 73% in 1997 (Martinez, 2003).

COMMON PRACTICES OF FOR-PROFIT HMOS

In their quest for profits above all else, here are some of the common practices of for-profit HMOs that have led to widespread public and even legislative and judicial distrust. Unfortunately, some not-for-profit HMOs have at times emulated some of these practices in the competitive marketplace (Kuttner, 1998), as illustrated by Kaiser Permanente, California's largest HMO, which conducted a pilot program for two years whereby financial bonuses were given to clerks who spent the least amount of time on the telephone with patients and limited the number of physicians' appointments (Ornstein, 2002).

Selection of Enrollees

For-profit HMOs invariably seek out healthier enrollees to avoid the higher financial risk of providing care for the chronically ill. They often segment local markets by geography and type of employer (Robinson, 1999). Another example of cherry picking the market is the disenrollment of patients (e.g., of about 6 million seniors enrolled in Medicare + Choice HMOs, more than 2 million were dropped between 1999 and 2003) (Bodenheimer, 2003).

Incentives for Physicians

During the 1980s and early 1990s many for-profit HMOs were quite straightforward in attempting to manipulate physician practice through financial incentives which rewarded the physician for limiting visits, diagnostic studies, and hospitalizations. One such method was the placement of funds by an HMO into a hospital risk pool, which could be shared by hospitals and physicians at the end of the year if there were residual funds in the pool (Bodenheimer & Grumbach, 2002, p. 50). The obvious ethical problems involved by such a bonus system brought increased professional and public concern (American Medical Association, 1995) as well as passage by a number of states of "patient protection" laws (Kuttner, 1998; Shalgian,

1999). More recently, HMOs have developed more acceptable bonus systems that reward quality of care.

Intrusions Upon Physicians Autonomy

For-profit HMOs have intruded into the physician-patient relationship and physician prerogatives in clinical decision making in a number of ways. These are some examples:

- "Gag clauses" in physicians' contracts restrict communication between physicians and their patients, including fully informed consents and consideration of diagnostic or therapeutic alternatives. A typical example of such a gag clause is: "Physicians shall agree not to take action or make any communication which undermines or could undermine the confidence of enrollees, potential enrollees, their employers, their unions, or the public in . . . the quality of . . . health care coverage" (Misocky, 1998).
- Physicians' claims of medical necessity are denied every day, initially by nonphysician reviewers, and later become matters of dispute between treating physicians, "experts" appointed by the HMOs, or the HMO's medical director. In their cost containment roles, these medical directors are in effect practicing medicine without seeing the patient, often across state lines, with just a telephone, rubber stamp and pen (Peeno, 1996). When challenged, HMOs typically respond that they are not practicing medicine or restraining care, just making coverage decisions.
- Use of actuarial, not clinical, guidelines for length of hospital stays that have no clinical or scientific basis, and are often only half as long as average hospital stays within a national database of 2,400 hospitals (e.g., 1 day for a hospital admission for a child with asthma vs. a national average of 2.2 days) (Martinez, 2000).

Denial of Services

Medical directors of for-profit HMOs are typically expected to deny at least 10% of approval requests, and have financial incentives to do so by receiving bonuses if they exceed that rate. They have various methods to achieve that goal, including medical underwriting to avoid high-risk individuals or groups, development of procedural barriers to approval, and revising contract benefits (Peeno, 1997, 1998). A recent study of coverage denials in a mixed-model HMO showed that patients scoring lower on physical functioning were more than twice as likely to be denied services as other patients. They also rated the quality of their health plan lower and had less trust in their own primary care physicians (Pearson, 2003).

The 1999 book *Making a Killing: HMOs and the Threat to Your Health* is filled with examples of unfortunate and often preventable outcomes as a result of denial of services by HMOs (Court & Smith, 1999). These are some other examples:

- inappropriate denial of emergency room services has been frequently documented (e.g., a 43% rejection rate by CIGNA in Pennsylvania in 1994) (Lippman, 1996)
- denial of corrective surgery for children with cleft palates, asserting that such surgery is cosmetic and not medically necessary (Rundle, 2003)
- denial of coverage of growth hormone therapy in children despite a 96% treatment approval rate by pediatric endocrinologists (Finkelstein, Silvers, Marreno, Neuhauser, & Cuttler, 1998)

As for-profit HMOs have been put on the defensive for such practices, a few have made some policy changes (e.g., United Healthcare decided to forgo pre-authorization review), but many critics of HMO abuses still call for federal legislation to assure responsible coverage by HMOs (Rose, 2000).

Undertreatment

There are many approaches to undertreatment and cost containment by for-profit HMOs, including denial of services, restrictive formula policies for prescription drugs, policies relating to hospital admission and length of stay, and others. These often result in compromised access to care and its quality. Four examples since the 1970s illustrate the extent of the problem:

- An administrator of a California HMO in the 1970s sent this written directive to providers: "Do as little as you possibly can for the PHP (prepaid health plan) patient." Later chart audits by the California Health Department found many instances of undertreatment (U.S. Senate, 1975).
- Undertreatment was common among for-profit HMOs during the 1980s. One example is a Florida based Medicare HMO (International Medical Centers, Inc.), where an administrator was fired after blowing the whistle to his superiors of 130 major quality problems (U.S. House of Representatives, 1988).

- More recently, a national study in 1999 showed that investor-owned HMOs scored worse than not-for-profit HMOs on all 14 quality indicators reported to the National Committee for Quality Assurance (e.g., a 27% lower rate of eye examinations for patients with diabetes and a 16% lower rate of appropriate drug treatment for patients after myocardial infarction) (Hellander, 1999).
- Medicaid HMOs in New Jersey are now rejecting 17-30% of claims for hospital stays, about three times as often as other managed care plans (Freudenheim, 2003).

Hiding Performance Data

A voluntary national system for reporting of quality assurance data has been in place since the mid-1990s. Accredited HMOs have been required since 1999 to have their performance data made public. A good idea has been rendered ineffectual, however, since most HMOs with poor quality of care withhold reporting of their scores. Published report cards by the National Committee for Quality Assurance (NCQA) are therefore biased toward higher scores and mislead the public as to the overall performance of HMOs across the country. About one-half of the 329 HMOs that reported data in 1997 did not report in 1998, while about one-quarter of HMOs that reported in 1998 failed to report in 1999 (McCormick, Himmelstein, Woolhandler, Wolfe & Bor, 2002). Nonreporters fall at the for-profit, investor-owned end of the spectrum (of the 228 quality reporting dropouts in 1998 and 1999, 60 were Prudential plans, 37 CIGNA, 17 United Healthcare, and 14 Humana) (Physicians for a National Health Program, 2000).

Fraud

In our deregulated and loosely monitored health care system, fraud is unfortunately widespread and accounts for enormous waste of health care dollars every year in the U.S. Investor-owned HMOs are a big part of the problem. Some fraud is flagrantly criminal, such as the collusion between Department of Social Services employees in Maryland in the mid-1990s, who accepted bribes from HMO marketing representatives in return for the names and other information about potential HMO enrollees. This information was then used by the HMOs to enroll and collect capitation fees without the "enrollees" knowledge (Maryland Office of the Attorney General, 1999).

Other fraud is more subtle as a result of a wide variety of abusive corporate policies and may be difficult to ferret out from the complex layers of businesses which separate payers from providers and their patients. Whether related to Medicare, Medicaid or other patient populations, corporate fraud ends up diverting capitation funds from care.

Below are some of the fraudulent practices that are well known to regulators, and which collectively are estimated to account for somewhere between 10% and 40% of total health care expenditures each year in the U.S:

- "falsification of new enrollee registrations (either fictitious patients or fictitious enrollments)
- kickbacks to primary care physicians for referrals of sicker patients to "out-of-network" specialists
- fraudulent subcontracts (for example, where no services are provided, or phony management contracts)
- failing to procure health practitioners so that no service is ultimately provided
- retaining exorbitant "administrative fees" and leaving inadequate provision for services
- assigning unreasonably high numbers of beneficiaries to providers of service, making adequate service impossible
- "bust-outs" (money goes in, no money goes out to the vendors, then the entrepreneur claims bankruptcy or simply disappears)
- withholding or unreasonably delaying payments to subcontractors, providers, or provider networks
- destruction of claims
- embezzlement of capitation funds paid by the state
- improper disenrollment practices (deliberately eliminating bad risks—persuading or forcing sicker patients to leave)
- disenrolling beneficiaries prior to hospital treatment (so hospital fees are paid under fee-for-service system), then re-enrolling them once they have recovered." (Sparrow, 2000).

SOME UNRESOLVED ISSUES

Three major issues about for-profit HMOs have been controversial for many years. Despite prolonged debate, they remain largely unresolved.

Are Investor-Owned HMOs Unethical?

For-profit HMOs are a product of the market-based system, and markets are fundamentally amoral (Kuttner, 1996). So the quick answer to this question is that the kinds of practices practiced widely by investor-owned HMOs, though often successful by business standards, cannot be justified on ethical grounds. If one has any doubts about this issue, this case example, by no means an anecdotal exception, makes the point:

> Dr. Robert Gumbiner was one of the early pioneers of HMO practice. He founded *FHP* as a staff-model HMO in Southern California during the 1970s. Its operations were based on the premise that all services would be more accessible if placed under one roof at reduced cost. In one of the mega-mergers in the late 1990s, FHP was consolidated with PacifiCare. The merger was contentious to the point of litigation. Dr. Gumbiner alleged that venture capitalists defrauded FHP shareholders of over $200 million by firing one-third of FHP physicians and dismantling its medical programs in order to cut costs and make it a more attractive purchase (Court & Smith, 1999, pp. 107–108). After more than 25 years experience in HMO practice, Dr. Gumbiner has come to the view that today's HMOs, which in many cases own no medical resources but merely contract with physicians and hospitals to provide care, should be regulated as public utilities (Gumbiner, 1997).

As an ethicist at the University of Notre Dame, Larry Churchill reminds us that we cannot expect much better from a market-based system where the commodification of health care distorts ethics and threatens equity:

> Market forces in health care do not solve the access problem. They aggravate it. They create still further fragmentation between the insured and uninsured, the employed and the unemployed, the sick and the well. But to be fair, markets were never designed to achieve equity in access. (Churchill, 1999).

Can Investor-Owned HMOs Be Held Accountable?

Of all the abuses of for-profit HMOs, those dealing with appeal mechanisms after denial of treatment requests have been a flashpoint for the most controversy. Most states have laws on the books preventing corporations from practicing medicine (Court & Smith, 1999, p. 135). HMOs for years claimed that, as a "corporate person," they were making coverage decisions, not practicing medicine. They also shielded themselves with the federal Employee Retirement Income Security Act of 1974 (ERISA). ERISA was enacted before the advent of managed care, and governs private, company-sponsored health plans. Although patients can sue their health plans under ERISA for denial of benefits, they can recover only the costs of the benefits denied, not damages. ERISA does not apply to health insurance provided by government employers or churches, nor to beneficiaries of Medicare or Medicaid. ERISA has pre-empted state regulation of managed care organizations for many years, hamstringing regulators from challenging illegitimate denial of services by many HMOs.

As abuses by for-profit HMOs have drawn increased scrutiny and public backlash in recent years, there have been legislative and judicial responses to the problem, which now at least partially improve the opportunities for patients and their physicians to obtain fair coverage. Here are some examples of this progress:

- There are now external review mechanisms in place for review of HMO coverage decisions in more than 40 states (Pollitz, Crowley, Lucia, & Bangit, 2002) and their legal standing was upheld by the U.S. Supreme Court in the 2000 case, *Rush Prudential HMO Inc. vs. Moran.*
- Texas passed legislation in 1997 becoming the first state in the country to allow HMOs to be taken to court for alleged corporate medical negligence, including claims for damages for negligence and quality-of-care violations (Court & Smith, 1999, p. 133).
- The U.S. Supreme Court in a 2000 case held that some coverage decisions involve both interpretation of an insurance contract and the exercise of a medical judgment about medical diagnosis and treatment (Pegram vs. Herdrich, 2000)
- A 2002 decision by the Missouri Supreme Court ruled that utilization review decisions by HMOs *do* constitute the practice of medicine, thereby holding medical directors of HMOs accountable for their coverage decisions (Rice, 2002).
- In April 2003, the U.S. Supreme Court ruled unanimously that states can force HMOs to open their networks to physicians who agree to the network's terms (Anderson, 2003).
- Also in 2003, the U.S. Court of Appeals for the 2nd Circuit ruled that patients have the right to sue health insurers that refuse to authorize medically necessary treatment (Frieden, 2003).

Each year in the U.S., there are more than 250,000 appeals made by privately insured HMO enrollees (Gresenz, Studdert, Campbell, & Hensler, 2002). Although the legal landscape is changing and now brings some protections to patients, the for-profit HMO industry still places many procedural barriers in the appeals process and lobbies against patient bills of rights in Congress. The right to sue HMOs over contractual as well as medical necessity disputes has been the most controversial part of proposed legislation to strengthen patients' rights; the provisions were killed in the 107th Congress in 2002, and still have a questionable future (Rosenbaum, 2003).

Can Quality Assurance Be Provided by Investor-Owned HMOs?

Based on the foregoing, it might appear that quality assurance in an investor-owned HMO is an oxymoron. As we have seen, voluntary reporting to the National Committee for Quality Assurance does not work when poor-quality HMOs withhold their performance data. The IPA model HMO, involving many providers in different practice settings, lacks the structure for a coherent system of quality assurance. In addition, the emphasis by investor-owned HMOs on short-term profits in the next two or three quarters works against their active, long-term commitment to and investment in effective screening and prevention programs. One would have to conclude that a national mandatory reporting system for performance data will be needed before there can be any reasonable expectation of reliable quality assurance information for investor-owned HMOs.

CONCLUDING COMMENTS

The rapid growth rate of for-profit HMOs seen during the 1990s came to an end by the turn of the century as managed care became tarnished by HMO abuses and large employers lost confidence in its potential for cost containment. The motivation and practices of for-profit HMOs have been called into question by public, legislative, and judicial responses to their excesses. Inflation of health care costs has returned as a major problem, and these costs are being passed along to consumers by HMOs, other insurers and employers. Robert Kuttner, a well-known health care analyst, draws this conclusion about the market-based system, which fostered the abuses of for-profit HMOs:

For more than a decade, "market-driven health care" has been advertised as the salvation of the American health care system. In the 1990s, entrepreneurs succeeded in obtaining the easily available cost savings, at great profit to themselves and their investors. By the late 1990s, however, pressure to protect profit margins had led to such dubious business strategies as the avoidance of sick patients, the excessive micromanagement of physicians, the worsening of staff-to-patient ratios, and the outright denial of care. In an industry driven by investor-owned companies, the original promise of managed care—greater efficiency in the use of available resources and greater integration of preventive and treatment services—has degenerated into mere avoidance of cost. (Kuttner, 1999)

That these trends have gone unchecked is indicated by the finding by Weiss Ratings, a Florida-based independent research firm, that the nation's HMOs reported an 81% increase in profits in 2002 over 2001, attributed to higher premiums and more restrictive policies (Rose, 2004).

REFERENCES

American Medical Association (AMA) (1995). Council on Ethical and Judicial Affairs: ethical issues in managed care. *Journal of the American Medical Association, 273,* 330.

Anderson, M. (2003, April 3). States can force HMOs to open networks to doctors. *The New York Times,* A2.

Bodenheimer, T. S. & Grumbach, K. (2002). *Understanding health policy: A clinical approach (pp. 73–75).* New York: Lange Medical Books/McGraw-Hill.

Bodenheim, T. S. ((2003). The dismal failure of Medicare privatization. Senior Action Network, San Francisco, California.

Churchill, L. R. (1999). The United States health care system under managed care: How the commodification of health care distorts ethics and threatens equity. *Health Care Analysis, 7,* 393.

Court, J. & Smith, F. ((1999). *Making a Killing: HMOs and the Threat to Your Health.* Monroe, ME: Common Courage Press.

Duff, C. (1998, June 25). Americans tell government to stay out—except in case of health care. *The Wall Street Journal,* A9, A14.

Finkelstein, B. S., Silvers, J. B., Marrero, U., Neuhauser, D., Cuttler, L. (1998). Insurance coverage, physician recommendations, and access to emerging treatments: Growth hormone therapy for childhood short stature. *Journal of the American Medical Association, 279,* 663, 1998.

Freudenheim, M. (2003, Feb. 19). Some concerns thrive on Medicaid patients. *The New York Times,* C1.

Frieden, J. (2003). Practice Trends: Policy & Practice. A patient's right to sue. *Family Practice News, 33,* 54.

Gresenz, C. R., Studdert, D. M., Campbell, N. Hensler, D. R. (2002). Patients in conflict with managed care: A profile of appeals in two HMOs. *Health Affairs (Millwood)*, 21, 189.

Gumbiner, R. (1997). FHP: The evolution of a managed care health maintenance organization, 1993–1997, Volume II. Berkeley: University of California Press.

Hellander, I. (1999, July 12). Quality of care lower in for-profit HMOs than in non-profits. PNHP news release.

Kovner, A. R., & Jonas, S. (Editors). *Health Care Delivery in the United States.* New York: Springer Publishing Company, 1999, p. 47.

Kuttner, R. (1996, July-Aug). Taking care of business. *The American Prospect*, 29, 28.

Kuttner, R. (1998). Must good HMOs go bad? The search for checks and balances. *The New England Journal of Medicine*, 338, 1635.

Kuttner, R. (1999). The American health care system: Wall Street and health care. *The New England Journal of Medicine*, 340, 664.

Lippman, H. (1996). The game plans play with ER bills. *Business and Health*, 14, 20.

Martinez, B. (2000, Sept. 14). Care guidelines used by insurers face scrutiny. *The Wall Street Journal*, B1, B4.

Martinez, B. (2003, Jan. 16). HMOs grip is easing doctors say. *The Wall Street Journal*, D4.

Maryland Office of the Attorney General (1999). News release, June 13, Baltimore, Maryland, p. 1.

McCormick, D., Himmelstein, D. U., Woolhandler, S., Wolfe, S. M., Bor, D. H. (2002). Relationship between low quality-of-care scores and HMOs subsequent public disclosure of quality-of-care scores. *Journal of the American Medical Association*, 288, 1484.

Misocky, M. (1998). The patients' bill of rights: Managed care under siege. *Journal of Contemporary Health Law Policy*, 15, 72.

Nader, R. (1999). In J. Court & F. Smith, *Making a killing: HMOs and the threat to your health.* Monroe, ME: Common Courage Press.

Ornstein, C. (2002, May 19). Kaiser clerks paid more for helping less. *Los Angeles Times.*

Pearson, S. D. (2003). Patient reports of coverage denial: Association with ratings of health plan quality and trust in physician. *American Journal of Managed Care*, 9, 238.

Peeno, L. (1996). A physician answers questions about denial of care in managed care corporations. *Citizen Action.*

Peeno, L. (1997, Dec. 2). A Day in the Life of a Company Doctor. Excerpted from a talk before the Ad Hoc Committee to Defend Health Care. Boston, Massachusetts.

Peeno, L. (1998, Mar. 9). Approved or denied—how HMOs decide what care you need. *U.S. News and World Report*, 124(9).

Phillips, D. F. (1998). Erecting an ethical framework for managed care. *Journal of the American Medical Association*, 280, 2060.

Physicians for a National Health Program (PNHP) (2002). Quality reporting dropouts in 1998 and 1999, press release. September 20.

Pollitz, K., Crowley, J., Lucias, K., & Bangit, E. (2002, May). Assessing state external review programs and the effects of pending federal patients' rights legislation. Menlo Park, CA: Henry J. Kaiser Family Foundation.

Rice, B. (2002, June 7). When an HMO denial is practicing medicine. *Medical Economics, 100,* pp. 100–103.

Robinson, J. C. (1999). *The Corporate Practice of Medicine: Competition and Innovation in Health Care.* Berkeley, CA: University of California Press.

Rose, J. R. (2000, Jan. 24). Utilization review: Skeptical reaction to United Healthcare's "we trust doctors' gambit. *Medical Economics, 30.*

Rose, J. R. (2004, Feb. 6). Focus on Practice. HMO coffers overflow. *Medical Economics,* p. 19.

Rosenbaum, S. (2003). Managed care and patients' rights. *Journal of the American Medical Association, 289,* 906.

Rundle, R. L. (2003, Feb. 19). HMO denial of crucial care is rare. *The Wall Street Journal.*

Rush Prudential HMO Inc v Moran, No. 00-1021 (SCT 2002).

Shalgian, C. (1999). A brief history of patient protection legislation. *Bulletin of American College of Surgery, 84,* 8.

Somers, A. R., & Somers, H. M. *Health and Health Care: Policies in Perspective.* Germantown, MD Aspen Systems Corporation, 1977, p. 222.

Sparrow, M. K. (2000). *License to steal: How fraud bleeds America's health care system (71, 106–107).* Boulder, CO: Westview Press.

Starr, P. (1982). *The social transformation of American medicine.* New York: Basic Books.

U. S. House of Representatives (1988). 45th Report by the Committee on Government Operations, April 14. Medicare Health Maintenance Organizations: The International Medical Centers Experience. Washington, DC: U.S. Government Printing Office.

U.S. Senate (1975). Prepaid Health Plans. Hearings before the Permanent Subcommittee on Investigations, Committee on Government Operations, March 13 and 14. Washington, DC: U. S. Government Printing Office.

Chapter 4

THE HEALTH INSURANCE INDUSTRY

Illness is an unpredictable risk for the individual family, but we know fairly accurately how much illness a large group of people will have, how much medical care they will require, and how many days they will have to spend in hospitals. In other words, we cannot budget the cost of illness for the individual family but we can budget it for the nation. The principle must be to spread the risk among as many people as possible and to pool the resources of as many people as possible . . . The experience of the last 15 years in the United States has, in my opinion, demonstrated that voluntary health insurance does not solve the problem of the nation. It reaches only certain groups and is always at the mercy of economic fluctuations... Hence, if we decide to finance medical services through insurance, the insurance system must be compulsory.

Henry Sigerist, MD
Director, Johns Hopkins University,
Institute of the History of Medicine

The above observations by Dr. Sigerist in 1944 were thought by many at the time to be radical, even revolutionary, ideas. Today, almost 60 years later, they are well grounded in fact and experience, though still denied by a powerful and well-heeled private insurance industry and many proponents of the market-based system. The battle over voluntary versus compulsory health insurance, as well as business versus social goals of health insurance, has been waged in the U.S. for over 90 years. Although private interests have always won out, there have been four efforts to enact national health insurance since 1912, and the controversy continues as a result of today's failing health care system.

This chapter has four goals: (1) to present some historical perspective on the evolution of health insurance in the United States; (2) to briefly describe the structure of today's health insurance coverage, both private and public; (3) to outline some common practices of investor-owned health insurance companies not in the public interest; and (4) to discuss some pressing, but still unresolved policy issues concerning the future of health insurance in this country.

HISTORICAL PERSPECTIVE

The problems of limited access to health care, and its increasing costs, were hotly debated issues even before the advent of health insurance. Under Theodore Roosevelt's leadership, the Progressive Party made national health insurance (NHI) a platform plank in the presidential election campaign of 1912. Despite the energetic efforts of various reform groups from 1912 to 1917, however, an alliance between employers and organized medicine defeated the proposal in 1917 (Somers & Somers, 1977; Starr, 1982).

During the Great Depression, the increasing costs of medical care, especially of hospitalization, again became a major political issue. For many families, bills for medical care had grown to one-third or even one-half of their income (Starr, 1982). In 1930, 97% of the nation's work force had no health insurance (Lear, 1962). The Committee on the Costs of Medical Care (CCMC) recommended that the costs of medical care should be managed on a group payment basis through the use of insurance or taxation or both (Falk, 1983). The Social Security Act was passed in 1935 as a key part of President Franklin D. Roosevelt's New Deal, and federal funds were made available to local health departments for maternal and child health services (Rosenblatt & Moscovice, 1982). National health insurance was favored by Roosevelt and might have been included in the Social Security Act, but he withdrew it in the face of strong opposition from organized medicine (Starr, 1982, pp. 1266–1270). The newly emerged not-for-profit Blue Cross was being promoted as an alternative to compulsory health insurance (Rothman, 1991, 1993). Blue Cross promised that its coverage would:

> . . . eliminate the demand for compulsory health insurance and stop the reintroduction of vicious sociological bills into the state legislature year after year—Blue Cross plans are a distinctly American institution, a unique combination of individual initiative and social responsibility. They perform a public service without public compulsion. (Rothman, 1991).

Blue Cross was first created on January 1, 1930 by the Baylor University Hospital in Dallas, Texas as an insurance plan covering hospitalization for public school teachers. So, in its early years, it had every right to claim its central commitment to the public interest through community service. The concept spread rapidly in many states through the initiative of hospitals. In 1939 the first Blue Shield plans were developed by physicians' organizations in California and Michigan, at first to cover fees of surgeons and other hospital-based specialists (Andrews, 1995). By providing coverage at discounted rates for hospitals and physicians, Blue Cross and Blue Shield (BCBS) plans enabled insured patients to have access to medical care and at the same time keep hospital beds open (McNerney, 1996).

Noting the early success of Blue Cross plans, many commercial insurance companies entered the health insurance business during the 1930s. From the start their plans set limits on benefits, which were often custom-tailored to the desires of each employer. World War II brought the U.S. out of the Depression and into a severe labor shortage in a wartime economy. Wage stabilization rules were established by the federal government, and many companies granted health benefits to their employees in lieu of additional wages in order to recruit and retain workers. IRS rulings further propelled the growth of employer-based health insurance by making the costs of health insurance tax-exempt to employers (Somers & Somers, 1977, pp. 109–111; Andrews, 1995). By the end of the war in 1945, about 25% of the population had some kind of health insurance, mostly for hospitalization (Labor Research Association, 1947).

President Roosevelt again proposed NHI as part of an "economic bill of rights" in his 1944 State of the Union address. Following his death in 1945, President Harry Truman put forward such a plan to be administered through the Social Security system (Truman, 1945). After an intense public and legislative debate, it was defeated by strong opposition led by the American Medical Association (AMA), the American Hospital Association (AHA), and the insurance industry. The only surviving remnants of the NHI proposal were amendments to the Social Security Act, passed in 1950, which provided for federal "vendor payments" to the states as matching funds for medical care of welfare recipients (Somers & Somers, 1977).

In addition to the rapid growth of employer-based voluntary health insurance, the 1940s also saw the advent of prepaid group practice. Henry Kaiser started his not-for-profit HMO in 1942 to provide medical care for workers in his shipyards. Kaiser clinics grew rapidly in California during the 1940s, and were soon joined by other not-for-profit HMOs, such as Group Health Cooperative of Puget Sound (Andrews, 1995).

Commercial companies expanded into the group and individual health insurance market throughout the 1950s. By 1951, they had surpassed Blue Cross in enrollment and there were 800 commercial carriers by 1961 with 40 million individual enrollees (Andrews, 1995). However, only one-quarter of the population had health insurance of any kind and two-thirds of people over 65 years of age had no hospital insurance (Kolko, 1962). As the costs of health care continued to rise and access to care decreased for many millions of Americans, the stage was set for the passage of Medicare and Medicaid in 1965. These new public programs were strongly opposed by the AMA (Campion, 1984) while the AHA and Blue Cross joined forces to support their passage. Hospitals were assured that Blue Cross would process their claims for hospital services, and the rules on costs were both generous and vague (Andrews, 1995, p. 16).

While Medicare and Medicaid provided access to health care for many millions of disadvantaged Americans, they ushered in an extended period of health care inflation. Initial federal budget estimates projected a $10 billion outlay for Medicare in 1990, which turned out to be about $100 billion (Ginsberg, 1999). The 1970s and 1980s were halcyon years for hospitals and physicians, with most of their services paid for by open-ended cost reimbursement and professional fee schedules. New efforts to contain health care costs were needed. As we saw in the last chapter, managed care and for-profit HMOs were promoted as market strategies to contain costs. President Nixon put forward a "play or pay" employer mandate proposal in the early 1970s, under which employers would either offer acceptable coverage to their employees or pay a tax that would finance their coverage from an insurance pool that would also cover the unemployed (Rivlin, 1974). Several alternative proposals approaching universal coverage were hotly debated in Congress in 1973, but all fell short of consensus as Watergate and the Vietnam war took center stage (Rivlin, 1974; Iglehart, 1973, 1974). Government undertook other initiatives to limit expenditures such as the *diagnostic-related groups (DRG)* system for prospective payment of hospital services, enacted in 1982.

By the 1990s, there were more than 1,200 health insurers in the country. Most were for-profit and many were investor-owned. The failed Clinton Health Plan (CHP) of 1994, in its attempt to provide universal coverage through the private insurance industry as well as public programs, exposed divided interests among insurers as well as business. The agendas of the big insurers (i.e., Prudential, Metropolitan Life, Aetna and CIGNA) differed from those of many hundreds of small insurers represented by the Health Insurance Association of America (HIAA). Large employers could support employer mandates, while many small employers could not. Amid the crossfire of warring interests, the CHP ended up pleasing almost nobody, and the complex 1,342-page bill was dead on arrival in Congress. It was opposed by every special interest in the health care industry, and would probably have been a disastrous program anyway. As a political sellout to the private insurance industry, it was dubbed by cynics as the "Health Insurance Preservation Act" (Gordon, 1995).

The last years of the 20th Century brought the return of surging health care inflation, the realization that managed care and other cost containment strategies were ineffective, and the erosion of public safety net programs despite the addition of some new ones, such as the Children's Health Insurance Program (CHIP), established in 1997. (Kuttner, 1999b). Urged on by stakeholders in our market-based system, public policy continued its reliance on the market under the mantra of increasing consumer choice (and cost-sharing). Table 4.1

TABLE 4.1. Some Historical Highlights of Health Insurance in the U.S.

1912–1917	First attempt to enact National Health Insurance (NHI) defeated by business, organized labor, and American Medical Association (AMA)
1930s	Emergence of private health insurance for hospitalization NHI considered as part of Social Security Act, but withdrawn due to opposition by AMA
1940s	Growth of employer-based health insurance Emergence of prepaid group practice through not-for-profit HMOs (e.g., Kaiser Permanente, Group Health Cooperative of Puget Sound) Third attempt to enact NHI defeated (1946–1948) by coalition of AMA, American Hospital Association (AHA), the insurance industry, and other business interests
1950s	Expansion of for-profit commercial health insurance industry
1960s	Medicare and Medicaid programs established in 1965 Advent of first for-profit, investor-owned HMOs
1970s	Fourth attempt to establish universal coverage; alternative proposal fell victim to more pressing issues of Watergate and Vietnam War
1980s	Continued inflation of health care costs Market-based attempts to contain costs by managed care and tightening of reimbursement policies by government
1990s	Defeat of Clinton Health Plan, a flawed private-public proposal, which had little support after intense debate Children's Health Insurance Program (CHIP) established in 1997 Insurers gain dominance over providers

summarizes some historical highlights of the evolution of health insurance over the last 90 years.

TODAY'S HEALTH INSURANCE MARKET

The health insurance market is complex and split into three basic segments—large group, small group, and individual. Since each state has its own regulations for the insurance industry, the U.S. health insurance market is further fragmented into 150 different state-level markets (Hall, 2000; Kleinke, 2001). Employer-based health insurance covers about two-thirds of the nation's workforce. Large investor-owned insurance companies dominate the group market while Blue Cross-Blue Shield (BCBS) plans account for the largest share of the individual market.

As we have already seen in earlier chapters, large corporations often cross over into other parts of the health care system in their efforts to increase overall market share. About a dozen national managed care organizations control almost one-half of the HMO and preferred provider organization (PPO) industries. PPOs are looser-knit than HMOs, and include physicians who agree to accept fee-for-service reimbursement, typically on a discounted basis. In a recent national study by the AMA, in one-half of states at least one insurer controls more than 30% of the HMO/PPO market (Frieden, J., 2002). Thus, there tends to be much less competition in the market than one might expect or hope. A recent report by Inter Study observed that competition between the HMO and PPO industries "may actually be described as competition between national firms that offer a variety of business lines and will emphasize or de-emphasize them depending on current wants and needs of employers and consumers" (Chollet, 1997).

The original concept of not-for-profit, socially responsive health insurance, as pioneered by Blue Cross in the 1930s, was based on community rating, whereby the same coverage and premiums are offered to enrollees throughout the covered community regardless of individual risk. Community rating has long since given way to actuarial risk-rated health insurance, thereby enabling insurers to avoid unfavorable risks (i. e., people who most need health insurance). The profit motive has taken over the health insurance industry, and almost one-half of the nation's BCBS plans have converted to for-profit status (Song, 2003). The national Blue Cross association has permitted for-profit takeovers of their plans since 1994. Indianapolis-based

Anthem and California-based Wellpoint Health Networks, with plans in 11 states, are now the largest owners of BCBS plans. (PNHP, 2002). Conversions of not-for-profit insurers to for-profit status inevitably raises premiums and makes health insurance less affordable for many, but it can bring a windfall in new tax revenue to fiscally beleaguered states (Song, 2003; Cowan & McKinley, 2003). That for-profit versus not-for-profit status makes a big difference is illustrated by the experience in California where Kaiser (not-for-profit) spent 96% of every premium dollar on health care in 2000, while Blue Cross (for-profit) spent only 76% on patient care (Benko, 2002).

The health insurance industry, now mostly for-profit, is bloated with middlemen, bureaucracy and high administrative overhead. The extent of fragmentation, inefficiency, and administrative waste becomes clear in a study of more than 2,000 depressed patients in greater Seattle who were found to be covered by 189 different plans with 755 different policies (Grembowski et al., 2000). The impact of this kind of inefficiency elsewhere in the system, such as administrative overhead for physicians and other providers, is enormous and adds cumulatively to the cost of health care. One recent estimate placed the nation's expenditure for private insurance and government administrative costs at $111 billion, not including administrative costs incurred by hospitals and other health care providers or by individuals as they enroll, disenroll, re-enroll, or change insurance coverage and plans (Davis, 2003).

For the last several years, the health insurance industry has been passing along double-digit increases in premiums to employers and consumers, all the while blaming others in the health care system (especially hospitals) for unabated inflation of health care costs. A 2003 report by Goldman Sachs projects similar premium increases for at least another two years (Foundation for Taxpayer and Consumer Rights, 2002). The Federal Employees Health Benefits Plan (FEHBP), which covers federal employees as the largest employer-sponsored health plan in the country and touted by many as a model of efficiency, saw a premium hike over 13% in 2002, while the University of Miami was hit with a 45% increase from its insurer, United Healthcare (Physicians for a National Health Program, 2002a). Meanwhile, health insurers' profits grew by an average of 25% in 2001 (Terry, 2003), and United Health Group, the nation's largest health insurer, reported that 2002 fourth-quarter net income surged by 53% and earnings-per-share growth is projected at 22% for 2003 (United Health profits, 2003). High levels of CEO compensation further contribute to the spiraling costs of health insurance. A study by Families USA

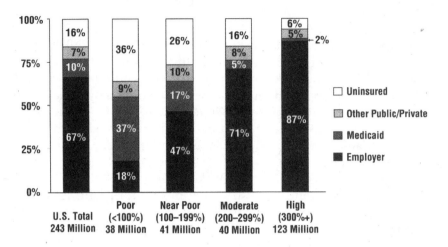

FIGURE 4.1 Health insurance coverage of the non-elderly by poverty level, 2000.

Source: DHHS 2002: Commission on Medicaid and the Uninsured. Reprinted with permission. *Health Insurance Coverage in America: 2000 Update.*

found, for example, that the average compensation for top executives of United Health Group was over $14 million in 2000, plus $119 million in unexercised stock options (Frieden, 2002).

As the cost of health insurance continues to escalate, employers tend to pass along these increases to their employees. As Figure 4.1 shows, many lower-income working families cannot afford employer-based insurance even if offered by their employers and many millions are ineligible for Medicaid. The average premium cost for a family of four now exceeds $9,000 per year (Appleby, 2004). For uninsured people seeking coverage in the more expensive individual market, a majority cannot afford coverage, especially in families with at least one member in fair or poor health status (Table 4.2).

Current trends in the health insurance market are based on the premise that consumers will benefit from more choice among more flexible plans and that costs can be contained more effectively if consumers take more responsibility for their own health care spending. These plans offer a complex menu of premiums, copayments and deductibles, and employees are encouraged to shop for their own plans, increasingly with a defined contribution from their employers. In order to keep premiums affordable, however, the plans often reduce benefits, increase patient cost sharing, or exclude higher-risk patients. Here are just three examples of these new plans from both the private and public sector:

TABLE 4.2. Health Insurance Take-Up Rates Among the Nonelderly Population, by Type of Insurance, Self-Reported Health Status, and Income, 2000–2001

	Employer coverage take-up rate		Nongroup coverage take-up rate	
	Persons In families with at least one member who reports fair or poor health status	Persons In families in which all members report being In good, very good, or excellent health	Persons In families with at least one member who reports fair or poor health status	Persons In families in which all members report being In good, very good, or excellent health
All persons	82.6%	91.4%	11.3%	30.0%
Below poverty	53.4	67.5	1.2	9.3
100–199 percent of poverty	74.6	74.6	5.7	13.4
200–399 percent of poverty	86.6	92.5	20.1	29.9
400 percent of poverty or more	92.8	95.7	33.2	50.7

Source: Pauly, M. V., & Nichols, L. (2002). The non-group insurance market: Short on facts, long on opinions and policy disputes. *Health Affairs* W332, October 23. Reprinted with permission.

Notes: The nonelderly population includes those under age sixty-five. The nongroup take-up rate is computed with nongroup candidates (those who do not have access to employer or public coverage, as explained in Exhibit 1) as the denominator.

- Health Partners has a Web-based tool allowing employees to choose a customized benefit plan, combined with an employer's defined contribution, among three network sizes and benefit packages; the plan uses actuarial pricing to minimize adverse selection (Gabel, Lo Sosso, & Rice, 2002).
- Blue Cross in Massachusetts is now marketing a PPO that charges individuals up to $5,000 and families up to $12,500 in deductibles before insurance coverage takes effect; although some preventive services are exempted from the deductible, emergency room services, specialist care, and surgery are all subject to the deductible (Kowalczyk, 2002).
- The new "Enhanced Medicare" plans being promoted by the Bush Administration offer choice among various plans, each with a limited prescription drug benefit, but all costing more for less coverage under contracts with the private insurance industry (The White House, 2003).

Although market-based health insurance serves the interests of the insurance industry very well, it discriminates against the sick and lower-income people. While the RAND Health Insurance Experiment found some years ago that patients with less insurance used less care, they also found that those same patients did not use less appropriate or necessary care (Siu, et al., 1986). Cost containment on that premise is therefore invalid. The private, voluntary health insurance market has clearly failed to provide comprehensive coverage at affordable costs, especially for people most in need of coverage. That should come as no surprise, as reflected by the observation by J. D. Kleinke, an executive with a health care information technology company and author of the book *Oxymorons: The Myth of the U.S. Health Care System*:

> The splintering of the national health insurance market into 150 different submarkets, compelled by competitive market forces and state-based regulation, defeats the entire purpose of insurance. It encourages health insurers to pursue young, healthy workforces and price-discriminate against older ones. The result is a competitive pricing spiral that ensures that those who need insurance most are those most likely to be priced out of the market. This represents another health care market failure that ultimately benefits no one.(Kleinke, 2001).

Despite all of the evidence for inequity and inefficiency in the private health insurance market, the debate continues. This is illustrated by this recent comment by Tom Scully, until recently the head of the

Centers for Medicare and Medicaid Services (CMS) and formerly a board member of a large for-profit dialysis company and president of a for-profit health industry trade group:

> The notion of a healthcare market is something of a mirage, given the dominant role of Medicare as a healthcare payer… only when the agency's role as a price fixer is modified will there be true competition that benefits consumers. (Fong, 2003).

Even though the Congressional Budget Office estimates that private health plans under Medicare will cost 8-12% more than traditional fee-for-service Medicare, Scully still hopes that "once we're getting to the point where more local insurance companies make decisions and drive behavior, the entire Medicare system will be much more efficient" (Reinhardt, 2003).

COMMON PRACTICES OF THE CORPORATE HEALTH INSURANCE INDUSTRY

Everyday practices within the large private health insurance industry reflect the business ethic and are mostly legal, although carefully avoiding state regulations in some cases. The issue here is not to condemn the industry for malintent or sharp business practices, but to question whether this is the best, most efficient, and most equitable way to manage and finance our country's health care.

Re-Underwriting

Medical underwriting, whereby higher premiums are charged to individuals or groups at higher risk of being sick, was considered unethical before the 1970s (Kuttner, 1999a). Today re-underwriting, typically on an annual experience basis, is the norm throughout the industry. The overriding goal is to maximize profits for insurers and their shareholders while minimizing the financial risk and the "loss ratio," the percentage of each premium dollar paid out in claims. Table 4.3 lists risks commonly used by commercial insurers in this process (Light, 1992). Table 4.4 shows the denial rate in the individual market for seven medical problems based on a 2001 report. One large insurer routinely raises its premium by 37% at the time of annual renewal for its least healthy patients or those with claims, and imposes other across-the-board increases (Terhune, 2002a).

TABLE 4.3. Risks Used by Commercial Insurers to Adjust Health Policies

Higher Premium

Allergies
Asthma
Back strain
Hypertension (controlled)
Arthritis
Gout
Glaucoma
Obesity
Psychoneurosis (mild)
Kidney stones
Emphysema (mild to moderate)
Alcoholism/drug use
Heart murmur
Peptic ulcer
Colitis

Exclusion Waiver

Cataract(s)
Gallstones
Fibroid tumor (uterus)
Hernia (hiatal/inguinal)
Migraine headaches
Pelvic inflammatory disease (PID)
Chronic otitis media (recent)
Spine/back disorders
Hemorrhoids
Knee impairment
Asthma
Allergies
Varicose veins
Sinusitis (chronic or severe)
Fractures

Denial

Acquired immunodeficiency syndrome (AIDS)
Ulcerative colitis
Cirrhosis of fiver
Diabetes mellitus
Leukemia
Schizophrenia
Hypertension (uncontrolled)
Emphysema
Stroke
Obesity (severe)
Angina (severe)
Coronary artery disease
Epilepsy
Lupus
Alcoholism/drug abuse

Source: Light, D. W. (1992). The practice and ethics of risk-rated health insurance. *Journal of the American Medical Association, 267,* 2503. Reprinted with permission.

TABLE 4.4. Denial Rate for Individual Health Insurance Applicants With Specified Health Conditions/Histories, 2001

Condition/history	Denial rate (60 applications)	Number affected by health condition
Seasonal allergies (hay fever)	8%	36 million
History of knee injury	12	5 million
Asthma	15	17 million
Breast cancer survivor	43	8.4 million[a]
Depression	23	19 million
Hypertension, overweight, smoker	55	69 million (obesity)
		64 million (hypertension)
		47 million (smokers)
HIV/AIDS	100	800,000–900,000

Source: Pollitz, K., et al. (2002). How accessible is individual health insurance for consumers in less-than-perfect health? Menlo Park, CA: Henry J. Kaiser Family Foundation, Reprinted with permission.

[a]Survivors of cancer of all types.

Carve-Outs

This is another approach used by insurers to limit their financial risk and deliver the least care. Often applied to mental health services, in a typical situation an HMO contracts to insure the employees of a large corporation, then subcontracts to a for-profit behavioral health company, which sets up various barriers and limits to care. Examples include limits on visits to psychiatrists by time (often 20 minutes) and number, not having providers in counties being served, and premature discharges from hospitals without arrangements for adequate follow-up care (Munoz, 2002).

Bait and Switch

After individuals enroll in a health plan based on its network of hospitals and physicians, insurers frequently add new restrictive policies in fine print, such as surcharges of as much as $400 per day for top-tier hospitals or new copayments of hundreds of dollars for each cancer radiation treatment. Jamie Court, executive director of the Foundation for Taxpayer and Consumer Rights in Santa Monica, California, makes this observation:

> Insurance, an agreement that for a fixed sum a company will pay for the costs if serious illness or injury strikes, has become a process of

"disinsurance," turning the promise of protection into little more than a coupon book. (Court, 2002).

Short-Term and Incomplete Coverage

A new and highly profitable niche has opened up in the health insurance market in recent years—short-term policies targeting healthy people. These plans don't cover pre-existing conditions and offer no continuing protection (Chaker, 2002). A recent example of a limited plan is that developed by the American Association of Retired Persons (AARP) in partnership with United Health Group aimed at people too young for Medicare (between 50 and 64 years of age). This plan would pay less than $8,000 toward a cardiac bypass operation, hardly enough to qualify for the term "insurance policy" (The Washington Post, 2003). Other limited benefit plans now being offered to employees of Wal-Mart Stores, Inc. and McDonald Corporation, cap annual benefits at only $1,000 (Terhune, 2003).

Cancellation of Policies

Although some regulations are in place which restrict insurers from dropping coverage of individuals on the basis of an unprofitable loss ratio, insurers can withdraw from a market, as many Medicare+Choice HMOs have done (Waldholz, 2002), or cancel policies for an entire group. For example, 100,000 enrollees in the Mid-South Health Plan were given six months to find other coverage, and were often unsuccessful if sick or unable to afford other plans (Morrison & Wolfe, 2001).

False-Front Non-Profit Groups

Insurers frequently set up nonprofit associations as false fronts for their own for-profit marketing activities. In most states, such association health plans (AHPs) are exempt from state rate-setting regulations, and are allowed to offer minimal benefits and excessive cost-sharing with enrollees. A typical example of this scam is a 76% premium increase for thousands of families pegged to annual renewal dates (Terhune, 2001). A 2004 report by Families USA, a consumer-advocacy group based in Washington, D.C., found that many AHPs misrepresent their benefits to sell these policies at low rates, then make steep premium increases after enrollment (Terhune, 2004).

Out-of-State Sales

Some insurers establish an administrative base in a state with lax regulations in order to avoid state rate-setting regulations. In Florida, where premium increases are occasionally disallowed, 13 of 21 individual insurance companies do business through out-of-state groups (Terhune, 2002b). Association health plans, now being promoted by business interests, would allow small businesses to band together to offer health insurance across state lines, and thereby exempt from state regulation of benefits, rates, or payment to providers (Frieden, 2003).

Hidden Brokerage Costs

Brokerage costs within the private health insurance industry account for enormous and invisible sums each year in the U.S. There are about 50,000 brokers, agents, and consultants across the country charging commissions from 3% to as much as 20% of the total cost of plans sold (Robertson, 1999). An Internet-based agency, EHealth Insurance, in partnership with 135 insurance companies, takes a 20% broker's fee for all health insurance policies sold over the Internet, plus another 10% commission for any policy holders who renew their coverage, even if not renewed through Ehealth (Tep, 2002).

Automatic Reductions of Physician Reimbursement

More than 450 health insurance plans across the country use one of several software programs made by McKesson Corporation of San Francisco to automatically reduce payments to about 700,000 U.S. physicians (Martinez, 2002). Litigation has been brought by physician groups in a number of states charging that standard billing codes have been changed without transparency or disclosure. Multiple suits have been consolidated into a RICO suit against eight defendants— Aetna, Anthem Blue Cross and Blue Shield, Cigna, Coventry Health Care, Humana, PacifiCare Health Systems, United Healthcare, and Well-Point—charging them with violating federal racketeering law by conspiring to reduce, delay, and deny payments to physicians. The case is pending, and the U.S. Supreme Court has agreed to hear an appeal by United Healthcare and PacifiCare that the racketeering claims should be arbitrated (Rose, 2002; Flaherty, 2003). In separate settlements, Hartford-based Aetna agreed to a settlement of $170 million while promising more clarity and disclosure of its coverage and payment policies (Treaster, 2003), and Cigna agreed to a $540 million settlement (Physicians Financial News, 2004).

Fraud

Since 1993 the federal government has recovered more than $400 million in settlements from insurance companies making false Medicare claims (McGinley, 2002). Blue Cross/Blue Shield plans serve as fiscal intermediaries for the Medicare program across the country, and have been successfully prosecuted for a number of fraudulent practices, including falsification of audits, administrative costs, and number of claims processed (Sparrow, 2000). The U.S. Department of Labor currently has pending over 100 civil and 17 criminal investigations that involve alleged fraud by multiple health plans sold to employers in a number of states (Wysockie, 2002). A 2004 report by the General Accounting Office identified widespread scams in every state involving more than 15,000 employers and 200,000 policyholders; unlicensed insurance companies were found to offer cheap policies, collect millions in premiums, then refuse to pay claims (Pear, 2004).

SOME UNRESOLVED POLICY ISSUES

Several major interrelated policy issues will need to be addressed before any meaningful long-term health care reform becomes likely. Unfortunately, these are issues of an ongoing debate perpetuated, in part, by stakeholders in the present market-based system. Since the debate tends to become mired in rhetoric and technical details, many legislators and policy-makers find it difficult to see the forest for the trees.

Should Medical Underwriting Be Banned?

This question exposes core economic, political, and moral differences across a wide ideologic chasm of strongly held beliefs. As a way of spreading risk, insurance can be most effective when the risk pool is large, and the many subsidize the few. Since about one-half of health care expenses are incurred by 5% of the population and 70% by 10% of the population, an actuarial approach to risk rating (as opposed to community rating) eliminates the opportunity for younger, healthier people to subsidize older, sick people (Kuttner, 1999a; Aaron, 1996). Insurers see sick people as medical and financial risks, they maximize profits by avoiding coverage of these individuals, which then shifts costs to those most in need of insurance and often least able to pay for it.

The American health insurance industry has come to think that risk rating is fair, contending that risk-rated insurance is more efficient and a better value for enrollees (Schramm, 1988; Stone, 1990). This position is bolstered by the libertarian argument that it is unjust for one individual or group to be required to pay for the needs of another (Nozick, 1974). The polar opposite view, supported by a large body of evidence, is that risk rating discriminates against disadvantaged minorities, the chronically ill, and older individuals, as well as groups that include many such individuals. Risk-rated health insurance drives up overall costs and makes insurance less affordable for those most in need (Kuttner, 1996b; Hadley, Steinberg, Feder, 1991; U.S. General Accounting Office, 1991). This last dynamic has led Donald Light, Professor of Comparative Health Care Systems at the University of Medicine and Dentistry of New Jersey, to this conclusion:

> Risk rating leads to the inverse coverage law; the more people need coverage, the less coverage they are likely to get or the more they are likely to pay for what they get (Light, 1992, p. 2504).

The President's Commission on Ethics in Medicine in 1983 took a firm position that a morally fair health care system should assure access to services that minimize disadvantages and suffering due to illness (President's Commission, 1983).

Returning to our question, strong arguments can be marshalled that risk-rated health insurance is unfair and morally unjust, and that community rating would be preferable public policy. However, as long as we have a large and powerful private health insurance industry, the odds of returning to community rating appear to be small. Medical underwriting of individual health insurance is permitted in 45 states and the District of Columbia (Pollitz & Sorian, 2002). State regulatory policies vary widely from one state to another and can be readily avoided by insurers. In addition, the current political climate favors states' prerogatives over new federal regulations and our society still favors individualism over collective action, wherever possible. Since actuarial risk-rating is likely to prevail in health insurance, that leads us to the next question.

Can the Voluntary Private Health Insurance Industry Be Effectively Regulated in the Public Interest?

Despite concerted efforts by federal and state regulators over the years, much of the evidence points to a negative answer to this important question. Here is how these efforts toward regulation have sorted out.

At the federal level, the Employee Retirement Income Security Act of 1974 (ERISA), originally intended to protect pension plans, soon became a major loophole in states' efforts to regulate abuses by health insurers. Under ERISA, all self-funded employer health plans were exempt from state regulation, as were beneficiaries of Medicare, Medicaid, and insurance provided by government employers. And, as we saw in the last chapter, ERISA has pre-empted state regulation of managed care organizations for many years.

The Health Insurance Portability and Accountability Act of 1996 (HIPAA) corrected some of the abuses in the health insurance marketplace, especially in the group market. New protections were brought to consumers with regard to pre-existing conditions, availability of coverage from small employers, discrimination based on health status, and renewability (Atchinson & Fox, 1997). One big loophole in HIPPA, however, is its avoidance of regulating the amounts of premium increases as policies are renewed in the individual market (Patel & Pauly, 2002). In fact, an individual in one state incurred a premium increase of 2000% after a change in health status. In addition, many states are not receptive to federal intrusion into their regulatory responsibilities, and Congress did not appropriate funds for public education, oversight, and enforcement (Pollitz, Topay, Hadley, Specht, 2000).

The Mental Health Parity Act of 1996 (Domenici-Wellstone Bill) was another well-intended federal initiative to redress disparities and inequities in the provision of mental health services. Its effectiveness was limited, however, since health plans that provided mental health coverage could impose days per annum and visit time limitations for such services or drop coverage altogether (Frank, Kovanagi, & McGuire, 1997).

It is well documented that some Medicare managed care plans have pursued favorable risk selection for many years (Lichtenstein, Thomas, Adams-Watson, Lepowski, & Simone, 1991; Riley, Lubitz, & Rabey, 1991; Porell & Turner, 1990; Brown, 1993; U.S. General Accounting Office, 1997; Neuman, Maibach, Dusenbury, Kitchman & Zupp, 1998). Although in violation of federal regulations, a 1995 study found that almost one-half of Medicare beneficiaries were asked about their health status before enrollment (U.S. Department of Health & Human Services, 1995). It has been shown that a single question "In general, compared with other people your age, would you say your health is: excellent, very good, good, fair, or poor?" can screen out a five-fold difference in future health care costs between the excellent and poor categories (Bierman, Bubolz, Fisher, Wasson, Buboly 1999). Two health insurance markets that unraveled as a result of adverse selection during the 1980s and 1990s were the mental health care market under the Federal Employees Health Benefits Program, and the individual markets in New York and New Jersey (National Center for Policy Analysis, 1994; Tooman, 2001).

Although many states have adopted some HIPAA provisions, states' regulation of health insurance continues to be inconsistent and often ineffectual. Many insurers exploit this variability by shopping for states with the least regulatory obstacles. State portability laws, where they are in effect, still trump HIPPA. If state regulators attempt to force employers to offer more benefits, some employers may escape to the self-insurance exemption under ERISA or drop coverage entirely (Kleinke, 2001, p. 189). Health insurers have found other ways to circumvent state laws, including the creation of group trusts whereby individual policies are issued under a group master policy (Hall, 2000). And where states attempted to enforce strict rating rules, premiums were increased to such an extent that many policy holders could no longer afford coverage. In Washington State, for example, premiums went up by 71% and individual coverage was available in only 3 of 39 counties (Locke, 2000).

Can the Private Health Insurance Industry Ever Be More Efficient and a Better Value than a Public System?

Given the administrative complexity, large overhead, and profit margins of an enormous private health insurance industry which shifts costs without containing them, the industry's track record alone negates any claims to increased efficiency or value. Comparisons with Medicare amplify the point. Medicare, covering 40 million people age 65 or older, spends about 98 cents of every funded dollar on patient care through its standard benefit plan, as compared with about 80 cents for private health plans (Kleinke, 2001, p. 195). While imperfect and incomplete in its coverage, Medicare is able to provide essential health care services for an older population regardless of health status, while containing costs better than private plans (Boccuti &

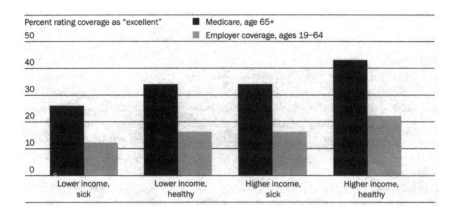

FIGURE 4.2 Predicted rating of health insurance coverage, by health, poverty, and insurance status, 2001.

Source: Davis, K., et al. (2002). Medicare versus private insurance: rhetoric and reality. *Health Affairs,* Web exclusive, October 9, 2002. Reprinted with permission.

Moon, 2003). A 2001 study by the Commonwealth Fund found that Medicare coverage, compared with private employer-based coverage, is much more likely to be rated excellent across all income and health status categories, as shown in Figure 4.2 (Davis, Schoen, Doty, Tenney, 2002).

A growing number of analysts of the health insurance market have recognized the structural problems of the private employer-based insurance system, which, after all, is more an accident of history than a well thought-out financing system for the nation's health care (Bodenheimer & Sullivan, 1998; Fuchs, 2002; Kleinke, 2001; Kuttner, 1999b). Humphrey Taylor, chairman of the Harris Poll at Harris Interactive in New York City, predicts the inevitable collapse of employer-based insurance as a result of a death spiral of adverse selection, spurred on ironically by the trend toward more consumer choice, and the increasing use of defined contribution plans by employers and insurers (Taylor, 2002). If one still harbors any faith in the social responsibility of the for-profit private health insurance industry, it is disavowed by this recent statement by Dr. John Rowe, chairman and CEO of Aetna, one of the country's largest health insurance companies:

In 2002, Aetna improved its financial performance. This success was built on a seven-point reduction in the medical cost ratio (MCR), as well as lower administrative costs. This decline in MCR was driven by three factors: reduction of membership with historically higher

MCRs...premium increases... and changing contracts and benefits. (Aetna, 2003).

CONCLUDING COMMENTS

We can now add 60 more years of experience to the assessment of voluntary health insurance made by Dr. Sigerist in 1944, after just 15 years of experience. In 75 years the problem has not changed. With health insurance splintered into many small risk pools and a large, private, mostly for-profit insurance industry with many parasitic middlemen, the original social contract pioneered by Blue Cross in the 1930s is in tatters. Many Blue Cross and Blue Shield plans, which today serve about 85 million Americans in every market (large employers, small employers, and individual) and in every state (Serota, 2002), are for-profit, and more are hoping to convert from not-for-profit to for-profit status. The original community-rating ethic has for the most part disappeared. As health insurance becomes more unaffordable for millions of Americans and as the numbers of uninsured continue to rise, stakeholders in the present system advocate incremental changes, which have already proved ineffectual over the years. Thus, the private insurance market has failed the public interest. The issue is not that the insurance industry is evil as it succeeds in its business venture. The issue is that it is bad public policy to base the population's health care on an increasingly unfair and unsustainable financing system. Major reform will be needed to renew the social contract of health insurance. Both the politics and the policy alternatives will be addressed in Part III.

REFERENCES

Aaron, H. J. (1996). Health care reform: The clash of goals, facts, and ideology. In V. R. Fuch (Editor), *Individual and social responsibility: Child care, education, medical care, and long-term care in America.* Chicago: University of Chicago Press.

AARP offers a plan, but the experts aren't buying it. (2003, Feb. 11) *Washington Post.*

Aetna (2003, Feb. 11) Aetna reports fourth quarter and full-year 2002 results. Press release.

Andrews, C. (1995). *Profit Fever: The drive to corporatize health care and how to stop it (pp. 3–8).* Monroe, ME: Common Courage Press.

Appleby, J. (2004, March 17). Health insurance premiums crash down on middle class. *USA Today*, p. B1.

Atchinson, B. K., & Fox, D. M. (1997). The politics of the Health Insurance Portability and Accountability Act. *Health Affairs (Millwood), 16*(3), 146, 1997.

Author, A. A. (2003). United Health's profits soar. *Physicians Financial News, 21*(3), 913.

Benko, L. B. (2002, May 13). Managed care. Shakeup in California. *Modern Healthcare,* p. 32.

Bierman, A. S., Bubolz, T. A. Fisher, E. S., Wasson, J. H. (1999). How well does a single question about health predict the financial health of Medicare managed care plans? *Effective Clinical Practice, 2*(2).

Boccuti, C., & Moon, M. (2003). Comparing Medicare and private insurers: Growth rates in spending over three decades. *Health Affairs (Millwood), 22*(2), 230.

Bodenheimer, T., & Sullivan, K. (1998). How large employers are shaping the health care marketplace. *New England Journal of Medicine, 338*, 1084.

Brown, R. S., Clements, D. G., Hill, J. W., Retchin, S. M., Bergeron, J. W. (1993). Do health maintenance organizations work for Medicare? *Health Care Finance Review, 15*, 7.

Campion, F. D. (1984). *The AMA and U.S. Health Policy since 1940.* Chicago: Chicago Review Press.

Chaker, A. M. (2001, May 7). A pinch hit on health coverage. *The Wall Street Journal,* p. D6.

Cholet, D. (1997). Mapping state health insurance markets: Structure and change in the states' group and individual health insurance markets, 1995–1997 Available at *(www.statecoverage.net/mapping.pdf*

Court, J. (2002). Insurance: You pay, they bait and switch. *Los Angeles Times.*

Cowan, A. L. & McKinley, J. C. Jr. (2003, February 1). Critics say Albany wastes Empire Blue Cross profits. *The New York Times,* p. A18.

Davis, K. (2003, March 10). Time for change: The hidden cost of a fragmented health insurance system. Testimony of Karen Davis, President, The Commonwealth Fund before the United States Senate Special Committee on Aging.

Davis, K., Schoen, C., Doty, M., Tenney, K. (2002, Oct. 9). Medicare versus private insurance: Rhetoric and reality. *Health Affairs*—Web exclusive. pp. W311–323.

U.S. Department of Health and Human Services. (1995). *Beneficiary perspectives on Medicare risk HMOs.* Washington, DC: Author.

The White House Executive Summary. (2003, March 4). President's framework to modernize and improve Medicare. Falk, I.S. (1983). Some lessons from the fifty years since the COMC Final Report, 1932. *Journal of Public Health Policy, 4*(2), 139.

Flaherty, M. (2003). Health plans facing pressure to disclose policies on payment. *Physicians Financial News, 20*(1), 1.

Fong, T. (2003, March 2). Things aren't getting better. *Modern Healthcare.* pp. 6–7.

Foundation for Taxpayer and Consumer Rights (2002). FTCR calls for health care rate regulation. News release. Santa Monica, CA: Author.

Frank, R. G., Kovanagi, C., McGuire, T. G. (1997). The politics and economics of mental health "parity" laws. *Health Affairs (Millwood), 16*(4), 108.

Frieden, J. (2002). Vital signs. *Family Practice News, 32*(3), 1.

Frieden, J. (2003). Not subject to state regulations: Novel insurance bill may skirt prompt pay rules. *Family Practice News, 43*(17), 73.

Fuchs, V. (2002). What's ahead for health insurance in the United States? *The New England Journal of Medicine, 346,* 13. Gabel, J. R., Lo Sosso, A. T., Rice, T. (2002). Consumer-driven health plans: Are they more than talk now? *Health Affairs (Millwood),* Web exclusives, W398.

Ginsberg, E. (1999). Ten encounters with the U.S. health sector, 1930–1999. *Journal of the American Medical Association, 282,* 1665, 1999.

Gordon, C. (1995). *The Clinton Health Care Plan: Dead on Arrival.* Westfield, NJ: Open Magazine Pamphlet Series.

Grembowski, D. E., Diehr, P. Novak, L. C., Roussel, A. F., Morton, D. P., (2000). Measuring the "managedness" and covered benefits of health plans. *Health Services Research, 35*(3), 707.

Hadley, J., Steinberg, E. P., Feder, J. (1991). Comparison of uninsured and privately insured hospital patients: Condition on admission, resource use, and outcome. *Journal of the American Medical Association, 265,* 374.

Hall, M. (2000). The geography of health insurance regulation: A guide to identifying, exploiting, and policing market boundaries. *Health Affairs (Millwood), 19*(2), 173.

Iglehart, J. K. (1973). Consensus forms for National Insurance plan, proposals vary widely in scope. *National Journal Reports, 5,* 1855–1863.

Iglehart, J. K. (1974). Compromise seems unlikely on three major insurance plans. *National Journal Reports, 6,* 700. Name, N. N. (2002). Insurance monopoly: Policy and practice. *Family Practice News,* p. 21.

Kleinke, J. D. (2001). *Oxymorons: The myths of the U.S. health care system (p. 192).* San Francisco: Jossey-Bass. Kolko, G. (1962). *Wealth and power in America (p. 118).* New York: Praeger Publishers.

Kowalczyk, L. (2002). High—deductible HMO plans pushed. *The Boston Globe.*

Kuttner, R. (1996a). *Everything for sale: The virtues and limits of markets.* Chicago: University of Chicago Press. Kuttner, R., (1999b). The American health care system: Health insurance coverage. *New England Journal of Medicine, 340,* 163.

Labor Research Association. (1947). *Labor Fact Book 8.* New York: International Publishers.

Lear, W. J. (1963). *Medical care and family security (p. 209).* Englewood Cliffs, NJ: Prentice-Hall.

Lichtenstein, R., Thomas, J. W., Adams-Watson, J., Lepowski, J., Simone, B. (1991). Selection bias in TEFRA at-risk HMOs. *Medical Care, 29,* 318.

Light, D. W. (1992). The practice and ethics of risk-rated health insurance. *Journal of the American Medical Association, 267,* 2503.

Locke, G. (2000, March). Health insurance coverage: Every citizen's risk. Policy Brief 2000. Olympia, WA: Governor's Executive Office.

Martinez, B. (2002, Nov. 27). CIGNA to settle suit over cuts in doctor bills. *The Wall Street Journal*, p. A3.

McGinley, L. (2002, June 26). General American to pay $76 million in Medicare case. *The Wall Street Journal*, p. A2.

McNerney, W. C. (1996). Big question for the Blues: Where to go from here? C. Rufus Rorem award lecture. *Inquiry, 33*, 110.

Morrison, A. B., & Wolfe, S. M. (2001, February). Outrage of the month: None of your business. *Public Citizen's Health Research Group Health Letter*, p 11.

Munoz, R. (2002, May 22). How health care insurers avoid treating mental illness. *San Diego Union Tribune*.

National Center for Policy Analysis. (1994, June 13). Federal Employee Health Plan: Model for reform, Brief Analysis No. 107. Washington, DC: Author.

Neuman, P., Maibach, E., Dusenbury, K., Kitchman, M., Zupp, P. (1998). Marketing HMOs to Medicare beneficiaries. *Health Affairs (Millwood), 117*, 132.

Nozick, R. (1974). *Anarchy, state and utopia*. Oxford England: Blackwell Scientific Publications.

Patel, V., & Pauly, M. V. (2002, Aug. 28). Guaranteed renewability and the problem of risk variation in individual health insurance markets. *Health Affairs*—Web exclusive, p. W284.

Pear, R. (2003, March 3). Inquiry finds sharp increase in health insurance scams. *New York Times*, p. A12.

Physicians Financial News. (2004, Mar. 15). Judge approves $540 million Cigna settlement.

PNHP (2002a, January). Physicians for a National Health Program, Chicago, Illinois: Data update January, p. 7.

PNHP (2002b). Data Update. Physicians for a National Health Program. Chicago, Illinois: Data update, Fall, p. 6.

Pollitz, K., (2001). How accessible is individual health insurance for consumers in less-than-perfect health? Menlo Park, CA: Henry J. Kaiser Family Foundation, Inc.

Pollitz, K., Topay, N., Hadley, E., Specht, J. (2000). Early experience with "new federalism" in health insurance regulation. *Health Affairs (Millwood), 19*(4), 7.

Pollitz, K., & Sorian, R. (2002, Oct. 23). Ensuring health security: is the individual market ready for prime time? *Health Affairs*- Web exclusive, p. W373.

Porell, F.W., & Turner, W. M. (1990). Biased selection under an experimental enrollment and marketing Medicare HMO broker. *Medical Care, 28*, 604.

President's Commission for the Study of Ethical Problems in Medicine and Behavioral Research (1983). *Securing Access to Health Care*. Washington, DC: Author.

Reinhardt, U. W. (2003). Interview. The Medicare world from both sides: A conversation with Tom Scully. *Health Affairs (Millwood), 22*(6), 74.

Riley, G., Lubitz, J., Rabey, E. (1991). Enrollee health status under Medicare risk contracts: An analysis of mortality rates. *Health Services Research, 26,* 173.

Rivlin, A. M. (1974, July 21). Agreed: Here comes national health insurance. *The New York Times,* p. 174.

Robertson, K. (1999, Sept. 13). Are health plan brokers paid too much? *Sacramento Business Journal.*

Rose, J. R. (2002, Nov. 22). Practice beat: A court battle with the muscle of 600,000 doctors behind it. *Medical Economics,* p. 15.

Rosenblatt, R. A., & Moscovice I. S. (1982). *Rural health care (p. 33).* New York: John Wiley.

Rothman, D. J. (1991). The public perception of Blue Cross, 1935–1965. *Journal of Health Politics, Policy and Law, 16*(4), 671.

Rothman, D. J. (1993). A century of failure: Health care reform in America. *Journal of Health Politics, Policy and Law, 18*(2), 271.

Schramm, C. J. (1988). Insurers advocate HIV testing. *AIDS Patient Care.* February pp. 4–6.

Serota, S. (2002, Oct. 23). The individual market: A delicate balance. *Health Affairs*-Web exclusive, p. W377.

Sigerist, H. E. (1944). Medical care for all the people. *Canadian Journal of Public Health, 35*(7), 258.

Siu, A. L., (1986). Inappropriate use of hospitals in a randomized trial of health insurance plans. *The New England Journal of Medicine, 315,* 1259.

Somers, A. R., & Somers H. M. (1977). *Health and health care: Policies in perspectives.* Germantown, MD: Aspen Systems Corp.

Song, K. M. (2003, Jan. 23). Hospitals to sue Premera to halt for-profit switch. *Seattle Times,* p. A1.

Sparrow, M. K. (2000). *License to steal: How fraud bleeds America's health care system (pp. 74–75).* Boulder, CO: Westview Press.

Starr, P. (1982). *The social transformation of American medicine (pp. 252–253).* New York: Basic Books.

Stone, D. A. (1990). AIDS and the moral economy of insurance. *American Prospect, 1,* 62.

Taylor, H. (2002). How and why the health insurance system will collapse. *Health Affairs (Millwood), 21,* 195.

Tep, R. (2002, Nov. 21). Click here for coverage. *Forbes.com.*

Terhune, C. (2001, Nov. 21). Non-profit groups that tout insurance have hidden links. *The Wall Street Journal,* p. A1.

Terhune, C. (2002a, April 9). Health insurers' premium practices add to profit surge, roil customers. *The Wall Street Journal Online.*

Terhune, C. (2002b, April 9). Insurers avoid state regulations by selling via groups elsewhere. *The Wall Street Journal,* p.A20.

Terhune, C. (2003, May 14). Thin cushion. Fast-growing health plan has a catch: $1,000–a-year cap. *The Wall Street Journal,* p. A1.

Terry, K. (2003). Where has all the money gone? *Medical Economics,* January 19, p. 72.

Terhune, C. (2004, March 11). Report raps association insurance. *The Wall Street Journal*, D3.

Tooman, L. (2001, July). New Jersey's health insurance disaster. *Health Care News.* Chicago: Heartland Institute. Treaster, J. B. (2002, May 23). Aetna agreement with doctors envisions altered managed care. *New York Times,* p. A1.

Truman, H. S. (1945). A national health program: Message from the president. *Social Security Bulletin, 8*(12).

U.S. General Accounting Office (1991). Canadian health insurance: Lessons for the United States. Publication GAO/HRD-91, 90. Washington, DC: Author.

U.S. General Accounting Office (1997). Fewer and lower cost beneficiaries chronic conditions enroll in HMOs. Washington, DC: Author.

Waldholz, M. (2002, Oct. 3). Prescriptions: Medicare seniors face confusion as HMOs bail out of program. *The Wall Street Journal*, p. D4.

Wysockie, B. (2002, oct. 2). Bogus insurers leave patients with big bills. *The Wall Street Journal*, p. D1.

Chapter 5

THE PHARMACEUTICAL INDUSTRY

> Essential medicines save lives and improve health for millions of people around the world. But millions more have little or no access to safe, high-quality medicines. This huge gap between the potential to save lives and the reality for millions of poor people for whom medicines are unavailable, unaffordable, unsafe, or improperly used must be bridged.
>
> *Gro Harken Brundtland, MD*
> *Director-General, World Health Organization*

Prescription drugs have become a central and increasing part of what medical technology can contribute to modern health care, in many instances replacing surgery or other treatment modalities. Drug therapy is essential to the health, and often survival, of many millions of people. The soaring costs of prescription drugs in the unregulated American market (National Institute for Health Care Management, 2002a), however, are pricing prescription drugs beyond the reach of a growing part of the population. While one-third of people in developing countries have no access to essential medicines, tens of millions of Americans also lack such access. Thus, the core issue identified by Dr. Brundtland of the World Health Organization, the gap between potential therapy and access in the real world, has become an urgent issue in the U.S. as well (Brundtland, 2002).

This chapter has four goals: (1) to briefly describe the structure and practices of the pharmaceutical industry in the U.S. market; (2) to discuss the extent to which prescription drugs have become unaffordable for Americans, together with the backlash by purchasers and consumers to escalating drug costs; (3) to describe certain practices of the pharmaceutical industry that are more in its own self interest than the public interest; and (4) to consider some controversial policy issues concerning prescription drugs.

THE MOST PROFITABLE OF ALL INDUSTRIES

The investor-owned pharmaceutical industry tops all other industries in the U.S. in profits. In 2000, a time of recession, the top 10 U.S. drug companies increased their profits by 33% while the overall profits of Fortune 500 companies fell by 53% (Public Citizen Report, 2002). After relaxation of federal anti-trust regulations in 1994, there was a surge in mergers and acquisitions throughout the industry. Marketing goals appear to drive companies to mergers more than scientific reason (Harris & Fuhrmans, 2002). Today 50 companies control about two-thirds of the world's pharmaceutical market, while just five large pharmaceutical corporations take in almost one-half of the total profits of the wealthiest drug companies (DeMoro, 2003).

Since 1994, prescription drug costs have almost doubled as a proportion of U.S. health care expenditures, and drug industry profits are three times greater than the average of all other industries (DeMoro, 2003). Retail spending on prescription drugs in the U.S. almost doubled in just four years between 1997 and 2001, with increases of about 18% each year (prescription drug expenditures, 2002).

The pharmaceutical industry has for many years jealously guarded its prerogatives to set prices and has fought hard against attempts by government or other purchasers to set prices. Drug patent laws in this country extend a 17-year monopoly to drug manufacturers, who then use the unregulated U.S. market to set prices in order to maximize profits. Prices for prescription drugs are regulated, typically by government, in Europe, Japan, and many other countries. The average price for prescription drugs around the world is just one-quarter of the U.S. monopoly price (Baker, 2001).

The $400 billion a year pharmaceutical industry, after almost 10 years of double-digit growth, is starting to experience counter pressures which may rein in some of its profits. Industry trends in the last decade include declining numbers of new drugs coming to market, increased purchasing power by insurers and government programs, and many drugs going generic after patent expirations (Harris, 2002). Despite these trends, however, Pfizer still posted a 137% increase in net income in the fourth quarter of 2002 (Hensley & Burton, 2003).

Although generic drugs are priced lower than brand-name drugs, cost savings to patients are starting to disappear there as well. Prices for generic drugs are rising almost twice as fast as branded drugs over the last two years. The generic drug industry is undergoing consolidation, and often raises prices as high as the market will bear. The prices of some generic drugs has recently been raised by their manufacturers by as much as 1,000%. Lucrative markets are then added all along the distribution chain, including wholesalers, pharmacy benefit managers, and pharmacists. The prices of some generics has increased to the point where some insurers don't even try to switch patients from their brand-name counterparts (Freudenheim, 2002a).

The pharmaceutical industry is quick to defend its pricing practices as essential to fund its research and development costs. It asserts that innovations in drug therapy will be stifled if price controls are put in place. This is an old argument, advanced as early as the 1960s, and the industry's claims do not stand up to scrutiny. More than 40 years ago, Senator Estes Kefauver (D-TN) led an investigation by the Senate Judiciary Committee's Subcommittee on Antitrust and Monopoly. The investigation found that drug prices far exceeded those warranted by research and production costs, with U.S. prices much higher than overseas. Reforms such as shortening drug patents to only three years and compulsory licensing, were proposed but they were quickly killed in Congress under a lobbying assault by the industry (Mintz, 2001).

The pharmaceutical industry has greatly exaggerated the costs of research and development (R&D) of its products for many years. During the 1960s, the drug industry spent four times as much on promotion as on research (Mintz, 2001). A 1998 study of the disposition of sales revenue of the eight largest research-based pharmaceutical companies shows that R&D expenditures accounted for just more than one-third of marketing and administrative costs (see Figure 5.1). (Deutsche, 1999; Reinhardt, 2001). A 2002 report by *Families USA* showed that executive compensation within the pharmaceutical industry is a very large part of its cost of doing business; as an example, the former chairman and CEO of Bristol-Myers Squibb was paid $74.9 million in that year, plus stock options valued at another $76 million (*Families USA*, 2002).

While drug manufacturers often claim that it costs them $800 million to bring any new drug to market, this claim loses credibility on several counts. Public Citizen sets that figure closer to $110 million and notes that over 55% of the studies leading to the discovery and development of the top five selling drugs in 1995 were done at taxpayers expense with National Institutes of Health (NIH) funding (Lueck, 2001). A 2001 report found that only two of Bristol-Myers Squibb's top 10 drugs were developed in-house. Moreover, recent years have seen a decline in the number of new drugs reaching the market, and most of those that do are not breakthroughs but "me-

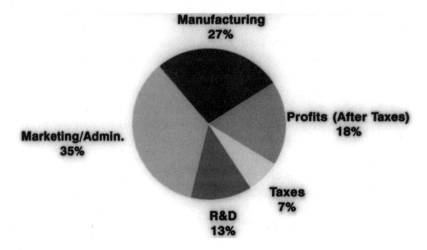

FIGURE 5.1 Drug companies' cost structure.

Source: Slide Set Show; 2002 edition. Physicians for a National Health Program (2002). Retrieved from *www.pnhp.org* Reprinted with permission.

too" drugs with minimal pharmacological change and maximal marketing hype (Angell & Relman, 2001). A 2004 example is Pfizer's "new" drug Caduet, which combines two of its top-selling drugs (Lipitor, a cholesterol-reducer and Norvasc, for high blood pressure (Hensley, 2004). The nonprofit National Institute for Health Care Management (NIHCM) estimates that 85% of drugs approved by the FDA between 1989 and 2000 were modified versions of existing drugs (*USA Today,* 2002).

In the U.S., drug manufacturers are free to set their prices without regulation. They generally establish their "average wholesale price" (AWP) as a basis for negotiation with purchasers. It is often unclear to purchasers how AWPs are calculated. AWPs are published by drug-price compendiums such as the Red Book and the National Drug Data File. The AWP does not reflect any discounts that may be obtained by intermediaries, such as pharmacy-benefit managers or group purchasing organizations, which then sell the drugs to health plans, pharmacies, medical groups, and others (Gencarelli, 2002; Iglehart, 2003; U.S. General Accounting Office, 2001).

In effect, then, pharmaceutical manufacturers enjoy many government protections and subsidies, including a large amount of publicly-funded research, 17-year patent protection from competitors, the freedom to set their own prices, and the ability to deduct expenses of R&D and marketing (Angell & Relman, 2001). In addition, the industry pays less taxes than all other U.S. industries (16% versus 27% as the all-industry average) (Congressional Research Service, 1991). The profitability of the unregulated U.S. market has been a major factor attracting large European pharmaceutical corporations to move their R&D bases to this country (e.g., Swedish Pharmacia from London to New Jersey in 1995 and Swiss Novartis to Cambridge, Massachusetts in 2003) (*The Wall Street Journal*, 2002).

INCREASING UNAFFORDABILITY OF PRESCRIPTION DRUGS

Average retail prices for prescription drugs have more than doubled over the last 10 years (Barry, 2002), and as we have just seen, the costs of generics are also rising rapidly (Freudenheim, 2002b). Prescription drugs have become unaffordable for many millions of Americans, especially the underinsured, the uninsured, and those on Medicare and Medicaid. Figure 5.2 shows the proportions of these populations which were unable to fill a prescription in the last year because of cost (Center for Studying Health System Change, 2002).

As expected, the uninsured are the hardest hit by rising drug prices. Since the 1950s, through a longstanding practice of differential

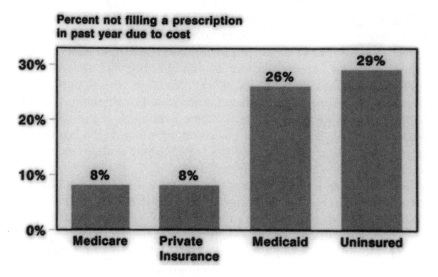

FIGURE 5.2 Millions can't afford prescriptions.
Source: Slide Set Show; 2002 edition. Physicians for a National Health Program (2002). *www.pnhp.org*. Reprinted with permission.

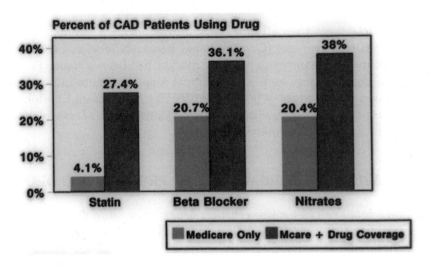

FIGURE 5.3 Seniors without drug coverage forgo cardiac medications.
Source: Federman, A. D., et al. (2001). Supplemental insurance and use of effective cardiovascular drugs among elderly Medicare beneficiaries with coronary health disease. *Journal of the American Medical Association, 286,* 1732. Retrieved from *www.pnhp.org* Reprinted with permission.

pricing, cash buyers at pharmacies (the majority of purchasers) pay the highest, undiscounted prices (Frank, 2001). The elderly and individuals with chronic illness and disabilities are likewise hard hit by the cost of their medications. Six of ten Medicare beneficiaries have had no drug coverage at all (Laschober, et al., 2002). Lanoxin is the most common drug used by the elderly; although it is an old drug, its price rose about seven times the inflation rate in 1998 (Publications and Reports, 2000). Figure 5.3 shows marked differences among Medicare patients with and without drug coverage in terms of statin, beta blocker, and nitrate use (Federman, et al., 2001). Many patients taking multiple medications for chronic diseases now find themselves forced to skip doses or stop taking some medications altogether (Prescription drug access, 2002).

Soaring prices of prescription drugs have led to a backlash by insurers, employers, and government at both state and federal levels. WellPoint Health Networks (parent of Blue Cross in California) has been mailing coupons to 400,000 members to help them buy Alavert, a nonprescription version of Claritin, in an effort to avoid the use of more expensive antihistamines (Freudenheim, 2002b). A growing number of employers are deciding, if they continue to offer employer-based health insurance at all, to do so by defined contribution plans, whereby costs are shifted to employees beyond a set annual amount. More than one-half of large employers have adopted three-tier copays to encourage use of generic drugs (Langreth, 2003). Many states have taken steps to reduce costs of pharmaceuticals for their residents, including efforts to establish preferred drug lists and organizing to extract deeper discounts for Medicaid enrollees (Freudenheim, 2003a). The state of Maine enacted legislation to obtain about a 20% discount on retail drug prices for its Medicaid program and to establish barriers to sales of drugs in the state by any manufacturers refusing to participate in the program (Greenberger, 2003) At the federal level, Centers for Medicare & Medicaid Services (CMS) is now refusing to pay for some drugs not considered superior to equivalent, less expensive drugs (e.g., Nexium versus Prilosec) (Pear, 2003a).

Consumers are also revolting against escalating drug prices by use of mail-order pharmacies, which often offer discounts (Carroll, 2002), and by purchase of drugs over the Internet from Canadian pharmacies (Peterson, 2002). Some insurers are even beginning to cover prescription drugs purchased from Canada (Lueck, 2002). Major savings can be gained by these means. For example, in March of 2003 Tamoxifen for breast cancer could be purchased by Canadian mail order for little more than 25% of the cost of U.S. mail order (Barry, 2003).

All of these efforts by purchasers to press drug manufacturers to lower their prices have met with a reactive backlash from the pharmaceutical industry itself. Its trade organization, PhRMA, has brought suits against states' programs to discount drugs. It has lobbied Congress aggressively to curtail Medicare coverage decisions based on cost-effectiveness of drugs and price controls. Glaxo-Smith Kline cut supplies to Canadian pharmacies that sell to Americans on the Internet, and then was boycotted by senior citizen groups south of the border (Barry, 2003; Sailant, 2003). At the same time, the drug industry has attempted to improve its public image through various means, including offers of free trials of prescription drugs (Parker-Pope, 2002), discount cards for low-income seniors (Waldholz, 2002a), and funding case workers for disease management programs for Medicaid beneficiaries (also a marketing strategy for their drugs) in exchange for exemption from states' requirements of discounts (Peterson, 2003b).

According to the AARP Public Policy Institute, U.S. prescription drug prices, both wholesale and retail, are about 70% higher on average than in Canada (Gross, 2003). As a result of this continuing battle over drug prices in the U.S., the marketplace is chaotic and faces an uncertain future. The U.S. Supreme Court ruled by a 6–3 vote in June

2003 against an injunction sought by the drug industry, thereby supporting the initiatives by Maine and other states to use their purchasing clout to obtain discounted drug prices for their Medicaid beneficiaries (Lueck, Greenberger, Rundle, 2002). As lawsuits fly back and forth between states and the drug industry, mail-order pharmacies are growing fast, purchases of Canadian drugs on the Internet continue to increase, and more Canadian pharmacies are establishing U.S.-based storefronts. One example, Best Canadian Prescription Service, has already opened 20 sites across the U.S., with outlets planned in all states by the end of 2003 (*Practice Trends*, 2003).

As the pharmaceutical industry attempts to ward off efforts within the U.S. to lower drug prices, it has also prevailed upon the Bush Administration to seek to *raise* prices of drugs in other countries and prevent imports of lower-cost drugs to the U.S. The goals now being pursued by U.S. trade negotiators as part of our Free Trade Agreements are to: "(1) restructure internal markets to raise prices on patented drugs, (2) extend patent protection and data exclusivity to delay generic competition, and (3) block cheap exports to the U.S." "Free trade" in this policy is really a misnomer—it really means free from competition over prices (Light & Lexchin, 2004).

COMMON PRACTICES OF THE DRUG INDUSTRY

Despite growing public and legislative concern about unabated increases in the cost of prescription drugs, the pharmaceutical industry continues to pursue a primary focus on profits. While this is good business practice and meets the interests of drug companies and their shareholders, the public interest is often left behind, as illustrated by the following common industry practices.

Misleading Advertising and Marketing

As we have already seen, marketing expenditures by drug companies far exceed their R&D expenditures. Marketing by the drug industry is indeed a large and growing business. Although detailing and giving samples to physicians account for about 80% of total promotional spending, direct-to-consumer (DTC) advertising is also a large and growing marketing strategy (Rosenberg, 2003).

Much of the DTC marketing presents a distorted case for treatment, overstating benefits and downplaying risks. There are many examples of intentional deception in advertising content, such as promoting Celebrex (a well-known arthritis medication) as risk-free for peptic ulcer, and OxyContin for pain control without stating potential life-threatening risks (Adams, 2003; Wolfe, 2001a). The FDA has found that some drug companies repeatedly violate drug marketing laws in their advertising, and some even continue DTC ads while under review by the FDA for violations. DTC advertising has been growing rapidly since 1997 when the FDA relaxed restrictions on the practice. Over 8 million Americans request and receive prescription drugs each year after seeing or hearing DTC ads, so the risks of deceptive advertising are substantial (Pear, 2002).

An especially common practice by many drug companies is the promotion of "me too" drugs as a "breakthrough" when they are no better and hardly different from older drugs (e.g., Nexium versus Prilosec, Clarinex versus Claritin). This kind of advertising has been called a "smoke and mirrors" technique—smoke for a false breakthrough, and mirrors for slightly rearranged isomers in the new drug's chemical structure. Only about one-third of drugs approved by the FDA between 1989 and 2000 were new molecular entities (National Institute for Health Care Management, 2002b). One recent report from the Health Research Group of Public Citizen found that of seven pairs of drugs, six had no therapeutic advantage over their predecessors, and one was more toxic than the original (Wolfe, 2003).

Creation of "Disease" Through Biased "Research"

The boundaries between marketing and legitimate drug research frequently become blurred when conflicts of interest permeate the ranks of investigators. One example, which clearly shows that the line has been crossed into the area of phony "research," is instructive. Pfizer brought the blockbuster drug Viagra to market in 1998. Since then more than 17 million men have filled prescriptions as a treatment for erectile dysfunction, with sales of $1.5 billion in 2001 (Pfizer, Inc., 2001). In order to build a similar market among women, Pfizer took the lead in organizing an international effort to define and treat female sexual dysfunction. With a consortium of drug company sponsors, a series of consensus development conferences was held for invited corporate-friendly investigators and drug company marketing representatives. Handpicked participants in "closed session" discussions produced a new definition and classification of female sexual dysfunction including disorders of desire, arousal, orgasm, and pain (Special supplement, 1998; Moynihan, 2003).

Some of the investigators published a paper in the *Journal of the American Medical Association* on the prevalence and predictors of this new "disease," concluding that 43% of women between 18 and 59 years of age had one or more symptoms of sexual dysfunction, including lack of desire, anxiety about performance, or problems with lubrication. This figure was based upon a survey asking respondents whether they had experienced any of seven such problems for two months or more during the previous year (Laumann, Park, & Rosen, 1999). Two of the authors later disclosed close links to Pfizer (Moynihan, 2003), and the 43% figure has since been widely cited in marketing materials (Berman, Berman, & Goldstein, 1999; Cooke, 2002). Almost all of the investigators have financial interests or other relationships with sponsoring drug companies. As these "investigators" continue to pursue building a new market for a female equivalent of Viagra, leading independent sex researchers have called into question their definition and reported prevalence of female sexual dysfunction (Bancroft, 2002; Seagraves, 2001; (Tiefer, 1996, 2000).

Delayed or Inaccurate Reporting of Risks

It is not uncommon for an initially popular drug to be withdrawn from the market as its toxicity and risks become better known from wider use. Litigation may then follow as the events and decisions leading up to its withdrawal are brought to light. Two current examples illustrate how drug firm executives can underestimate risks or delay warnings of risks in an effort to continue profitable marketing of their drugs.

The cholesterol drug Baycol was withdrawn from the market in 2001 after causing about 100 deaths worldwide linked to a muscle disorder (rhabdomyolysis) with secondary renal failure. Bayer, its manufacturer, withdrew the drug only after the FDA raised serious concerns about it. More recently, newly disclosed company documents show that some senior executives were aware of these serious and life-threatening risks, but continued to promote the drug without clarifying the risks (Peterson & Berenson, 2003).

Another similar example involves Warner-Lambert and its diabetes drug, Regulin. It was withdrawn from the U.S. market in 2000 after generating over $2 billion in sales. Since then, it has become clear from internal company documents that company executives minimized the risks of liver damage from the drug. The drug was linked to scores of liver-related deaths over the three years it was on the market. During that period, the company continued to promote Regulin as safe, failed to warn physicians that monitoring of liver function tests would not prevent some deaths from liver failure, and even offered to indemnify prescribing physicians nationwide against liability if they were sued for use of the drug (Willman, 2002).

Aggressive Marketing to Physicians

There are about 88,000 pharmaceutical sales representatives in the U.S. , more than one for every eight practicing physicians, detailing their products to physicians (Relman & Angell, 2002). The drug industry spends about $12 billion each year on this effort (Wolfe, 1996), which can be variously viewed as marketing or educational. Typically physicians see a drug sales representative about once a week. Interactions between physicians and drug representatives can take place under varied circumstances, including medical offices, hospitals, teaching conferences, symposia, and other continuing medical education (CME) activities. A recent initiative by some drug companies involves the drug representative "shadowing" the physician in the office, even in the examination room. One drug company pays participating physicians for their time and obtains consents from involved patients (Fox News, 2003). Invariably, the drug representatives bring gifts in the form of samples, free meals, or funding for travel and lodgings to attend symposia at resorts.

The drug industry considers these interactions to be educational and in the interests of patients through their use of about $10 billion a year in free samples (Frieden, J., 2002). Experience has proven, however, that there is no free lunch. Conflicts of interest permeate these interactions, sometimes in subtle and easily denied ways. Many physicians, for example, keep stores of starter samples in their offices and give them out to needy patients. The downside however, is that since samples are usually more expensive brand name drugs, patients may not be able to afford continuing such medications, and may later require a change to a less expensive drug.

A systematic review was published in 2000 reporting the results of all available studies of the interactions between drug industry representatives and physicians. It conclusively documented that these interactions effectively lead to increased prescribing of sponsors' drugs as well as new requests by physicians to add these drugs to hospital formularies (Wazana, 2000).

Excesses in drug marketing have sparked public and regulators' concerns in recent years as the sales pitch has often been extended to include all-expense-paid outings at golf, ski, or other resorts. In reaction to these kinds of excesses, many physicians refuse to see drug representatives or set up clear restrictions to these interactions. Vermont has enacted legislation requiring disclosure of any gifts to physicians valued over $25 (Johannes, 2002), and the federal government is developing new guidelines to rein in excessive marketing practices (Rawe, 2002). A large gray area for potential marketing abuses remains, however, as illustrated by these examples:

- The drug industry funds more than 40% of continuing medical education (CME) activities in the U.S., up from 17% in 1994, according to the Accrediting Council for Continuing Medical Education (Hensley, 2002)
- A 1995 study found that 11% of statements by drug representatives were inaccurate, and always in favor of the drugs being detailed (Ziegler, Lew, & Singer, 1995)
- Pfizer has recently agreed to pay $430 million to resolve criminal and civil charges that it paid physicians to prescribe its top selling Neurontin (approved for treatment of seizures), for other nonapproved, off-label uses, including bipolar disorder, migraine, and attention deficit disorder (Harris, 2004).

Invisible Marketing and Profiteering Along the Distribution Chain

It is often difficult for purchasers to determine how manufacturers set prices for their drugs. It is also difficult to understand how prices are manipulated along the distribution chain, where invisible discounts and kickbacks are common. There are two ways by which drug companies can market their products below the radar screen of public awareness. In the first instance, drug companies pay pharmacies to send letters to patients promoting their drugs. One drug store in Florida, for example, contracted with a drug company to contact 150,000 patients over a six-month period by means of its own prescription drug records. Typical payments to pharmacies range from 85 cents to $1.50 per letter and $2.00 to $3.50 per telephone call (Armstrong & Zimmerman, 2002). Another practice involves "health newsletters" as point-of-purchase ads which are wrapped into warning labels given to patients when they pick up their prescriptions. These ads, paid for by the drug companies, now involve more than one-half of all prescriptions filled by chain drug stores across the country (Armstrong & Zimmerman, 2002).

Another area of invisible profit taking along the distribution chain involves the large business of pharmacy-benefit managers (PBMs). Over the last 10 years, almost all large employers in the U.S. have delegated the management of drug benefits for their employees to

TABLE 5.1. How Generic Drugs Yield Big Profits

Example: A 30-day prescription of generic Prozac	
Patient's copayment to pharmacy	$ 5.00
Pharmacy-benefit manager's payment to pharmacy	$ 2.50
What the manufacturer charges pharmacy for the prescription	$ 1.50
Pharmacy's profit	$ 6.00
(Patient's copayment plus PBM's payment minus manufacturer's price)	
PBM bill to patient's employer	$13.00
PBM's profit	$10.50
(PBM bill to employer minus payment to pharmacy)	

Source: Martinez, B. (2003). Rx for margins. Hired to cut costs, firms find profits in generic drugs. *The Wall Street Journal,* March 31, A1.

one of four major PBMs. These companies have created electronic networks for automated purchasing and billing, and four PBMs claim to control the drug benefits of over 200,000 people (Martinez, 2003). PBMs are hired by large payers to cut the costs of prescription drugs, but there is widespread evidence that they ultimately end up driving costs up through a complex maze of undisclosed rebates, fees, and payments between drug firms, PBMs, and pharmacies. Table 5.1 details how a 30-day prescription for the common generic antidepressant, Prozac, ends up with a high charge to the employer and a sizable profit for the PBM (Martinez, 2003). PBMs have been so aggressive in negotiating discounts with pharmacies that the price of some common generic drugs end up lower than patients' copayments. Thus even with copayments of $5 or $10, there is a hidden profit to the PBM and/or pharmacy unbeknownst to consumers (Martinez, 2002). PBMs are running a thriving business, but neither employers nor patients are realizing savings. The largest publicly traded PBM, Advance PCS, reported earnings growth of 44% for the last 9 months of 2002 compared with the previous year (Martinez, 2003).

Some drug companies use PBMs to market their own drugs against competitors. Typically, these are more expensive, brand-name drugs, so here again the costs to patients and payers will tend to be higher than less expensive alternatives. The second largest PBM in the country, Merck Medco (now Express Scripts) is involved in litigation alleging that it was paid more than $3 billion in rebates from drug manufacturers in the late 1990s to promote the sales of certain drugs. Investigators have documented that Medco has vigorously promoted Merck drugs over other drugs and has effectively raised Merck's sales to Medco mail-order clients compared with its national market share (Medco sales of Merck drugs for hypertension and heart failure were 50% higher) (Freudenheim, 2003b).

Gaming the Patent System

Drug patent laws provide manufacturers with a 17-year monopoly on their drugs and are a key element in the profit potential of the drug industry in the U.S. market. Drug companies defend their patents as essential to innovation and their R&D. As we found with marketing practices, however, this claim becomes less compelling as the numbers are scrutinized. Dean Baker, codirector of the Center for Economic and Policy Research, points out that patent protection to U.S. drug companies amounted to about $79 billion in 2000 (75% of U.S. expenditures on prescription drugs that year, with the average free market price overseas just 25% of U.S. prices). Only about $22.5 billion was spent by the U.S. drug industry on research that year, with another $28 billion being paid by the NIH, other federal agencies, universities, private foundations, and charities. As a result, consumers pay more than three and a half dollars to drug companies for every dollar spent on drug research (Baker, 2001).

Drug companies have developed elaborate strategies to extend their patents and monopolies beyond the 17 years, or to block other companies from acquiring competitive patents. Those strategies include setting up diversionary patents on nonessential details of a drug's main patent, filing of new patents for "new" uses of old drugs, and filing a "citizen petition" against generic competition (Public Citizen, 2001). All of these create a legal minefield for competitors, since federal law automatically delays the entry of competing drugs into the market for at least 30 months whenever patent-holding companies file such lawsuits (*Los Angeles Times,* 2002). Another ploy used by some manufacturers to buy more time on their expiring patents is to request patent extension of six months for testing of their drugs in children. The FDA estimates that pediatric patent extensions bring in revenues at least 40 times the costs of such testing to the parent drug companies (Green, 2002).

Blocking Generic Competition

Although Congress passed the Drug Price Competition Act in 1984 in an effort to encourage competition between brand-name and generic drugs as well as increased use of generics, it has proven to be ineffective. Instead, here is what we find in the marketplace. In 2000 Abbott Laboratories contracted to pay a generic competitor (Geneva Pharmaceuticals) $4.5 million a month (up to $101 million over the term of the contract) *not* to bring its generic to market (Ivins, 2001). Bristol-Myers paid $670 million to settle litigation concerning its efforts to block generic competition for two of its best-selling drugs, the cancer drug Taxol and the anti-anxiety drug Buspar (Harris, 2003). More recently, some pharmaceutical companies are licensing some brand-name drugs to selected generics makers as a way to undermine plans of rival generics makers to copy these drugs. (Abboud, 2004).

A renewed effort was made by Congress in 2002 to achieve some containment of escalating drug costs through increased use of generic drugs, but it was blocked by an intense lobbying campaign by the drug industry. The Senate passed the Greater Access to Affordable Pharmaceuticals Act (by a vote of 78 to 21), but the bill died in the House. If enacted, it would have given generic drug companies more opportunity to challenge inappropriate brand patents and would have prohibited more than one 30-month extension of a contended patent (CONGRESSWATCHDOG, 2002).

Fraud

Beyond the above of practices, outright fraud is, unfortunately, far from rare in the drug industry. These examples make the point:

- Two large pharmaceutical companies incurred $725 million in criminal fines in 2000, while another six companies were fined $335 million to settle charges of price-fixing of vitamins (Physicians for a National Health Program (PNHP, 2001)
- Medicare was overcharged $1.9 billion in 2001 for 24 common prescription drugs (Department of Health and Human Services, 2001)
- Bayer agreed to a Medicaid fraud settlement of $257 million in 2003, pleading guilty to a criminal charge of engaging in a scheme to overcharge for its drug Cipro (Peterson, 2003a).
- Between 1997 and 2001, there were more than 500 advertisements for prescription drugs targeting physicians or patients which were found to violate FDA laws and regulations, generally by overstating benefits and minimizing risks (Wolfe, 2001b).

SOME CONTROVERSIAL POLICY ISSUES

As many millions of Americans find prescription drugs increasingly unaffordable and as the political debate about health care heats up during the 2004 presidential election campaign, three policy issues stand out concerning the drug industry.

Should direct-to-consumer advertising (DTCA) be banned?

Proponents of DTCA, led by the drug industry's trade group PhR-MA, argue that DTCA serves an important educational purpose in informing patients about the latest advances in drug therapy and prompting them to discuss their health problems with physicians. Proponents also suggest that DTCA may encourage patients to discuss diet and preventive services with their physicians, and that it can contribute to a better informed public and less geographic variability in prescribing patterns (Holmer, 2002; Weissman, Blumenthal, Silk, Zopert, Newman et al., 2003).

Critics of DTCA contend that DTCA raises overall spending on prescription drugs (since higher volumes of more expensive brand drugs are filled) and leads in many cases to inappropriate use of medication, that misleading and unbalanced information is presented to consumers, and that the FDA has been ineffective in regulating the accuracy of such advertising (Weissman, 2003; Wolfe, 2002b).

There are a number of recent studies of DTCA which confirm critics' concerns. One study found that 87% of the content of these ads gave only vague, qualitative descriptions of benefits of treatment, with only 13% including data and none mentioning cost (Woloshin, Schwartz, Tremmel, & Welch, 2001). A 2003 report of a large national study of more than 1,000 physicians and 2,500 patients found that one-half of DTCA-prompted requests for specific drugs were viewed by the physicians to be clinically inappropriate (with 69% of inappropriate requests still being prescribed); four of ten physicians thought that DTCA damaged the time efficiency of visits, and they felt pressured to prescribe (Murray, Lo, Pollack, Donelan, & Lee, 2003); only 6% of DTCA-prompted visits triggered a request for some type of preventive care (Murray, Lo, Pollack, Donelan, & Lee, 2004). Investigators from the General Accounting Office have found that inaccurate DTC ads often run their full course before the FDA can warn the manufacturer of a marketing violation (Pear, 2002).

While there is strong evidence that DTCA should be banned, as it has been in some countries (e.g., Australia), the drug industry lobbies hard for its continuance and it is still supported by the government. It brings in added revenue to drug companies, but the almost $3 billion a year spent on it has not been shown to result in improved clinical outcomes.

How Can Public Policy Best Meet Goals of Efficiency, Access, and Equity in the Use of Prescription Drugs?

The pharmaceuticals market is extremely complex, and rising drug prices and spending pose an ongoing challenge to all health care systems around the world. Each country tries to balance three basic goals—expenditure control, access, and cost-effectiveness. There is no perfect policy anywhere for this continuing challenge, but many other countries achieve these goals far better than the U.S. (Maynard & Bloor, 2003).

In an excellent review of policy alternatives, Alan Maynard and Karen Bloor, leading researchers on this subject based at the University of York in England, summarize international experience with the three categories of possible strategies—influencing patients, influencing providers, and regulating industry. There is much that policymakers in the U.S. can learn from this experience. (Maynard & Bloor, 2003).

Influencing patients. Copayments and cost-sharing have been shown to contain some spending on drugs, but especially for lower income populations (e.g., Medicaid in the U.S.), are associated with adverse health outcomes (Appleby, 2002; Soumerai, Avora, Ross-Degnan, Gortmaker, 1987; Soumerai, McLaughlin, Ross-Degnan, Casteris, Bollini, 1994; Prescription drug access, 2002). Another trend, increasingly common in Europe since the late 1990s, is the policy of governments to switch some prescription drugs to over-the-counter (OTC) status, thereby shifting costs from government to patients. Competition has been encouraged in the United Kingdom by a 2000 ruling making price-fixing for OTC drugs illegal (Office of Fair Trading, 2001).

Influencing providers. Feedback to physicians on prescribing patterns, clinical guidelines, limited drug lists, and generic substitution are the most common approaches taken in Europe. Explicit budget controls and financial incentives to physicians for cost-effective prescribing have been of limited use and value. Of these approaches, the use of a limited list of cost-effective drugs, if monitored, appears to be an effective strategy (Maynard & Bloor, 2003).

Regulating industry. Three approaches have been tried by a number of countries in an effort to contain pharmaceutical costs—price controls, profit controls, and cost-effectiveness controls. Mechanisms to control prices vary considerably from one country to another, but over the last ten years, systems of "reference pricing" have seen increasingly common use, especially in Europe, . Reference pricing (RP) requires patients to pay the difference between retail prices at pharmacies and the reference price set by the insurer or government payer, which is the price of a therapeutic cluster of drugs considered clinically equivalent in the treatment of a given illness (Kanavos & Reinhardt, 2003). RP has achieved only short-term cost savings in a number of countries (Ioannides-Demos, Ibrahim, McNeill, 2002), but as a means of cost sharing with patients through defined contribution plans of employers it is being proposed by some for the U.S., perhaps even for Medicare (Huskamp, Rosenthal, Frank, & Newhouse, 2000). Other analysts observe that RP may not constrain drug spending, and has not yet demonstrated improvements in clinical outcomes, health status, or total system costs (Kanavos & Reinhardt, 2003). The United Kingdom has attempted to control profits through its Pharmaceutical Price Regulation Scheme (PPRS), but it offers little incentive to manufacturers to be efficient and has been of limited effectiveness (Maynard & Bloor, 1997). Australia pioneered cost-effectiveness controls through its Pharmacy Benefits Scheme (PBS), which requires manufacturers to submit evidence of costs and effects of its drugs (Australian Department of Health, 2002). Economic data are now also being used in many countries in Europe to inform pricing and reimbursement decisions (Maynard & Bloor, 2003).

Based on the experience of other countries and the realities and problems within the U.S. pharmaceutical market, the following approaches would appear to merit serious consideration by policymakers:

- Ban DTCA, unless the accuracy of its ads can be effectively regulated by the FDA and cost information included
- Further encourage generic substitution for brand-name drugs, and require transparency of price setting by manufacturers of both brand-name and generic drugs
- Require drug research to compare new drugs with alternative drugs, not just with placebos
- Introduce cost-effectiveness data into reimbursement decisions of payers as well as into marketing and education of providers
- Clear the way for states to establish preferred-drug lists and negotiate discounted drug prices with manufacturers, as many states have been trying to do despite the vigorous opposition of the drug industry (Freudenheim, 2003a)

Is a Prescription Drug Benefit Under Medicare Good Public Policy?

For many, the quick answer to this question, is "of course, why not!" This is a complex issue, however, with the devil in the details. Several other questions need to be asked, for example: how would it be implemented, by whom, and for whom? How would the pharmaceutical market be regulated to constrain costs and avoid expensive "me too" drugs? Can health benefits thereby be achieved for Medicare beneficiaries?

This issue has taken center stage on the domestic agenda as public demand and political pressure have mounted for some kind of prescription drug benefit under Medicare, fueled by the failure of Congress to enact a plan over the previous six years. After a long and bitter debate in Congress, the Medicare Prescription Drug, Improvement and Modernization Act of 2003 was finally passed by a narrow margin in November 2003. The bill was fought from the right as an expensive entitlement, and from the left as too limited a benefit favoring special interests over patients. In order to gain enough support for passage, the final bill of 678 pages ended up as a "Christmas tree" with many provisions unrelated to the prescription drug benefit tacked on, including provisions to increase reimbursement to hospitals and physicians, to raise reimbursement rates in rural areas, to experiment with further privatization of Medicare, and to study the role of specialty hospitals. As a result, additional support was gained for other reasons, as illustrated by some Democratic senators from rural states crossing party lines to vote for the bill (Pear, 2003b).

The new Medicare legislation is complex. How it will sort out is not entirely clear, since many of the rules governing its implementation are not yet written. Highlights of the bill are summarized in Table 5.2 (McGinley & Lueck, 2003; Pear & Hulse, 2003).

In the aftermath of the 2003 Medicare bill's passage, the Bush Administration and most Republicans claimed victory thinking they had stolen a crucial issue from the Democrats as the 2004 election cycle went forward. Democrats vowed renewed legislative efforts to improve the prescription drug benefit, protect the traditional Medicare program, and repeal the most contentious provisions of the bill. The AARP, which threw its weight behind the bill in its last stages, came under fire from many of its own members and consumer advocacy groups for selling out to special interests. AARP defended its decision claiming the bill was a "flawed but important first step"

**TABLE 5.2. Highlights of the Medicare Prescription Drug,
Improvement and Modernization Act of 2003**

Feature	Description
Drug Discount Card	Medicare beneficiaries eligible in May 2004 to buy a prescription drug card, which is expected to lower costs by about 15%
Drug Benefits	Starting in 2006, Medicare recipients can enroll in new benefit for prescription drugs. They pay average monthly premiums of $35, and a $250 annual deductible. The government pays 75% of costs, up to $2,250. Gap in coverage ('donut') between $2,250 and $3600 annual drug costs. Government pays 95% of costs after out-of-pocket annual expenses reach $3,600.
Retiree Coverage	Corporations offering qualified drug coverage will receive 28% tax exempt payments for drug costs between $250 and $5,000.
Low-Income Beneficiaries	In 2004 and 2005, low-income beneficiaries will receive an annual subsidy of $600 to reduce drug costs further. Starting in 2006, the premium deductible and coverage gap will be waived for beneficiaries with incomes up to $12,123 a year; in order to qualify for this subsidy, individuals can have no more than $6,000 in assets.
Administering the Drug Benefit	Private companies, including pharmacy benefit managers and PPOs, will administer the drug benefit, and will receive about $12 billion in subsidies.
Competition With Traditional Medicare	Starting in 2010, traditional government-run Medicare will compete directly with private plans in up to six metropolitan areas where at least 25 percent of Medicare beneficiaries are in private plans. If traditional Medicare's cost is more than private health plans, its beneficiaries will have to pay higher premiums.
Drug Imports From Canada	The ban on importing prescription drugs is continued unless the Department of Health and Human Services certifies their safety, which the department has refused to do for many years.

TABLE 5.2. *(continued)*

Feature	Description
Health-Related Tax Savings Accounts	People with high-deductible health insurance policies—$1,000 a year for individuals, $2,000 for couples—will be allowed to shelter income from taxes.
Means Testing	Beginning in 2007, higher-income seniors earning more than $80,000 per year will be required to pay higher Medicare Part B premiums for physician services.
Physician Payments	Planned cuts in physician payments in 2004 and 2005 will be canceled and instead a 1.5% increase is planned for each year.
Rural Health	About $25 billion is earmarked to increase payments to rural hospitals and physicians, among others.
Home Health Care	Payments to home health agencies will be cut, but copayments from patients will not be required.

(Toner, 2003), but critics pointed AARP's involvement in the insurance business as a possible motivation for its support of the bill. About 60% of AARP's revenue is derived from insurance-related ventures, including the sale of Medigap policies and sales of its membership list (about double its revenue from members' dues) (Drinkard, 2003).

Is the 2003 Medicare bill good public policy? Despite the claims of its supporters, the following points would suggest that it is not:

- Without any price controls built into the system, the prescription drug benefit will bring many billions in new profits to the pharmaceutical and insurance industries with very little accountability, while drug prices for many seniors will remain increasingly unaffordable.
- The experiment with privatization of Medicare through Medicare + Choice HMOs over the last 10 years has already been a failure (Bodenheimer, 2003). Medicare PPOs have indicated that they will not participate unless government subsidies cover their greater administrative costs and still yield a profit. $14 billion in subsidies were earmarked to cover the higher costs of the insurance and managed care industries, a figure that was later revised to $46 billion (Pear, 2004), hardly qualifying as "competition" with the traditional, not-for-profit Medicare program (Public

Citizen, 2003). True competition would involve a level playing field without subsidies.

- The more healthier and affluent seniors are siphoned off to private Medicare plans, the more Medicare itself is made vulnerable to adverse selection. A "death spiral" of Medicare would be the ultimate outcome as the traditional program confronts the increased costs of sicker and lower-income seniors who are least able to afford higher levels of cost sharing.
- Private pharmacy benefit managers (PBMs) will select the drugs to be covered under this plan, with no transparency or public accountability. They are unlikely to gain more than 10% or 15% discounts from standard reference or retailers' prices of covered drugs (Abboud & Hensley, 2003).
- The government is expressly prohibited from using its purchasing power, as it does so effectively within the Veterans Administration, to achieve deeply discounted drug prices for Medicare beneficiaries.
- According to a recent analysis by Consumers Union, only 22% of projected drug costs over the next 10 years will be covered by the Medicare prescription drug benefit (Shearer, 2003).
- Large subsidies will be provided to employers as incentives for them to continue to provide a drug benefit, but there is no assurance that they will do so. Even if they do, it will be through expensive private PBMs or health plans.
- The Congressional Budget Office estimates that 3.8 million retirees will have their private drug coverage reduced or eliminated (Pear, 2003a).
- More than 6 million elderly people now receiving drug coverage under Medicaid will lose that coverage (Pear, 2003a).
- Medicare approved drug discount cards will probably not obtain more than 10% to 15% discounts. There is evidence that rising drug prices have already eroded savings from discount cards, with the prices for many top-selling drugs up 20% or more since mid-2001, when plans for drug discount cards were announced. (Martinez, 2004). Seniors with annual incomes below $12,000 will receive only $600 on their cards to cover the costs of their medications, far below the needs of many such patients (Abboud & Hensley, 2003; Lueck, 2003).
- As drug prices continue to escalate without cost controls, many seniors will find the Medicare prescription drug benefit to be of limited value. Seniors with annual drug costs of $4,000 to $5,000

will have to pay more than two-thirds of those costs out of pocket (Pear & Hulse, 2003). By the eighth year of the program in 2013, their deductible and coverage gap will have grown by 78% (Sherman, 2003).

Even before the addition of a prescription drug benefit to Medicare, the program's annual expenditures were expected to double to almost $500 billion by 2012 and to account for 25% of the federal budget by 2025 (Lockhead, 2003). These fiscal realities are even more challenging in view of federal deficit projections for many years into the future, tax cuts, and doubling of the Medicare population to almost 80 million by 2030 as the baby boom generation reaches eligibility for the program (Rovner, 2003). Most Democrats favor a prescription drug benefit for all seniors as part of traditional Medicare, while most Republicans prefer a more restrictive program with higher deductibles, available especially through the private sector, privatization, and dismantling of Medicare as an entitlement program. The recently enacted Medicare prescription drug benefit is the largest and most important change to Medicare since its advent in 1965, with the potential to bankrupt the program since cost containment is not built in and further privatization is being promoted. As a result, we can look forward to many more political battles and fiscal crises in coming years over the future of Medicare.

CONCLUDING COMMENTS

Costs and spending on prescription drugs continue to soar in the U.S. without any semblance of cost containment. The pharmaceuticals market is overpriced, under-regulated, and nonsustainable in the long run. Even as the drug industry seeks to build its image through "feel good" ads and discount cards for some low-income people, it battles all efforts by government or large purchasers to contain prices. As the cost of pharmaceuticals takes up a growing part of state and federal health budgets, as well as those of employers and insurers, a backlash is underway. Unfortunately, however, most of the countertrends so far lead to further cost shifting to patients, and a growing part of the population cannot afford essential drug treatment. The drug industry still enjoys many protections and subsidies from government and needs to be held more accountable to the public interest. We will consider this issue further in Parts II and III of this book.

REFERENCES

Abboud, L. & Hensley, S. (2003, Nov. 26). Drug-discount cards to have 'ifs'. *The Wall Street Journal*, p. D2.

Abboud, L. Drug makers use new tactics to ding generics. *The Wall Street Journal*, January 27, 2004: B1.

Adams, C. (2003, January 23). FDA asks maker of OxyContin to pull "misleading" print ads. *The Wall Street Journal*, p. D3.

Angell, M., & Relman, A.S. (2001, June 21). Prescription for profit. Available at *www.washingtonpost.com*

Appleby, J. (2002, January 28). Patients drop treatment due to costs. Co-payments too steep for some Medicare HMO clients. Available at *USA Today*.com

Armstrong, D., & Zimmerman, A. (2002, June 14) Drug makers find new way to push pills. *The Wall Street Journal*, p. B1.

Australian Department of Health. (2002, Feb. 20). Pharmaceutical benefits scheme. September 6, 2002 Available at *www.health.gov.au/pbs/committt.htm*

Baker, D. (2001, Jan. 29). Patent medicine. *The American Prospect*, pp. 34–35.

Bancroft, J. (2002). The medicalization of female sexual dysfunction: The need for caution. *Archives of Sexual Behavior, 31,* 451.

Barry, P. (2002, March). Ads, promotions drive up costs. *AARP Bulletin, 43*(3), 1, 17.

Barry, P. (2003, April). More Americans go north for drugs. *AARP Bulletin, 44*(4), 3–5.

Berman, J., Berman, L., Goldstein, I. (1999). Female sexual dysfunction: incidence, pathophysiology, evaluation and treatment options. *Urology, 54,* 385.

Bodenheimer, T. (2003, June). The dismal failure of Medicare privatization. Senior Action Network. San Francisco, California, 1.

Brundtland, G. H. Essential medicines: 25 years of better health. *JAMA* 2002: 288(24), 3102.

Carroll, J. (2002, March 29). Prescription drug spending jumps 17%. *The Wall Street Journal*, p. A3.

Center for Studying Health System Change. (2002, April). Washington, DC Issue Brief #51.

Congressional Research Service. (1999). December 13.

CONGRESSWATCHDOG (2002). Senate passed legislation opposed by the Administration would have provided significantly more price relief for consumers. Retrieved from CONGRESSWATCHDOG@citizen.org, October 22.

Cooke, R. (2002, oct. 27). There's gold in them thar pills. *Observer*.

De Moro, D. (2003, March). Health policy expert calls Pharma merger costs and profits major factor in health care inflation, reduced access to care. *RN Journal*, March. CNA website, Available at calnurse.org

Deutsche, B., & Brown, A. (1999, Oct. 11). *Pharmaceutical industry outlook: sobering up on drugs, Fig. 40.* New York: Alex Brown.

Department of Health and Human Services (2001), Sept. 20). Inspector General report. *The New York Times.* September 20.

Drinkard, J. (2003, Nov. 21). AARP accused of conflict of interest. *USA Today,* p. 11A.

Families USA (2002, July 17). Press release.

Federman, A. D., Adams, A. S. Ross-Degnan, D., Soumerai, S. B. Arinian, J. Z. (2001). Supplemental insurance and use of effective cardiovascular drugs among elderly Medicare beneficiaries with coronary heart disease. *Journal of the American Medical Association, 286,* 1732.

Fox News. (2003, Jan. 21). Shadowing by drug representatives in physicians' offices.

Frank, R. (2001). Prescription drug prices: Why do some pay more than others do? *Health Affairs (Millwood), 20*(2), 115.

Frieden, J. (2002). Policy and Practice. Where drug dollars go. *Family Practice News, 32*(16).

Frieden, J. (2003, Apr. 15). Practice trends. Cheap drugs for American seniors. *Family Practice News, 33*(8), 42.

Freudenheim, M. (2002a, Dec. 24). WellPoint to help customers purchase allergy medication. *The New York Times,* p. C2.

Freudenheim, M. (2002b, Dec. 27). As patents on popular drugs end costs for generics show a surge. *The New York Times,* p. A1.

Freudenheim, M. (2003a, Jan. 14). States organizing a non-profit group to cut drug costs. *The New York Times,* p. A1.

Freudenheim, M. (2003b, March 13). Documents detail big payments by drug makers to sway sales. *The New York Times,* p. C1

Gencarelli, D. M. (2002, June). Average wholesale price for prescription drugs: Is there a more appropriate pricing mechanism? National Health Policy Forum Issue Brief, No. 775. Washington, DC: George Washington University.

Green, M. (2002). *Selling out: How big corporate money buys elections, rams through legislation and betrays our democracy (p. 185).* New York: Regan Books.

Greenberger, R. S. (2003, Jan. 15). A prescription for change. Maine drug plan, awaiting high court review, may sway U.S. *The Wall Street Journal,* p. B2.

Harris, G. (2002, April 18). Dose of trouble. For drug makers, good times yield to profit crunch. *The Wall Street Journal,* p. A1.

Gross, D. (2003, June). Prescription drug prices in Canada. AARP Public Policy Interests.

Harris, G., & Fuhrmans, V. (2002, July 16). Alliances prove an iffy panacea for drug makers. *The Wall Street Journal,* p. C1.

Harris, G. (2003, Jan. 8). Bristol-Myers agrees to generics pact. *The Wall Street Journal,* p. A4.

Harris, G. (2004, May 14). Pfizer to pay over $430 million promoting drug to doctors. *New York Times*, p. C1.

Hensley, S. (2002, Dec. 4). When doctors go to class, industry often foots the bill. *The Wall Street Journal*, p. A1.

Hensley, S., & Burton, T. M. (2003, April 23). Big drug makers report increase in sales. *The Wall Street Journal*, p. B2.

Hensley, S. (2004, Feb. 3). Combination drugs marketed by Pfizer win nod. *The Wall Street Journal*, p. D4.

Holmer, A. F. (2002). Direct-to-consumer advertising: Strengthening our health care system. *The New England Journal of Medicine, 346*, 526.

Huskamp, H. A., Rosenthal, M. B., Frank, R. G., Newhouse, J. I. (2000). The Medicare prescription drug benefit: How will the game be played? *Health Affairs (Millwood), 19*(2), 8.

Iglehart, J. K. (2003). Medicare and drug pricing. *The New England Journal of Medicine, 348*, 1590.

Ioannides-Demos, L. L., Ibrahim, J. E,. McNeil, J. J. (2002). Reference based pricing schemes: Its effects on pharmaceutical expenditures, resource utilization, and health outcomes. *Pharmacoeconomics, 20*(9), 577.

Ivins, M. (2001, July). Drug companies can really make you sick. *Public Citizen's Health Research Group Health Letter*, p. 4.

Johannes, L. (2002, June 14). Vermont to require drug companies to disclose gifts. *The Wall Street Journal*, p. B2.

Kanavos, P., & Reinhardt, U. (2003). Reference pricing for drugs: Is it compatible with U.S. health care? *Health Affairs (Millwood), 22*(3), 16.

Langreth, R. (2003, March 31). The new drug war. Available at *Forbes*.com

Laschober. M. A., Kitchman, M., Neuman, P., Strabic, A. A. (2002). Trends in Medicare supplemental insurance and prescription drug coverage, 1996–1999. *Health Affairs (Millwood), 21*(2), 11.

Laumann, E., Park, A., Rosen, R. C. (1999). Sexual function in the United States: prevalence and predictors. *Journal of American Medical Association, 281*, 537, 1174.

Light, D. W., & Lexchin, J. (2004, Winter). The international war on cheap drugs. *New Doctor, 81*.

Lockhead, C. (2003, April 27). Should Medicare just say yes to prescription drugs? *San Francisco Chronicle*.

Los Angeles Times (2002, June 10). Editorial. Gaming the patent drug system.

Lueck, S. (2002, July 24). Drug industry exaggerates R&D costs to justify pricing, consumer group says. *The Wall Street Journal*, p. B6.

Lueck, S., Greenberger, R, Rundle, R. (2002, June 25). Court backs patient appeals in battle over HMO coverage. *The Wall Street Journal*.

Lueck, S. (2002, Oct. 21). Upstart Texas firm makes stir with cheap drugs from Canada. *The Wall Street Journal*, p. A1.

Lueck, S. (2003, Nov. 25). The new Medicare: How it works. *The Wall Street Journal*, p. D1.

Martinez, B. (2002, Sept. 12). Why that $5 drug is a bad deal: Co-payments outpace true costs. *The Wall Street Journal online*.

Martinez, B. (2003, March 31). Rx for margins. Hired to cut costs, firms find profits in generic drugs. *The Wall Street Journal*, p. A1.

Martinez, B. Drug-price surge may erode savings from Medicare card. *The Wall Street Journal*, p. B1.

Maynard, A., & Bloor, K. (1997). Regulating the pharmaceutical industry. *British Medical Journal, 315*, 200. Maynard, A., & Bloor, K. (2003). Dilemmas in regulation of the market for pharmaceuticals. *Health Affairs (Millwood), 22*(3), 31.

McGinley, L., & Leuck, S. (2003, Nov. 24). Senate democrats wage fight to block Medicare legislation. *The Wall Street Journal*, p. A1.

Frieden, J. (2002). Medicare minus choice. *Family Practice News, 32*(2).

Mintz, M. (2001, Feb.). Still hard to swallow. *The Washington Post* Outlook Section.

Moynihan, R. (2003). The making of a disease: Female sexual dysfunction. *British Medical Journal, 326*, 45.

Murray, E., Lo, B., Pollack, L., Donelan, K., Lee, K. (2003). Direct-to-consumer advertising: Physician views of its effects on quality of care and the doctor-patient relationship. *The Journal of the American Board of Family Practice, 16*, 513–524.

Murray E., Lo, B., Pollack, L., Donelan, K., Lee, K. (2004). Direct-to-consumer advertising: Public perceptions of its effects on health behaviors, health care and the doctor-patient relationship. *The Journal of the American Board of Family Practice, 17*, 6–18.

National Institute for Health Care Management Research and Educational Foundation. (2002a). Prescription drug expenditures in 2001: Another year of escalating benefits. *Medical Benefits, 19*(8), 4–5.

National Institute for Health Care Management Research and Educational Foundation. (2002b). *Changing patterns of pharmaceutical innovations.* Washington, DC: Author.

Office of Fair Trading. (2001, May 15). Price fixing of medicaments ends. Press release. London: England.

Parker-Pope, T. (2002, April 16). The latest craze in coupon clipping: Free trial offers for prescription drugs. *The Wall Street Journal*, p. D1.

Pear, R. (2002, Dec. 4). Investigators find repeated deception in ads for drugs. *The New York Times*, p. A22.

Pear, R. (2003a, April 21). U.S. limiting costs of drugs for Medicare. *The New York Times*.

Pear, R., & Hulse, C. (2003, Nov. 25). Senate removes two roadblocks to drug benefit. *The New York Times*, p. A1.

Pear, R. (2003b, Nov. 26). Sweeping Medicare change wins approval in Congress. President claims a victory. *The New York Times*, p. A1.

Pear, R. (2004, March 20). Medicare actuary gives wanted data to Congress. *The New York Times*, p. A8.

Petersen, A. (2002, Apr. 13). How to buy cheap drugs online. *The Wall Street Journal*, pp. D1, D2.

Petersen, M. (2003a, Apr. 17). Bayer agrees to pay U.S. $257 million in drug fraud. *The New York Times*, p. C1.

Peterson, M. (2003b, Apr. 23). Drug makers expand their Medicaid role. *The New York Times*, p. C1.

Peterson, M., & Berenson, A. (2003, Feb. 22). Papers indicate that Bayer knew of dangers of its cholesterol drug. *The New York Times*, p. A1.

Pfizer, Inc. (2001). Annual Report. Available at: www.pfizer.com/pfizerinc/investingannual/2001/p2001ar21.htmlPNHP (2001, May). Newsletter. Data Update. Physicians for a National Health Program. Chicago, p. 8.

PNHP Newsletter. Data Update. Physicians for a National Health Program. Chicago: May 2001, 8.

Prescription drug access: not just a Medicare problem. (2002, Apr.) HSC Issue Brief.

Prescription drug expenditures in 2001: another year of escalating costs. *Medical Benefits*, 19(8), 4, 2002.

Publications and Reports. Prescription drugs. Hard to swallow rising prices for America's seniors. *Health Affairs (Millwood)*, 19(1), 254, 2000.

Public Citizen Report, November 9, 2001.

Public Citizen Report. April 18, 2002. Full report available at *http://www.citizen.org/congressreform/drug_industry/profits/articles.ctm?ID=(416)*.

Public Citizen. (2003, Nov. 25). Press Release. Bush heads for bright lights and big dollars in Vegas, promoting special-interest backed Medicare and medical malpractice bills. Washington, D.C.

Rawe, J. (2002, Nov. 2). Health care. *Time Inside Business*, p. A15.

Reinhardt, U. E. (2001). Perspectives on the pharmaceutical industry. *Health Affairs (Millwood)*, 20(5), 136.

Relman, A., & Angell, M. (2002, Dec. 16). America's other drug problem. *The New Republic*.

Rosenberg, J. (2003, Jan. 15). New code sets boundaries for drug company "perks". *Physicians Financial News*, p. 29.

Rovner, J. (2003, april 8). Former federal officials raise concerns about Medicare prescription drug benefit. *Congress Daily.*

Sailant, C. (2003, Feb. 8)Senior groups begin a boycott of drug maker. *Los Angeles Times.*

Seagraves. E. (Ed). (2001). Historical and international context of nosology of female sexual disorders. *Journal of Sex & Marital Therapy*, 27(2), 81–245.

Shearer, G. (2003).Medicare prescription drugs: Conference Committee agreement asks beneficiaries to pay too high a price for a modest benefit. Washington, DC: Consumers Union.

Sherman, S. (2003, Nov. 26). Seniors to face increasing costs for drugs. *Seattle Post Intelligencer*, p. A3.

Soumerai, S. B., Avorn, J., Ross-Degnan, D., Gortmaker, S. (1987). Payment restrictions for prescription drugs under Medicaid: Effects on therapy, cost, and equity. *The New England Journal of Medicine*, 317, 550.

Soumerai, S. B., McLaughlin, T. J., Ross-Degnan, P. Casteris, C. S., Bollini, P. (1994). Effects of a limit on Medicaid drug-reimbursement benefits on the use of psychotropic agents and acute mental health services by patients with schizophrenia. *The New England Journal of Medicine*, 331, 650.

Special supplement. (1998). *International Journal of Impotence Research, 10*(suppl 2):S1-142. The Cape Cod conference: sexual function assessment in clinical trials. Hyannis, Mass: 30–31, May 1997.

Stolberg, S. A., & Freudenheim, M. (2003, Nov. 26). Sweeping Medicare change wins approval in Congress: President claims a victory. *The New York Times,* p. A1.

Tiefer, L. (1996). The medicalization of sexuality: Conceptual, normative, and professional issues. *Annual Review of Sex Research, 7,* 252–282.

Tiefer, L. (2000). Sexology and the pharmaceutical industry: The threat of co-optation. *Journal of Sex Research, 37,* 273–285.

Toner, R. (2003, Nov. 25). An imperfect compromise. *The New York Times,* p. A1.

U.S. General Accounting Office (2001). Report to Congressional committees. Medicare payments for covered outpatient drugs exceed providers' costs. (GAO-01–1118.) Washington, DC: Author.

USA Today. (2002). Pricey copycat drugs bring big profits, not new cures. Available at *www.usatoday.com/usatonline/20020531/4156073s.htm*

Waldholz, M. (2002, April 18). Prescriptions: New drug cards for seniors. PR ploy or great bargain? *The Wall Street Journal,* p. D5.

Wazana, A. (2000). Physicians and the pharmaceutical industry: Is a gift ever just a gift? *Journal of American Medical Association, 283,* 373.

The Wall Street Journal (2002, May 8). Editorial. The Novartis warning. p. A18.

Weissman, J. S., Blumenthal, D., Silk, A. J., Zapert, K. Newman, M., Listman, R. (2003). The effects of direct-to-consumer drug advertising. *Health Affairs (Millwood), 22*(2), 14.

Willman, D. (2002, July 1). Hidden risks, lethal truths. Warner Lambert won approval of Regulon after masking the number of liver injuries in clinical studies. *Los Angeles Times.*

Wolfe, S. M. (1996). Why do American drug companies spend more than $12 billion a year pushing drugs? *Journal of General Internal Medicine, 11,* 637.

Wolfe, S. M. (2001a, March). Outrage of the month. *Health Letter,* pp. 10–12.

Wolfe, S. M. (2001b, July). Outrage of the month. "Operation Cure All" wages new battle in ongoing war against Internet health fraud. *Public Citizen's Health Research Group Health Letter,* pp. 11–12.

Wolfe, S. M. (2003, March) Selling "new" drugs using smoke and mirror (images). *Health Letter,* pp. 2–5.

Wolfe, S. M. (2002a, August) Update on the illegal promotion of Gabapentin (Neurontin). *Health Letter,* pp. 3–5.

Wolfe, S. M. (2002b). Direct-to-consumer advertising: education or emotion promotion? *The New England Journal of Medicine, 346,* 524.

Woloshin, S., Schwartz, L. M., Tremmel, J., Welch, H. G. (2001). Direct-to-consumer advertisements for prescription drugs: What are Americans being sold? *Lancet, 358,* (9288) 1141–1146.

Ziegler, M. G., Lew, P., Singer, B. C. The accuracy of drug information from pharmaceutical sales representatives. *Journal of American Medical Association, 273,* 1296–1298.

Chapter 6

MEDICALLY RELATED
INDUSTRIES

Having considered five corporate health care industries in the last four chapters, with a particular focus on their roles in the increasing costs of health care, we now turn our attention to three quite different health care industries. The first two, the diagnostic/screening test and medical device/supply industries, are of special interest inasmuch as they are central to the assimilation of advancing medical technology in health care. The third, dietary supplements, has become an enormous industry, mostly below the radar screen of public awareness, and presents many of the same problems as the pharmaceutical industry. Although not dominated to the same extent by corporate interests as the other industries we have examined, it is included because of its expanding role in health care, its impact on health care costs, its hazards to public health, and the challenge it presents to oversight and regulation in the public interest.

This chapter has four goals: (1) to briefly describe the size, scope, and common practices of each of these industries; (2) to outline the process of adoption of these products, together with the extent of oversight of their marketing, use, and quality; (3) to discuss their potential hazards; and (4) to consider how increased oversight and regulation of these industries can advance the public interest.

DIAGNOSTIC AND SCREENING TESTS

This industry is rapidly growing and already accounts in some cases for faster escalation of health care costs than even the pharmaceutical industry. The diagnostic/screening test industry ranges from blood tests to high-technology radiologic imaging. These tests are increasingly being marketed directly to the public without a physician's referral. The producers of these products and services tend to be large health care corporations, for example, General Electric in the imaging industry. In 2001, the costs of high-technology imaging tests in the U.S. (e.g., CT, MRI, and PET) rose 23% compared with a 16% increase for prescription drugs (Rundle, 2003).

Several examples illustrate how these diagnostic/screening tests are successfully marketed to the public, often without any evidence of clinical effectiveness or value.

Diagnostic Blood Tests

Claiming that patients can be empowered and given ownership of their health by direct diagnostic testing without involvement of physicians, a number of companies have sprouted up around the country to market these services. Inter Fit Health, for example, is a national health screening group based in Houston, Texas that provides phlebotomists and medical assistants to draw blood from patients at corporations and in chain pharmacies. Testing companies frequently advertise on the Internet, either for specific tests or panels of tests (e.g., women's health profile, comprehensive wellness profile). Although many states require a physician's referral for such testing, the companies avoid that barrier by having physicians on staff who approve all requests without questions (Davis, 2002). Abnormal test results are stamped with a recommendation that patients consult their personal physician, but there is no mechanism to assure adequate medical followup (Lapp, 2002).

Imaging Procedures

Several kinds of imaging procedures illustrate how easy it is for profitable new technologies to achieve widespread use with little or no scientific validation and without any regard to their cost effectiveness.

Quantitative heel ultrasound appears to be too inaccurate for screening of women at low risk for osteoporosis (i.e., young, healthy women). While abnormal heel ultrasound has been shown to predict hip fractures in cohort studies of older women (Bauer et al., 1997), its value as a screening test in general populations has not yet been tested in clinical trials. Nevertheless, it is being actively marketed for general use as a screening test for osteoporosis at a cost of up to $110 for each test (Fenton & Deyo, 2003).

Computed tomography (CT) scans, including whole body and coronary heart scans, are now available at more than 100 centers around the country. One company tows scanners to rural areas in trucks, while another provides ultrasound examinations in mobile vans in 43 states (Fenton & Deyo, 2003). Many patients self-refer themselves for these diagnostic/screening examinations, which are generally not covered by insurers without strong clinical indications or referral from a physician. Patients pay $800 to $1,500 out-of-pocket for full-body scans, which are not endorsed by either the American College of Radiology or the FDA. The FDA has concerns about the lack of scientific and cost-effectiveness studies, radiation exposure (one full-body CT scan equals about 150 chest x-rays), and the risks to patients of follow-up care chasing false positives (Pennachio, 2002). Whole-body CT is being vigorously promoted as a screening test for cancer without any scientific basis. Increasingly, these tests are being marketed on a direct-to-consumer basis by radio, television, print media, and the Internet (Lee & Brennan, 2003; Haas, 2001). Another current craze is the coronary heart scan, for calcium in coronary arteries, which, at a cost of $200 to $500, has a positive predictive value of only 13% for obstructive coronary disease (Fenton & Deyo, 2003). It has also been found to be ineffective in motivating patients to improve their cardiovascular risk (O'Malley, Feuerstein, & Taylor, 2003).

The latest technological "advance" in screening is the PET scan, which is being marketed as a means to detect cancer and other diseases (including Alzheimer's disease) at an earlier stage than other tests. Hospitals and imaging centers are hurrying to install these machines at a cost of $1 to 2.5 million each (North Carolina will soon have 20 such scanners). Although Medicare refuses to reimburse these scans because they have not been clinically proven to be effective, they are spreading rapidly around the country, often on testing trucks and vans. Operators typically charge $2,500 to $3,000 per examination. As a result, there is now a feeding frenzy among ancillary vendors such as the specialty pharmacy companies that make the radioactive tracer. "PET specialists" are vigorously marketing these studies to physicians and providers, estimating that they can break even financially with only two or three scans a day (Rundle, 2003).

Diagnostic imaging including CT, MRI and PET scans, is now approaching $100 billion-a-year industry in the U.S., according to a 2004 report of the Blue Cross Blue Shield Association. There is widespread evidence of entrepreneurship and overuse of this technology, especially in single-specialty group practices and specialty hospitals. Between 1999 and 2002, the average use of diagnostic imaging across the country increased at almost three times the rate of overall use of physicians' services (Abelson, 2004). Health plan executives at many

Community Tracking Study (CTS) sites believe that this trend has increased health care costs without evidence to date that quality of care is being improved. (Casalino, Phem, Bazzoli, 2004).

Hazards

There still have been no rigorously conducted studies showing that earlier detection of disease through these high-technology diagnostic and screening techniques improves patient outcomes. What is known is that they are costly to the consumer, not effective for general screening, and often lead to further diagnostic workup without clinical benefit. Michael Grodin, Director of the Law, Medicine, and Ethics Program at Boston University, has this to say of scans in asymptomatic people:

> Scanning an asymptomatic person is a fishing expedition. For every abnormal entity found, there may be 100 more. It does no more than make patients anxious. The bottom line: It's a bad idea to reassure patients inappropriately, and it's a bad idea to give information that's not helpful. Scans should only be done for clinical indications. (Pennachio, 2002).

His bioethicist colleague, George Annas, adds this wry comment "A well patient is someone who hasn't been sufficiently worked up"(Pennachio, 2002).

False positive as well as false negative results are common with widespread use of these self-referred screening procedures, each with their own particular hazards. False positives lead to the risks and costs of further clinical workups, together with anxiety for patients and their families along the way. False negative results (especially common with imaging procedures without the use of radioactive dye) in self-referred populations may give patients false reassurance and encourage them to continue unhealthy life styles. In reaction to the spread of these technologies without scientific validation by their entrepreneurial promoters, some professional organizations have called attention to the inflationary impact of their widespread use on costs of care, arguing that "a just health care system cannot accept such developments, even if the market would allow it" (Lee & Brennan, 2003; Vastag, 2001).

MEDICAL DEVICE AND SUPPLY MANUFACTURERS

A recent market update prepared by the Center for Medicare and Medicaid Services (CMS), Office of Research, Development and

Information on the medical device and supply industry provides a broad overview of the $74 billion a year industry. Medical devices comprise a wide range of products, including cardiac pacemakers, coronary stents, implantable defibrillators, hip and knee replacements, lasers, and respiratory/patient monitoring equipment. Medical supplies include such items as surgical instruments, syringes, and wound dressings. The market is dominated by very large health care corporations, led by Medtronic, Inc. for medical devices and Johnson & Johnson for medical supplies. The largest 2% of 6,000 U.S. medical device companies accounted for almost one-half of the industry's sales in 2001 (Office of Research, Development & Information, 2002).

Wall Street analysts sees this industry as "sound, strong, and stable" for investors, noting promising new launches in 2003 of drug-eluting stents, cardiac resynchronization therapy (CRT) for congestive heart failure, and treatments to fuse the spine. Analysts carefully track the progress of FDA approval decisions as well as decisions by CMS for Medicare reimbursement. The industry is about as profitable as the pharmaceutical industry, and spends less on research and development (Office of Research, Development & Information, 2002).

FDA and reimbursement decisions are high-stakes decisions with major impacts on health care spending, and they call for objective review of the scientific basis and cost effectiveness of new technologies. The implanted cardiac defibrillator is a good example currently under review by CMS for Medicare reimbursement. Guidant, a leading manufacturer of this device, funded a recent study which concluded that widespread use of this device could reduce mortality for up to 300,000 patients in the U.S. at an annual outlay of over $3 billion. Under questioning by CMS concerning research methodology and conclusions of the study, Guidant revised the number of candidates for the device down to 7,000 to 10,000 patients ($175 to $250 million a year). Fortunately, the ultimate reimbursement decision will be informed by an advisory panel chaired by Dr. Harold Sox, editor of the *Annals of Internal Medicine* (McGinley & Burton, 2003).

More than 8,000 new medical devices are brought to market in the U.S. each year. That there is significant risk of harms and adverse outcomes from use of these devices is suggested by the fact that over 1,000 devices are recalled each year. This fact also raises the question of how these devices are regulated. Over 4,000 new devices are considered low-risk (Class I) each year, and are exempt from the requirement of FDA approval. Another 3,500 devices are considered medium-risk (Class II) and are approved for marketing by the FDA after manufacturers have demonstrated "substantial equivalence" to an existing marketed device; only 8% of these instances require clinical data. The FDA requires scientific clinical evidence that high-risk devices (Class III) are "safe and effective," and 50 to 80 of such devices are approved each year (Feigal, Gardner, & McClellan, 2003).

Device manufacturers are required to report device-related deaths, serious injuries, and certain malfunctions, and the FDA received over 120,000 such reports in 2002. Clinical facilities filed more than 2,500 reports of device-related serious injuries to the FDA, while health professionals and consumers made over 3,500 reports in 2002. Between 10 and 20 recalls each year involve high-risk devices. The extent of risk to the public from this industry is indicated by the long list of products which have been recalled—heart valves, implantable cardioverter defibrillators, knee and hip prostheses, hemodialysis equipment, infusion pumps, respirators, endoscopes, and others (Feigal, Gardner, & McClellan, 2003). Despite this threat to the health of the public, the capability of the FDA to regulate the medical device industry is being weakened rather than strengthened. With the intent to speed up the approval of new medical devices, Congress passed legislation in 2002 which permits device companies to partially fund safety reviews and allows the industry to hire private contractors to inspect manufacturing facilities for compliance with good manufacturing practices, and even review some devices for approval. As noted by Frank Clemente, director of *Public Citizen's Congress Watch*, this legislation involves conflicts of interest that amount to the fox guarding the henhouse (Clemente, 2002).

That more, rather than less, oversight is needed in this industry is also suggested by many conflicts of interest along the distribution chain between manufacturers and hospitals. Premier and Novation are two private, for-profit group purchasing companies that dominate the hospital supply business in the U.S. Each company uses its market power of more than 1,500 U.S. hospitals to negotiate large purchases from suppliers, but their financial dealings in this $34 billion a year supply industry have been called into question by investigators. Both companies are paid by the medical products companies that they are supposed to be evaluating objectively for product quality and value. For example, the country's largest maker of needles, Becton Dickinson & Company, paid $1 million in 2000 to Novation in "special marketing" fees in connection with a three-year contract for syringes and needles (Meier & Walsh, 2002). In the 2001 fiscal year, Premier, an affiliate of Bridge Medical, Inc., is reported to have received $307 million in fees from supplier companies. Full accounting of these transactions is often lacking to hospitals and investigators, and there is also evidence of profiteering through padding of salaries, expenses, and CEO compensation. Instead of saving money, Premier's spending increased by 84% over a recent three-year period, including increases of 53% in salaries and benefits just two years earlier (Walsh, 2002). As these kinds of arrangements have come to public attention, a backlash is underway, including some hospitals and clinics breaking longstanding ties with Premier and Novation, criticism of the industry in Congress, and a new bill in California intended to regulate the business practices of group purchasing organizations (Walsh & Bogdanich, 2003).

DIETARY SUPPLEMENTS

The dietary supplement industry is a large and rapidly growing business, minimally regulated, that poses a significant threat to the health of the public. Although it is largely decentralized with many smaller companies, some of the major drug companies have now moved into the market in force (e.g., Bayer, Johnson & Johnson, Boehringer, and American Home Products) (Moore, 2003). In 2001, nearly $18 billion was spent in the U.S. on dietary supplements, including more than $4 billion for herbs and other botanical remedies (*Nutrition Business Journal*, 2002). These products include vitamins, minerals, herbs and other botanicals, amino acids (e.g., L-tryptophan), and even hormones such as melatonin and the human sex hormone, DHEA. The biggest sales are accounted for by echinacea, gingko biloba, ginseng, garlic, and St. John's wort, but since dietary supplements enjoy no patent protection, their annual sales are no more than $200 million each (Moore, 2003).

This industry was deregulated when Congress enacted the Dietary Supplement Health and Education Act (DSHEA) of 1994, strongly lobbied for by the industry and loyal consumers. The DSHEA defined dietary supplements as a regulatory category separate from drugs and also created an Office of Dietary Supplements at the National Institutes of Health. Labeling and marketing were also liberalized by the DSHEA. Current FDA rules permit claims by manufacturers that their products affect the structure or function of the body as long as the manufacturer has "substantiating documents" on file. Claims such as "maintains a healthy circulatory system," "enhances muscle strength," or "for hot flashes" are allowed. Specific claims to treat diseases, however, are prohibited, such as "treatment for cancer" or "cures osteoporosis" (Barrett, 2003). Of more than 20,000 dietary supplements on the market, only 46 have undergone even a cursory review by the FDA. The FDA has been authorized to prescribe "good manufacturing practices," but has little role in actually reviewing the process (Moore, 2003).

The popularity of dietary supplements has boomed in recent years, catalyzed by a media blitz by the industry, its deregulation in 1994, the growth of interest in alternative and complementary medicine, and the increasing costs of prescription drugs. Most people incorrectly believe that the government is involved in regulation of the marketing, safety, and effectiveness of dietary supplements (Taylor, 2003). Despite the FDA's ban on disease claims, manufacturers of dietary supplements make false and unsubstantiated health and safety claims and present testimonials for their products on a regular basis through radio, TV, print and Internet media (Morris & Avorn, 2003). One such example is bee pollen, promoted for its curative and healing properties for a wide range of diseases, including respiratory tract infections, allergies, endocrine disease, and colitis (Rector-Page, 1992). Bee pollen is also touted as a cancer-preventive supplement, as well as for its strength enhancing and life extending properties (Wade, 1992). None of these effects have been substantiated.

Many dietary supplements are promoted as "natural" or "nontoxic" with the false and misleading suggestion that they are safe. Here are just three examples of false and unsubstantiated claims made on the Internet which have been challenged by the Federal Trade Commission (FTC) (Wolfe, 2001b):

- use of advertised herbal products can allow patients to cancel surgery, radiation, or chemotherapy
- St. John's wort is a safe treatment for AIDS
- Colloidal silver can prevent, treat, or cure many serious diseases

Many dietary supplements are not only expensive and ineffective, but may cause adverse drug interactions, such as the effect of St. John's wort in accelerating the metabolic degradation of many prescription drugs, including antiretroviral drugs, digoxin, and Coumadin (Moore, Goodman, Jones, Wisely, Serabjit-Singh, 2000). It is estimated that only 10% of serious adverse drug interactions are reported to the FDA (Office of the Inspector General, 2001). Many more thousands of reports are received by poison control centers, as shown in Figure 6.1 (Wolfe, 2001a). In instances where credible research has been done, many dietary supplements, including the top sellers, have been found either ineffective or of unknown effectiveness. Examples

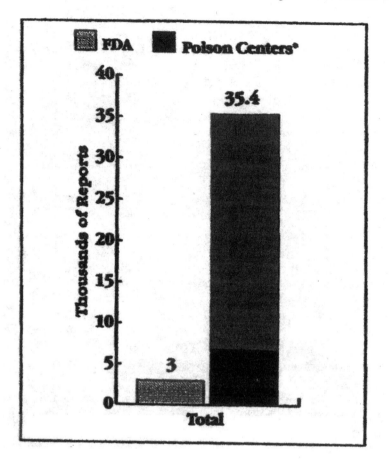

FIGURE 6.1 Adverse reaction reports for dietary supplements: FDA and National Poison Control Centers, 1994–1999.

Source: Wolfe, S. M. (2001). Outrage of the Month: Dietary supplements: The FDA should do more. *Health Letter, 17*(5), 11. Reprinted by permission.

include a 2002 report on ginkgo biloba and it effects on memory (Solomon, Adams, Silver, Zimmer, & De Veaux, 2002) and a 2001 assessment of echinacea and the incidence and severity of colds (Glasziou & Del Mar, 2001).

The case of ephedra illustrates well the politics and sorry state of the current regulatory process in the U.S. for dietary supplements, The industry estimates that 12 to 17 million Americans take over 3 billion doses of ephedra each year. It is heavily advertised for its promise to achieve long-term weight loss, increased energy, and enhanced athletic performance (Ives, 2003). Although representing less than 1% of sales of herbal supplements, it accounts for almost two-thirds of all adverse events reported to the FDA (Bent, Tiedt, Odden, & Shlipak, 2003). By 2003 the FDA had received over 16,000 reports suggesting possible links between the use of ephedra and strokes, cardiac arrhythmias, heatstroke, and psychotic episodes, as well as over 100 deaths (Pear & Grady, 2003). Metabolife, Inc., the leading maker of a weight-loss pill containing ephedra, caffeine, and several other herbs, has been under investigation by the Justice Department for having lied and underreported some 13,000 complaints which it received in recent years, including several hundred people requiring hospitalization and 80 incidents of serious injury or death (Hilts, 2002). By 2002, the U.S. Army, Air Force, and Marine Corps had all banned the sale of ephedra-containing products on their military bases worldwide (Wolfe, 2002b). Ephedra has also been banned by the National Football League, the NCAA, and the International Olympic Committee (*The New York Times,* 2003). In January, 2002, the Canadian government recalled all ephedra products "with labeled or implied claims for appetite suppression, weight-loss promotion, metabolic enhancement, increased exercise tolerance, body-building effects, euphoria, increased energy or wakefulness, or other stimulant effects" (Wolfe, 2002a). Yet, despite calls by the American Medical Association and other professional organizations to ban the product, and even after the highly publicized death of Baltimore Orioles pitcher Steve Bechler implicating ephedra products, the FDA, with the industry lobbying against a ban, still refused to ban these supplements, instead requiring only warning labels (Vinson, 2003). Finally, on December 30, 2003, when major manufacturers were no longer selling ephedra and after a total of 155 deaths had occurred from its use, the FDA did announce a ban on the product (Wolfe, 2004).

HOW CAN THESE INDUSTRIES BE BETTER REGULATED?

For all of these three industries, the foregoing provides solid evidence that our voluntary system of self-regulation is not adequate and that stronger oversight is required. In each instance, the early adoption and widespread use of these tests, treatments, and products raises health care costs. Many of them are of questionable clinical value, and some pose serious risks to patients. The marketing and safety claims of manufacturers within each industry need to be held accountable to scientific review. Clinical research should inform approval and reimbursement decisions, and it should not be biased by the funding sources of studies, potential conflicts of interest on the part of investigators, or political lobbying by manufacturers.

The FDA is presently too underfunded and understaffed to perform expanded reviews and ongoing oversight of these industries. For example, it has only three people to review and investigate reports of adverse reactions to dietary supplements, compared with 10 for veterinary drugs and 71 for prescription and over-the-counter drugs (Moore, 2003). Congressional action is needed to broaden the FDA's mandate for more effective regulation of all three of these industries. No federal agency now has authorization to regulate the use of high technology radiologic imaging equipment once it has been certified for marketing and distribution (Fenton & Deyo, 2003). Based on the frequency of recalls and adverse patient outcomes from the use of medical devices each year, the review and approval process by the FDA should be expanded. Further, since many herbs and botanical products act as drugs, they should be regulated as drugs, not as dietary supplements. A useful proposal for new legislation to regulate dietary supplements has been made by Donald Marcus and Arthur Grollman, with these recommendations:

1. Require registration of manufacturers with the FDA
2. Manufacturers should provide evidence of good manufacturing practices to the FDA, which, in turn, should have the authority to inspect their records and facilities
3. Premarketing approval should be required by the FDA, with manufacturers responsible for their products' safety
4. Manufacturers should be required to report all adverse effects promptly to the FDA
5. Labels should include a list of ingredients by both botanical and common names, as well as potential adverse effects and drug interaction warnings
6. The Department of Health and Human Services (DHHS) should organize expert panels to review the safety of dietary supplements modeled after the National Academy of Sciences Drug Efficacy Study (Marcus & Grollman, 2002)

In view of the profound effects on health care costs (as well as access to care) of many of these new technologies, a cautious and more deliberate approach to approval and reimbursement decisions is clearly in the public interest. That a societal perspective is also needed in these deliberations is well illustrated by the current debate on implantable cardiac defibrillators (Bigger, 2002; Donaldson, 2002;

Moss et al, 2002; Stecker & Pollack, 2002). In an industry-funded, unblinded study, Arthur Moss and his colleagues reported on a 20-month trial comparing outcomes with the defibrillator to usual care without one. A 5.6% absolute reduction in mortality was found in the defibrillator group. It was projected that up to 400,000 patients each year in the U.S. might benefit from this treatment (Moss et al., 2002). At a cost of $30,000 per cardiac defibrillator implantation (probably a low estimate in many cases), that would amount to a $12 billion expenditure by public and private payers each year, three times the estimated 2003 budget for the Centers for Disease Control and Prevention (CDC) (Donaldson, 2002). Demonstration of cost-effectiveness, not just efficacy, will therefore be required for such potentially costly draws on the national treasure.

CONCLUDING COMMENTS

The three medically related industries considered here reflect many similarities and parallels with the five industries discussed in the last four chapters. All aggressively pursue business goals without enough regard for the public interest, and are major cost inflators to the health care system. All resist price controls and regulation by government. We have found profiteering along the distribution chain, often without public awareness, ranging from the hospital supply industry to the pharmaceutical industry. Although still promoted by the current Administration and many in Congress, deregulation is failing to protect the public interest in terms of efficacy, safety, and quality of many health care products and services. In the next chapter, we will examine the collective impact of cost inflation by all of these industries on the overall health care system, the sustainability of the system, and the implications for access to and quality of care.

REFERENCES

Abelson, R. An M.R.I. machine for every doctor? Someone has to pay, *The New York Times*, March 13, 2004: A1.

Barrett, S. (2003). How the Dietary Supplement Health and Education Act of 1994 weakened the FDA. Retrieved May 13, from *www.quackwatch.org/02*

Bauer, D. C, Gluer, C. C., Cauley, J. A., Vogt, T. M., Ensrud, K. E, Genout, A. K. et al. (1997). Broadband ultrasound attenuation predicts fractures strongly and independently of densitometry in older women: A prospective study. *Archives of Internal Medicine, 157,* 629.

Bent, S., Tiedt, T. N., Odden, M. C., Shlipak, M. G. (2003). The relative safety of ephedra compared with other herbal products. *Annals of Internal Medicine, 138*, 468.

Bigger, J. T. (2002). Expanding indications for implantable cardiac defibrillators. *The New England Journal of Medicine, 346*, 931.

Casolino, L. P., Pham, H., & Bozzoli, G. (2004). Growth of single-specialty groups. *Health Affairs, 23*(2): 82–90.

Clemente, F. (2002, Oct. 18). Public Citizen decries conflict of interest created by new law regulating safety of medical devices. Public Citizen. Washington, DC.

Davis, R. J. (2002, Sept. 17). Aches and claims. Ordering up your own medical tests. *The Wall Street Journal*, p. D4.

Donaldson, R. M. (2002). Letter to editor. Implantable cardiac defibrillators. *The New England Journal of Medicine, 347*, 365.

The New York Times. (2003, Feb. 25). Editorial. Dangers of an herbal supplement. February 25, p. A28.

Feigal, D. W., Gardner, S. N. McClellan, M. (2003). Ensuring safe and effective medical devices. *The New England Journal of Medicine, 348*, 191, 2003.

Fenton, J. J., & Deyo, R. A. (2003). Patient self-referral for radiologic screening tests: Clinical and ethical concerns. *Journal of the American Board of Family Practice, 16*, p. 494–501.

Glaziou, P., & Del Mar, C. (2001). *Clinical evidence* (pp. 1068, 1071). London: BMJ Publishing Group.

Haas, N. (2001, Aug. 26). Scared sick: The $900 antidote. *The New York Times*.

Hilts, P. J. (2002, Aug. 16). U.S. in criminal inquiry on Metabolife product. *The New York Times*, p. C1.

Ives, N. (2003, May 17). Advertising. After a pitcher's death, marketers of dietary supplements try to dodge the taint of ephedra. *The New York Times*, p. C9.

Lapp, T. (2002). Direct-to-consumer tests: Just what the doctor didn't order. *Family Practice Report, 8*(8), 6.

Lee, T. H., & Brennan, T. A. (2003). Direct-to-consumer marketing of high-technology screening tests. *The New England Journal of Medicine, 346*, 529.

Marcus, D. M., & Grollman, A. P. (2002). Botanical medicines: The need for new regulations. *The New England Journal of Medicine, 347*, 2073.

McGinley, L., & Burton, T. M. ((2003, Feb. 12). Medicare panel to debate use of defibrillator. *The Wall Street Journal*, p. B1.

Meier, B., & Walsh, M. W. (2002, July 19). Medicine's middlemen. Questioning $1 million fee in a needle deal. *The New York Times*,

Moore, T. J. (2003). Big trouble in the health store. Retrieved May 13, from *www.thomasjmoore.com/pages/dietary—main.html*

Moore, L. B., Goodman, B., Jones, S. A., Wisely, J. B., Serabjit-Singh, C. J. (2000). St. John's wort induces hepatic drug metabolism through activation of the pregnane X receptor. *Proceedings of the National Academy of Science USA, 97*, 7500.

Morris, C. A., & Avorn, J. (2003). Internet marketing of herbal products. *Journal of the American Medical Association, 290,* 1505.

Moss, A. J., Zareba, W., Hall, W. I. Klein, H., Wilbur, D. I., Cannon, D.S. (2002). Prophylactic implantation of a defibrillator in patients with myocardial infarction and reduced ejection fraction. *The New England Journal of Medicine, 347,* 877.

Nutrition Business Journal. (2002, May/June). Annual industry overview VII.

Office of the Inspector General (2001). Adverse event reporting for dietary supplements. An inadequate safety valve. (Report no. OEI-01-00-00180). Washington, DC: Author.

Office of Research, Development & Information (2002, oct. 10). *Health care industry market update.* Washington, DC. O'Malley, P. G., Feuerstein, I. M., Taylor, A. J. (2003). Impact of electron beam tomography with or without case management on motivation, behavioral change, and cardiovascular risk profile: A randomized clinical trial. *Journal of the American Medical Association, 289,* 2215.

O'Malley, P. G., Fauerstein, I. M., & Taylor, A. J. (2003). Impact of electron beam tomography with or without case management on motivation, behavioral change, and cardiovascular risk profile: a randomized clinical trial. *Journal of American Medical Association, 289,* 2215.

Pear, R., & Grady, D. (2003, Mar. 1). Government moves to curtail use of diet supplement. *The New York Times,* p. A1.

Pennachio, D. L. (2002, Aug. 9). Full-body scans—or scams? *Medical Economics,* p. 62.

Rector-Page, L. G. (1992). *Healthy healing: An alternative health reference,* 9th edition. Sonora, CA: Health Healing Publications.

Rundle, R. L. (2003, May 6). PET scanners become new Rx for diagnostics. *The Wall Street Journal,* p. B1.

Solomon, P. R., Adams, E., Silver, A., Zimmer, I., De Veaux, R. (2002). Gingko for memory enhancement: A randomized controlled trial. *Journal of the American Medical Association, 288,* 835.

Stecker, E. C., & Pollack, H. A. (2002). Letter to editor. Implantable cardiac defibrillators. *The New England Journal of Medicine, 347,* 365.

Taylor H. Letter to the Editor. Inappropriate advertising of dietary supplements. *New England Journal of Medicine, 348,* 2255.

Vastag, B. (2001). *Annals of Internal Medicine's* Harold Sox, M.D., discusses physician charter of professionalism. *Journal of the American Medical Association, 286,* 3065.

Vinson, J. (2003). FDA hides behind Sen. Hatch's dietary supplement law, refuses to ban ephedra. *Public Citizen News, 23*(3), 1.

Wade, C. (1992). *Bee pollen and your health.* New Canaan, CT: Keats Publishers.

Walsh, M. W. (2002, June 7). A mission to save money: A record of otherwise. *The New York Times Online.*

Walsh, M. W., & Bogdanich, W. (2003, May 8). Two big buying groups settle lawsuit by needle maker. *The New York Times,* p. C1.

Wolfe, S. M. (2001). Outrage of the Month. Dietary supplements. The FDA should do more. *Public Citizen's Health Research Group Health Letter* 17(5), 11.

Wolfe, S. M. (2001a). Outrage of the Month. "Operation Cures All" wages new battle in ongoing war against Internet health fraud. *Public Citizen's Health Research Group Health Letter,* 17(7), 11.

Wolfe, S. M. (2002a, June 14). Public Citizen press release concerning HHS failure to ban ephedra or issue adequate warnings.

Wolfe, S. M. (2002b, Oct. 8). Testimony before Senate Governmental Affairs Committee's Subcommittee on Government Management.

Wolfe, S. M. (2004, Feb.) The FDA finally bans ephedra. *Worst Pills Best pills* Health Research Group. Public Citizen. pp. 9–10.

Chapter 7

IMPACT OF CORPORATE PRACTICES ON THE HEALTH CARE SYSTEM

The rise of a corporate ethos in medical care is already one of the most significant consequences of the changing structure of medical care. It permeates voluntary hospitals, government agencies, and academic thought, as well as profit-making medical care organizations. Those who talked about "health care planning" in the 1970s now talk about "health care marketing". Everywhere one sees the growth of a kind of marketing mentality in health care. And, indeed, business school graduates are displacing graduates of public health schools, hospital administrators, and even doctors in the top echelons of medical care organizations. The organizational culture of medicine used to be dominated by the ideals of professionalism and voluntarism, which softened the underlying acquisitive activity. The restraint exercised by those ideals now grows weaker. The "health center" of one era is the "profit center" of the next.

Paul Starr
The Social Transformation of American Medicine

In the last five chapters we have reviewed eight industries largely dominated by for-profit corporate interests, and have traced their inexorable inflationary effect on health care costs in this country. This journey has provided ample evidence that the concerns about a medical-industrial complex, expressed in 1980 by Arnold Relman (Relman, 1980), have come to pass, and Paul Starr's observation above (Starr, 1982) aptly describes today's culture in health care. It is now time for us to see how these trends affect the overall health care system and to assess whether, and how, cost containment can be achieved in health care.

This chapter has four goals: (1) to provide a brief overview of costs, access, and quality in the current system; (2) to estimate the extent to which for-profit corporate practices contribute to inflation of health care costs, and with what effects on access and quality of care; (3) to consider how sustainable the health care system is given current trends in the deregulated marketplace; and (4) to describe areas where major ongoing cost savings can be achieved if the health care system can be rebuilt around a not-for-profit service ethic.

COSTS, ACCESS, AND QUALITY IN OUR COLLAPSING HEALTH CARE SYSTEM

As the costs of health care continue to escalate, the inevitable effect is to decrease access to care for many millions of Americans. Moreover, quality of care is adversely affected, with increased spending producing less value to patients and their families through inefficiencies in our complex system. In the discussion which follows, we will examine each of these issues.

Increasing Costs

Double-digit annual increases in health care costs for active employees and retirees have been persistent in the U.S. since 1999. This is graphically shown in Figure 7.1 (Geyman, 2003). Average national per-capita health expenditures are $6,167 in 2004 or 15.5% of the GDP (Heffler, Smith, Keehan, Clemens, Zegga et al., 2004). The National Coalition on Health Care predicts that the average annual premium for employer-sponsored family health insurance will soar to $14,545 in 2006 (Simmons & Goldberg, 2003), and health care spending is projected to account for 17.7% of GDP by 2012. Hospital costs alone increased by almost 15% in 2002, and together with the costs of prescription drugs, account for the two largest components of health costs (Heffler, Smith, Keehan, Clemens, Won et al., 2003).

The impact of these cost increases on employers, workers, retirees, and their families is profound. General Motors spent about $5 billion in 2002 on health care for retirees and dependents, and its obligation for future retirees' health care have soared to over $63 billion (Hakim, 2004). Ford Motor Company now spends almost $600 million a year for current employees and more than three times that amount each year for retirees and their families. As a result, many employers are passing on more of these costs to employees, and are reducing health coverage for retirees or eliminating it altogether (Matthews, 2003). The California Public Employees Retirement System (CalPERS) is the nation's third-largest buyer of employee health benefits (behind the federal government and General Motors), spending $3.4 billion a year

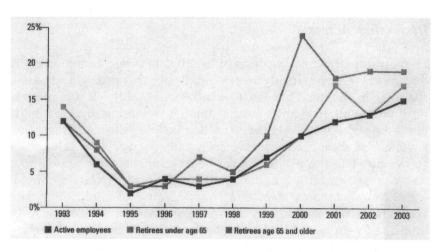

FIGURE 7.1 Average cost increases: 1993–2003.

Source: Towers Perrin. (2003). Health Care Cost Survey. In J. P. Geyman, The corporate transformation of medicine and its impacts on costs and access to care. *Journal of the American Board of Family Practice, 16,* 443. Reprinted with permission.

on health care. CalPERS has struggled with a 25% jump in HMO rates in 2003 (Colliver, 2003).

Americans spend much more per capita on health care each year than any other industrialized Western country (almost twice the per capita expenditures in Canada and nearly three times those in the United Kingdom in 2000) (Anderson, et al., 2003). Some might argue that this is because Americans seek and receive a higher volume of services than other countries. This question has been the subject of a number of studies which found that, on the contrary, aggregate utilization such as physician visits and hospital days per capita for the U.S. is less than in the UK and Canada and below the median for the Organization for Economic Cooperation and Development (OECD). One has to conclude that the main difference between the U.S. and other countries is higher prices (Anderson, Reinhardt, Hussey, Petroyon, 2003). The public recognizes this, as reflected by a 2002 study comparing public perspectives of noninstitutionalized sicker adults in the U.S. with those in four other countries. Americans listed the top two problems of our health care system as high cost and inadequate coverage of services (48% and 25%, respectively), much higher than in any other country (Blendon, Schoen, Des Roches, Osborn, Zappert, 2003).

Decreasing Access

The flip side of increasing costs of health care is decreasing access to that care. We have already seen examples of this problem in earlier chapters. In chapter 1 we discussed access of middle-class families to health care and, in chapter 5 we examined increasing unaffordability of prescription drugs. Almost 60 million people lack health insurance coverage at some point during each year (Pear, 2003a). Figure 7.2 shows by state the probability of being uninsured for populations under age 65 in 2001, ranging up to 26% in Texas (Institute of Medicine, 2003a). Medical debt is a leading cause of bankruptcy each year, and a recent study by the Access Project in Boston of 6,000 uninsured people in 18 states found that almost one-half of respondents were in debt to service providers. About one-quarter of these patients felt deterred by these bills to even return to "safety net" facilities (Survey, 2003). Moreover, as Figure 7.3 shows, even Americans with above average incomes also have more access problems than patients in Canada, the U.K., Australia, and New Zealand (Blendon, Schoen, Des Roches, Osborn, Scoles et al, 2002).

Health insurance, whether private or public, is the single most important requirement for adequate access to health care. Compared with the insured, the lack of health insurance is associated with less likelihood of having a regular source of primary care, delays in seeking care, higher rates of hospitalization for preventable or avoidable conditions, higher morbidity and mortality, and greater declines in health status (Institute of Medicine, 2001, 2002, 2003b; Baker, Sudano, Albert, Borawski, Dor et al., 2001). The Kaiser Family Foundation's Commission on Medicaid and the Uninsured has recently estimated that the nation's mortality rate for the uninsured could be reduced by 10 to 15% if they were to be extended health insurance, a figure that is comparable to the overall reduction of mortality in the U.S. over the past 40 years (Hadley, 2002).

Variable, Often Poor, Quality

Decreased access to care leads directly to poor quality of care in many ways, including lack of primary care, delay in seeking care, discontinuity of care, and denial of services. Although many still cling to the belief that the U.S. has the best health care system in the world (an idea propagated by the stakeholders in the present system), this cannot be defended on many counts. A 1998 RAND review

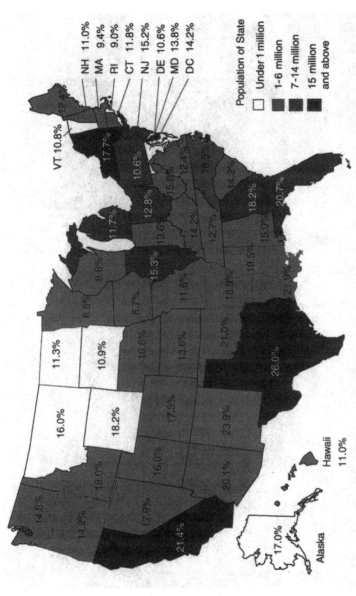

FIGURE 7.2 Probability of being uninsured for population under age 65, by state, 2001.

Source: Institute of Medicine. (2003). *A shared destiny: Community effects of uninsurance.* Washington, DC: National Academy Press. Reprinted with permission.

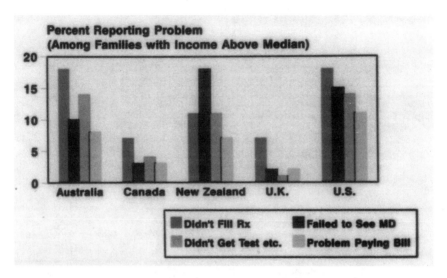

FIGURE 7.3 U.S. access is worse even for those with above average income.

Source: Blendon, R. J., et al. (2002). Inequities in health care: A five-country survey. *Health Affairs (Millwood), 21*(3), 182. Retrieved from *www.pnhp.org* Reprinted with permission.

(Schuster, McGlynn, Brook, 1998) of all available studies of quality of care reported the following unacceptable levels of care within the overall health care system:

- only 50% of people received recommended preventive care
- only 60% received recommended chronic care
- only 70% received recommended acute care
- 30% received *contraindicated* acute care
- 20% received *contraindicated* chronic care

While those who can afford it often receive high quality care, even they have to be concerned with another problem—too much care. Figure 7.4 shows high proportions of common medical and surgical procedures which are considered questionable or inappropriate according to a recent report of the Commonwealth Fund (2002). A 1999 report by the Technology Evaluation Center of the National Blue Cross and Blue Shield Association found that 10 of 28 evaluations showed drugs, devices, or procedures to be either lacking or uncertain in their effectiveness (Blue Cross and Blue Shield, 1999).

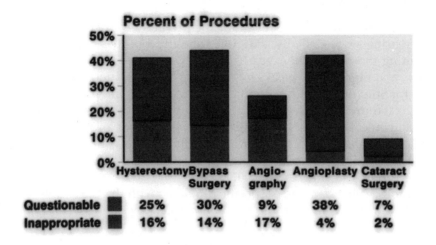

FIGURE 7.4 Unnecessary procedures.
Source: Commonwealth Fund. (2002). *Quality of care in the U.S. chartbook.* Retrieved from *www.pnhp.org* Reprinted with permission.

Comparison With Other Industrialized Nations

The U.S. health care system also performs poorly when measured against health care in other industrialized countries:

- The U.S. ranks last among 13 industrialized countries for low birth-weight percentages, neonatal and infant mortality overall, and years of potential life lost (Starfield, 1998)
- A weak primary care base places the U.S. last among 11 industrialized nations based on 11 criteria (Starfield, 1992)
- A 2000 study by the World Health Organization based on various indicators (including disability-adjusted life expectancy, child survival to five years of age, social disparities in care, and experiences with the health care system found the average ranking of the United States to be 15th out of 25 countries (Gray & Rowe, 2000)

By process measures as well, the U.S. health care system is not faring well. Providers and hospitals have to deal with the varied and often conflicting policies of over 1,200 private insurers. As a result, the administrative overhead in our health care bureaucracy is high, as illustrated by an average office overhead of 65% in family practice. A 2002 report by the Center for Studying Health System Change found that waiting times, even for the privately insured, are steadily increasing since 1997. By 2001, over one-third of these patients were waiting more than one week for a sick visit to see a physician when sick, and more than 3 weeks for a routine checkup appointment (Center for Studying Health System Change, 2002). An international study in 2000 found that 37% of U.S. physicians feel that external review of their clinical decisions to control costs is a major problem in their practices, about twice as high a percentage as in comparison countries, including Canada and the U.K. (Blendon, Schoen, Donelan, Osborn, Des Roches, et al., 2001).

Table 7.1 lists a range of specific problems with the U.S. health care system in terms of costs, access, and quality.

CONTRIBUTIONS OF CORPORATE HEALTH CARE TO INFLATION OF COSTS

The extent to which the profit motive of publicly held health care corporations drives up health care costs cannot be calculated with precision due to the complexity of the health care system, the multiple drivers of utilization, and the difficulties inherent in such calculations. Other factors admittedly drive up utilization and costs of care, including technological advances, an aging population with more chronic disease, bureaucracy in an inefficient system, and defensive medicine with increasing costs of malpractice insurance. Nevertheless, the unrestrained profit mission of corporate health care is certainly a dominant part of health care inflation without increase in value, as can be inferred from these examples of investor-owned companies, facilities, and providers compared with not-for-profit ones:

- *Acute hospitals*—Costs are 3 to 13% higher, with higher overhead, fewer nurses, and death rates 6 to 7% higher (Silverman, Skinner, Fisher, 1999; Woolhandler & Himmelstein, 1999; Yuan, Cooper, Einstadter, Cebul, Rimm, 2000). HCA, the largest national investor-owned hospital chain had accumulated $1.7 billion in civil fines and criminal penalties by the end of 2002 for such practices as falsification of patient records, billing for services not provided or not ordered by physicians, kickbacks for patient referrals, and fraudulent accountings; (*Associated Press,* 2002; Sparrow, 2000).
- *Rehabilitation hospitals*—Costs are 19% higher (Himmelstein, et al., 2001). Health South, the largest national chain of rehabilitation

TABLE 7.1. Some Major Problems of U.S. Health Care System

Increasing Costs of Care

Health care costs rising at double-digit levels over last 5 years (e.g., 16% in 2003), despite annual Consumer Price Index increases of only 2 to 3% (Towers Perrin, 2003).

Private health insurance rates are expected to increase by 20% in 2003 (Lee, 2002).

HMO premiums rose by 21% and 17% in 2002 and 2003, respectively, and are expected to increase by another 18% in 2004 (Bennett, 2003).

Profits of private health insurers in the U.S. averaged 25% in 2001 (Terry, 2003).

Average annual premium for employer-sponsored family health coverage is $9,160 in 2003, and is expected to surge to $14,545 by 2006 (National Coalition on Health Care, 2003).

Almost one-half of Americans report difficulty in affording health care, and a "medical divide" places those who earn less than $50,000 a year at a disadvantage (Marlis, 2002).

20% of the uninsured cannot afford the health insurance offered by their employers (Center for Studying Health System Change, 1999).

Administrative costs account for 31% of the nation's health care expenditures (Woolhandler, et al., 2003).

Decreasing Access to Care

According to the U.S. Census Bureau, 43.6 million Americans were uninsured over the entire year in 2002 (15.2% of the population), exceeding the aggregate population of 24 states (Pear, 2003a); almost 60 million are without health insurance at some point in the year (Pear, 2003a).

The proportion of Americans covered by employer-based insurance dropped from 63.6% in 2000 to 61.3% in 2002 (Pear, 2003b).

Consolidation and decreasing choice for employer-based insurance, e.g., Sears will offer just 35 HMOs nationwide in 2004, down from 220 five years ago (Simon, 2003).

Annual turnover rate of insurance coverage among the privately insured averages 17% to 20% (Cunningham & Kohn, 2000; Franks et al, 2003).

37% of applicants are denied insurance in the individual insurance market (Kaiser Family Foundation, 2001).

Although Medicaid covered 14 million people in poverty in 2002, 10.5 million others were uninsured in 2002 (U.S. Census Bureau, 2003).

Despite CHIP, the numbers of uninsured children did not change between 2000 and 2002, i.e., 8.5 million or 11.6% of all children in the U.S. less than 18 years of age (Pear, 2003b).

One in three Hispanics and one in five African Americans were without health insurance in 2002 (U.S. Census Bureau, 2003).

There is an increasingly fragile public safety net at a time of cutbacks and deficits at both state and federal levels.

TABLE 7.1. *(continued)*

Variable, and Often Poor, Quality of Care

Many factors lead to poor quality of care (e.g., denial of services, lack of primary care and continuity, unnecessary care, and neglect of psychosocial and quality-of-life issues) (Schiff, et al., 1994; Ansell & Schiff, 1987; Starfield, 1991; Leape, 1992).

Discontinuity of care resulting from health plan changes, e.g., a 2003 survey by the Kaiser Family Foundation found that one-third of employers changed health plans or insurance carriers in the last year (Fuhrmans, 2003); the first year after an insurance change is associated with higher costs, less chance of getting a mammogram, and increased risk of having an avoidable hospitalization (Franks, et al., 2003).

The uninsured and underinsured delay or avoid needed care and treatments, thereby experiencing higher death rates and worse clinical outcomes than their insured counterparts (Institute of Medicine, 2001).

The value of health capital foregone each year due to lack of health insurance coverage is estimated by the Institute of Medicine at between $65 and $130 billion (Institute of Medicine, 2003).

Due to limited access to medical technology for the care of heart attacks, cataracts and depression, more than $1.1 billion is lost each year from excess mortality and morbidity among the uninsured (Glied & Little, 2003).

A weak primary care base ranks the U.S. last among 11 industrialized nations by 11 criteria (Starfield, 1992).

The U.S. ranks last among 13 industrialized countries for low birth weight percentages, neonatal and infant mortality overall, and years of potential life lost (Starfield, 1998).

---

hospitals and surgicenters has been accused of adding at least $1.4 billion in false earnings (100 times the correct amount) between 1999 and 2003 in an Enron-type scandal (Norris, 2003).

- *Psychiatric hospitals*—National Medical Enterprises (now Tenet), one of nation's largest investor-owned chains of psychiatric hospitals, has paid out over $500 million in recent years to settle allegations of holding patients in locked wards against their will and paying kickbacks and bribes for patient referrals (Freudenheim, 1993).

- *HMOs*——Overhead is higher (25 to 33% for some of the largest HMOs), with worse scores on 14 of 14 quality measures reported to the National Committee for Quality Assurance (Freudenheim, 1993; Securities and Exchange Commission, 1999; Himmelstein, Woolhandler, Hellander, Wolfe, 1999)

- *Mental health centers*——80 programs were expelled by Medicare after investigations found that 91% of claims were fraudulent (Kuttner, 1999).
- *Nursing homes*—In their pursuit of maximal profits, for-profit nursing homes have been found to have lower staffing levels and lower quality of care. Beverly Enterprises, the largest investor-owned national chain of nursing homes, accumulated 1,000 violations of workers' rights in 1987 (Harrington, Woolhandler, Mullen, Carillo, Himmelstein, 2003)
- *Insurance industry*—Health insurer profits increased by an average of 25% in 2001 (Terry, 2003), while United Health Group, the country's largest health insurer, reported a fourth-quarter income surge of 53% in 2002 with projected growth in earnings per share of 22% for 2003 (United Health, 2003). Average compensation for top executives of United Health Group was more than $14 million in 2000, plus $119 million in unexercised stock options (Vital Signs, 2003). There are about 88,000 brokers, agents, and consultants in the private health insurance industry who charge hidden commissions ranging from 3% to as much as 20% of the total cost of plans sold (Robertson, 1999). The overhead charged by investor-owned Blues is over 26% compared with about 20% for commercial carriers, 16% for not-for-profit Blues and 3% for Medicare (Physicians for a National Health Program, 2002).

Similar patterns of profiteering are found throughout the supply side of health care, as reflected by these examples:

- *Pharmaceutical industry*—The top ten U.S. drug companies increased their profits by 33% in 2000, a time of recession, while the overall profits of Fortune 500 companies dropped by 53% (Public Citizen, 2002). The U.S. monopoly price for prescription drugs is about three times the average price for those drugs abroad (Baker, 2001). The industry has greatly exaggerated its costs of research and development for at least 40 years, pays less taxes than all other U.S. industries, and enjoys 17-year patent protection for its drugs (Mintz, 2001). Pfizer, the largest drug manufacturer in the world, posted a 137% increase in net income for the fourth quarter of 2002, still a period of economic slowdown (Hensley & Burton, 2002).
- *Diagnostic/screening imaging*—As we saw in the last chapter, expensive but lucrative high-technology imaging procedures such as full-body CT scans are being marketed vigorously to the public

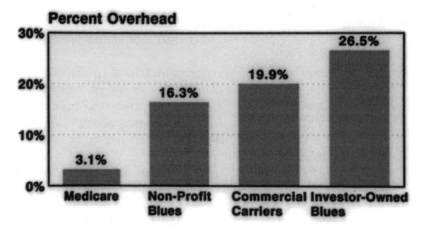

FIGURE 7.5 Private insurers' high overhead: investor-owned plans are worst.

Source: Physicians for a National Health Program (2002). Retrieved from *www.pnhp.org* Reprinted with permission.

with little oversight and without scientific basis. Their costs are then magnified by further diagnostic workups as a result of false positive results (Haas, 2001; (Lee & Brennan, 2003)

- *Medical devices*—Of the 8,000 new medical devices brought to market each year, more than 1,000 are recalled for being unsafe, and few are subject to review and approval by the FDA. This industry posted a net income margin of 16% in 2001, while spending almost four times as much on administration, sales, and marketing as on R&D. (Office of Research, Development & Information, 2002; (Feigel, Gardner, McClellan, 2003)
- *Medical supplies*—The medical supply industry also maintains a net profit margin of about 17% (Office of Research, Development & Information, 2002). The distribution chain to hospitals is dominated by for-profit group purchasing organizations which pad their expenses and maximize profits with minimal oversight or disclosure (Meier & Walsh, 2002; Walsh, 2002)

These examples are just the tip of the corporate self-interest iceberg. Collectively, even these few examples reach across all facets of health care from prevention and screening, to diagnosis and treatment. As we have seen, their proliferation is nearly unrestrained in the current deregulated business environment.

HOW SUSTAINABLE IS THE MARKET-BASED SYSTEM?

This may seem like a foolish, even unpatriotic, question in some quarters, especially among those who maintain a firm belief that the U.S. has the best health care system in the world. Even though market-based policies in health care have failed over many years to either control costs or address access and quality problems, there is a widespread belief among the public as well as in government and policy-making circles that the marketplace can resolve these problems. The myth that our "freely competitive" health care market can both function efficiently and regulate itself in the public interest is belied by its track record, as shown in the last five chapters. This should not come as a surprise. Robert Evans, a well-known health care economist at the University of British Columbia, has observed that market mechanisms give distributional advantages to particular groups, including providers, suppliers, and insurers, and more affluent and healthier people. He notes that providers, suppliers and higher-income citizens tend to support private financing of care, shifting the burden of care for the sick and uninsured to the public sector. Thus, the farther privatization goes, the greater the burden to finance and deliver care for lower-income people through a smaller risk pool (Evans, 1997).

This issue should not be considered on the basis of political ideology, but instead on the problems confronting the health care system and the resources available to sustain this system. Table 7.1 provides a snapshot of these problems. As of this writing, we are compelled to draw these conclusions in 2004:

- Double-digit cost increases are breaking the system and rendering health care increasingly unaffordable for at least one-half of the population. The status quo is, therefore, not sustainable.
- Health care inflation adversely affects access and quality of care. The present system is falling apart and requires major changes.
- The burden of care of a growing part of the population, especially those with chronic illness, disabilities, the elderly, and lower-income people, has seriously frayed whatever "safety net" still exists.
- Other domestic, security, and foreign policy priorities will constrain resources of federal and state governments to deal with a collapsing health care system.
- Growing state and federal deficits, together with continued inflation of health care costs, are certain to involve further

compromise of an already tattered safety net and will exacerbate access to and quality of care for much of the population; the Congressional Budget office now projects the nation's budget deficit to climb to $1.9 trillion by 2013, with a record budget deficit of $477 billion in 2004. (Andrews, 2004).

The urgency for major health care reform becomes obvious when the cold, hard facts are brought together in one place, as they are here. With many parts of the current system already underfunded (e.g., Medicare, Medicaid, CHIP), there is great risk that well-intended, incremental "reforms" will further destabilize the system. The addition of a Medicare prescription drug benefit is one good example, as we saw in chapter 5. The more it is tied mainly to the private sector, the more it will cost patients and the less value they will receive. The private sector will be the only winner. Without price containment in the pharmaceutical industry and without remedies of other pressing system problems, it could end up bankrupting the Medicare program.

Among the policy alternatives to be considered in Part III is a single-payer national health insurance program. Whether developed and implemented on a state-by-state basis or nationally, it would effectively shift the health care system from a profit-based market culture towards a not-for-profit, public-service culture.

POTENTIAL SAVINGS IF THE SYSTEM CAN BE REBUILT AROUND A NOT-FOR-PROFIT SERVICE ETHIC

For the sake of discussion, let's estimate how much money could be saved by such a change. There is good evidence that there is already plenty of money in our health care system to provide universal coverage for medically necessary health care services for all Americans— *if* our present resources can be reallocated to eliminate waste, duplication, and profiteering throughout the system. The U. S. already pays much more for health care than any other Western industrialized country yet gets less value from its poorly-performing system. The $1.6 trillion a year now being spent on U.S. health care is equivalent to $5,440 per year for every adult and child in the country. (PFN online, 2004). Whereas most people believe that we have a predominantly private system, that is no longer the case. As Woolhandler and Himmelstein recently demonstrated in a national study of health care financing, the government now pays 60% of total health care costs, including tax subsidies and public employees' health benefits. U.S. public expenditures for health care exceed total health care spending of every other country in the world except Switzerland. We are already paying for national health insurance and not getting it (Woolhandler & Himmelstein, 2002).

The key to achieving lasting cost containment of health care in this country, and to addressing access and quality problems, is the enactment of a system of social health insurance i.e., a single-payer system. In states where single-payer health insurance proposals have been studied, they have been found to provide universal coverage while saving money. In California, for example, where 21% of the population 65 years of age or younger are uninsured, single-payer proposals have been demonstrated to save the state about $8 billion of its $152 billion annual health expenditures, while providing every Californian with comprehensive coverage including prescription drugs, and vision and dental care (Kahn, Bodenheimer, Grumbach, Lingappa, Farey, et al., 2002). Cost savings of $118 million a year have been projected for a single-payer proposal in Vermont (Smith, 2001).

The largest cost saving to be achieved by single-payer national health insurance (NHI) would result from replacement of the wasteful for-profit private insurance industry by a single, publicly administered program, in effect Medicare for the entire population. As we saw earlier in Figure 7.5, the overhead of commercial carriers is about 20% and more than 26% for investor-owned Blues. If the existing 1,200 private insurance companies that use risk-rating to "cherry pick" the best risks and avoid the sick were replaced by a public system of national health insurace, it is estimated that over $280 billion would be saved each year (almost $7,000 for every uninsured American), while still providing universal coverage for medically-needed care (Himmelstein, Woolhandler, Wolfe, 2004). The current Medicare program is administered with an overhead of about 3%; even if this were to double under NHI, the cost savings from administrative simplification would be enormous.

A single-payer system could realize additional cost savings in a number of ways, including:

- bulk purchasing of drugs, medical devices and supplies by federal and state agencies
- coverage decisions based on clinical evidence of efficacy and cost-effectiveness, rather than marketing by suppliers and providers (e.g., no coverage for CT full-body screening scans)

- simplified administration for hospitals and providers (for example, a primary care physician's office overhead would very likely drop from 65% to 40% or less from not having to deal with hundreds of insurers and their differing policies)

Critics of the single-payer approach in defense of the market-based system, can be expected to make the following counterarguments to which I have added appropriate rebuttals:

- *"too simplistic a proposal"* (Then why have all other industrialized Western countries found it necessary to enact one or another form of social health insurance?)
- *"not the American way"* (Then is it the American way to leave out a growing part of the population from even basic health care, as has been well documented in preceding chapters?)
- *"NHI would stifle innovation"* (Drug and medical device manufacturers could still achieve more reasonable profit margins (e.g., 10% instead of 20%), while their prices are reduced by large group purchasing. New drugs are produced in Europe without large profit taking, and most U.S. drugs are "me too" drugs anyway) (National Institute for Health Care Management, 2002; Wolfe, 2003).
- *"this would result in rationing care"* (We are already rationing care, often in cruel ways, by income and class).
- *"the government can't be as efficient as the private sector"* (Despite its problems, the current Medicare program is actually more efficient, with lower overhead (3%), and more highly rated by its beneficiaries than private health insurance, as was found by surveys carried out by the Commonwealth Fund (see Figure 7.6) (Davis, Schoen, Doty, Tenney, 2002; Fuchs, 2002).

Restructuring U.S. health care along the lines of a public service model, while still preserving private practice of providers and the roles of private community hospitals, could be a stabilizing influence on other parts of the system which today are facing urgent problems of underfunding. These include public hospitals, academic medical centers, other teaching hospitals, trauma and burn units, community health centers, and other safety-net facilities. An expanded regulatory role for the FDA could more effectively review drugs and medical devices (as well as dietary supplements) in an effort to reduce the present substantial risks to the public posed by these products.

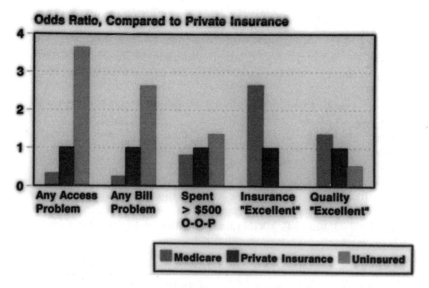

FIGURE 7.6 Medicare coverage is better than private.
Source: Physicians for a National Health Program (2002). Retrieved from *www.pnhp.org* Reprinted with permission.

CONCLUDING COMMENTS

The profit motive of corporate health care is a driving force in health care inflation, which is pricing health care beyond the reach of much of the U.S. population. The present expensive system is excessively fragmented, inefficient, bureaucratic and wasteful. Americans are not getting enough value for what they are paying. This system is not sustainable, nor should it be sustained without major reform. We will discuss reform alternatives, including single-payer national health insurance, in the last part of this book. The major impediment to needed reforms is, however, the powerful opposition of corporate stakeholders in the present system. For that reason, we need to shift gears and consider in the next four chapters how they defend and promote their interests.

REFERENCES

Anderson, G. F., Reinhardt, U. E., Hassey, P. S., Petroyan, V. (2003). It's the prices, stupid: Why the United States is so different from other countries. *Health Affairs (Millwood), 22*(3), 89.

Andrews, E. L. (2004, Jan. 22). Budget Office presents record deficit in '04 and sketches a pessimistic future. *New York Times,* p. A19.

Ansell, D. A., & Schiff, R. L. Patient dumping: Status, implications, and policy recommendation. *Journal of the American Medical Association, 257,* 1500.

Appleby, J. Health insurance premiums crash down on middle-class. *USA Today,* March 17, 2004: B1.

Associated Press. (2002). Hospital chain ends fraud case. Retrieved from *www.nytimes.com*

Baker, D. (2001, Jan. 29). Patent medicine. *The American Prospect,* p. 34.

Baker, D. W., Sudano, J. J., Albert, J. M., Borawski, E. A., Dor, A. (2001). Lack of health insurance and decline in overall health in late middle age. *The New England Journal of Medicine, 345,* 1106.

Bennett, J. (2003, June 24). HMO rates are expected to rise 18%. *San Francisco Chronicle.*

Blendon, R. J., Schoen, C., Donelan, K., Osborn, R., Des Roches, C., Scles, K., Davis, K., Binns, K., Zapert, K., (2001). Physicians' views on quality of care: A five-country comparison. *Health Affairs (Millwood), 20*(3), 233.

Blendon, R. J., Schoen, C., Des Roches, C., Osborn, R., Scoles, K. L., Zapert, K. (2002). Inequities in health care: A five-country survey. *Health Affairs (Millwood), 21*(3), 182.

Blendon, R. J., Schoen, C., Des Roches, C., Osborn, R., Zapert, K. (2003). Common concerns and diverse systems: health care experiences in five countries. *Health Affairs (Millwood), 22*(3), 106.

Blue Cross and Blue Shield (1999). Technology Evaluation Committee Reports, Chicago: No. 1–28.

Center for Studying Health System Change (HSC). (1999, (Oct.) Who declines employer-sponsored health insurance and is uninsured? Issue Brief 22,

Center for Studying Health System Change (HSC). (2002, Sept. 5). News release, September 5.

Colliver, V. (2003, May 15). CalPERS tries to cut HMO costs. *San Francisco Chronicle.*

Commonwealth Fund. (2002). *Quality of care in the U.S. chartbook.* New York: Author.

Cunningham, P. J., & Kohn, L. (2000). Health plan switching: Choice or circumstance? *Health Affairs (Millwood), 19*( ), 158.

Davis, K., Schoen, C., Doty, M., Tenney, K. (2002, Oct. 9). Medicare versus private insurance: Rhetoric and reality. *Health Affairs* Web exclusive, W311.

Evans, R. G. (1997). Going for the gold: The redistributive agenda behind market-based health care reform. *Journal of Health Politics, Policy & Law, 2292,* 427.

Feigal, D. W., Gardner, S. N., McClellan, M. D. (2003). Ensuring safe and effective medical devices. *The New England Journal of Medicine, 348,* 191.

Franks, P., Cameron, C,. Bertrakis, K. D. (2003). On being new to an insurance plan: Health care use associated with the first years in a health insurance plan. *Annals of Family Medicine, 1*(3), 156.

Freudenheim, M. (1993, Dec. 14). National Medical resolves last of insurance disputes. *The New York Times*, p. C5.

Fuchs, V. (2002). What's ahead for health insurance in the United States? *The New England Journal of Medicine, 346*, 13.

Furhmans, V. (2003, Oct. 15). The perils of switching. *The Wall Street Journal*, p. D1.

Geyman, J. P. (2003). The corporate transformation of medicine and its impacts on costs and access to care. *Journal of the American Board of Family Practice, 16*, pp. 443–454.

Glied, S., & Little, S. E. (2003). The uninsured and the benefits of medical progress. *Health Affairs (Millwood), 22*(4), 210.

Gray, B. H., & Rowe, C. (2000). Safety-net health plans: A status report. *Health Affairs (Millwood), 19*(1),185.

Haas, N. (2001, Aug. 26). Scared sick: The $900 antidote. *The New York Times.*

Hadley, J. (2002). Sicker and poorer: The consequences of being uninsured. Kaiser Commission on Medicaid and the Uninsured. May.

Hakim, D. (2004, Mar. 12). GM says costs for retiree care top $60 billion. *The New York Times*, p. C1.

Harrington, C., Woolhandler, S., Mullen, J., Carillo, H., Himmelstein, D. U. (2001). Does investor-ownership of nursing homes compromise the quality of care. *American Journal of Public Health, 91*(9), 1.

Heffler, S., Smith, S., Keehan, S., Clemens, M. K., Won, G, Zegga, M. (2003). Health spending projections for 2002– 201a. *Health Affairs (Millwood), 22*(2), 12.

Heffler, S., Smith, S., Keehan, S., Clemens, M. K., Zegga, M., Truffer, C. (2004, Feb. 11). Health spending projections through 2013. *Health Affairs* Web Exclusive Abstract.

Hensley, S., & Burton, T. M. (2003, Apr. 23). Big drug makers report increase in sales. *The Wall Street Journal*, p. B2.

Himmelstein, D. U., Woolhandler, S., Hellander, I., Wolfe, S. M. (1999). Quality of care in investor-owned vs. not-for-profit HMOs. *Journal of the American Medical Association, 282*, 159.

Himmelstein, D. U., Woolhandler, S., Hellander, I. (2001). *Bleeding the patient: The consequences of corporate health care.* Monroe, ME: Common Courage Press.

Himmelstein, D. U., Woolhandler, S., Wolfe, S. M. (2004). Administrative waste in the U.S. health care system in 2003: The costs to the nation, the states and the District of Columbia, with state-specific estimates of potential savings. *International Journal of Health Services, 34*(1): 79–86.

Institute of Medicine Committee on the Consequences of Uninsurance. (2001). *Coverage matters: Insurance and health care.* Washington, DC: National Academy Press.

Institute of Medicine Committee on the Consequencs of Uninsurance. (2002).

Health insurance is a family matter. Washington, DC: National Academy Press.

Institute of Medicine Committee on the Consequences of Uninsurance. (2003a). *A shared destiny: Community effects of uninsurance.* Washington, DC: National Academy Press.

Institute of Medicine (2003b). Committee on the Consequences of Uninsurance. *Hidden costs, value lost: Uninsurance in America.* Washington, DC: National Academy Press.

Kahn, J., Bodenheimer, T. S., Grumbach, K., Lingappa, V., Farey, K., McCanne, D. R. (2002). Single-payer proposal for California as analyzed by the Lewin Group. Available at *(www.healthcareoptions.ca.gov)*

Kaiser Family Foundation. (2001, June 19). Applicants denied insurance in the individual insurance market.

Kuttner, R. (1999). The American health care system: Wall Street and health care. *The New England Journal of Medicine, 340,* 664.

Leape, L. L. (1992). Unnecessary surgery. *Annual Review of Public Health, 13,* 363.

Lee, D. (2002, June 18). Health insurance rate hikes expected. *Los Angeles Times,* latimes.com June 18, 2002.

Lee T. H. & Brennan T.A. Direct-to-consumer marketing of high-technology screening tests. *The New England Journal of Medicine, 346,* 529.

Marlis, M. (2002, June). Family out-of-pocket spending for health services: A continuing source of financial insecurity. *Commonwealth Fund.*

Matthews, R. G. (2003, May 12). Life support: A retired steelworker struggles with a health insurance crisis. *The Wall Street Journal,* p. A1.

Meier, B., & Walsh, M. W. (2002, July 19). Medicine's middlemen. Questioning $1 million fee in a needle deal. *The New York Times.*

Mintz, M. (2001, Feb.). Still hard to swallow. *The Washington Post Outlook Section.*

National Institute for Health Care Management Research and Educational Foundation. *Changing patterns of pharmaceutical innovations.* Washington, DC: Author.

Norris, F. (2003, March 20). In U.S. eyes, a fraud particularly bold. *The New York Times,* p. C1.

Office of Research, Development & Information. (2002, Oct. 10). Center for Medicare and Medicaid Services. Health care industry market update. *Medical Devices & Supplies.*

Pear, R. (2003a, May 13). New study finds 60 million uninsured during a year. *The New York Times,* p. A20.

Pear, R. (2003b, Sept. 30). Big increase seen in people lacking health insurance. *The New York Times,* p. A1.

PFNewsline (2004). U.S. health spending surges to new high. *Physicians Financial News,* 22(2), 5.

Physicians for a National Health program (PNHP). (2002). Slide set (sources

Schramm, Blue Cross-conversion, Abell Foundation and CMS). Available from *www.pnhp.org*

Public Citizen Report (2002, April 18) Available at *http://www.citizen.org/congressreform/drug_industry/profits/articles.ctm?ID-(416)*

Relman, A. S. (1980). The new medical-industrial complex. *The New England Journal of Medicine, 303,* 963.

Robertson, K. (1999, Sept. 13). Are health plan brokers paid too much? *Sacramento Business Journal.*

Rose, J. R. (2003, Aug. 8). National Coalition on Health Care cost estimates of employer-sponsored family health coverage. *Medical Economics.*

Schiff, G. D., et al. (1994). A better quality alternative: Single-payer national health system reform. *Journal of the American Medical Association, 272,* 803.

Schuster, M. A., McGlynn, E. A., Brook, R. H. (1998). How good is the quality of health care in the United States? *Milbank Quarterly, 76*(4), 517, 509.

Securities and Exchange Commission (1999, apr. 12). SEC filings. *Best Week Life/Health Special* Report.

Silverman, E. M., Skinner, J. S., Fisher, E. S. (1999). The association between for-profit hospital ownership and increased Medicare spending. *The New England Journal of Medicine, 341,* 420.

Simmons, H., & Goldberg, M. A. (2003, May 19). Charting the cost of inaction. National Coalition on Health Care.

Simon, R. (2003, Oct. 15). Your health plan's new math. *The Wall Street Journal,* p. D1.

Smith, R. F. (2001, Nov. 2). Universal health insurance makes business sense. *Rutland Herald.*

Sparrow, M. K. (2000). License to steal: How fraud bleeds America's health care system. Boulder, CO: Westview Press. Starfield B. (1992). *Primary care: concept, evaluation and policy.* New York: Oxford University Press, 1992.

Starfield, B. (1998). *Primary care: balancing health needs, services, and technology.* New York: Oxford University Press.

Starfield, B. (1991). Primary care and health. A cross-national comparison. *Journal of American Medical Association, 266,* 2268.

Starr P. (1982). *The social transformation of American medicine.* New York: Basic Books.

Survey dispels myth of free care for uninsured. (2003). *Physicians Financial News,* 21 (4), 5.

Terry, K. (2003, Jan. 10). Where has all the money gone? *Medical Economics,* p. 72.

Towers Perrin. (2003). *2003 Health Care Cost Survey.* Available at *www.towersperrin.com*

United Health's profits soar. *Physicians Financial News, 21*(3), 913.

Vital signs. (2003). *Family Practice News, 32*(3), 1.

Walsh, M. W. (2002, June 7). A mission to save money: A record of otherwise. *The New York Times Online.*

Wolfe, S. (2003, March). Selling "new" drugs using smoke and mirror (images). *Health Letter,* p. 2.

Woolhander, S., Himmelstein, D. U., Angell, M., Young, Q. M., & Physicians Working Group for Single-Payer National Health Insurance. (2003). Proposal of the Physicians'Working Group for single-payer national health insurance. *Journal of the American Medical Association, 290,* 798.

Woolhandler, S., & Himmelstein, D. U. (1999). When money is the mission—the high costs of investor-owned care. *The New England Journal of Medicine, 341,* 444.

Woolhander, S., Campbell, T., Himmelstein, D. U. (2003). Costs of health care administration in the United States and Canada. *The New England Journal of Medicine, 349,* 768.

Woolhander, S., & Himmelstein, D. U. (2002). Paying for national health insurance—and not getting it. *Health Affairs (Millwood), 21*(4), 20.

Yuan, Z., Cooper, G. S., Einstadter, D., Cebul, R. P., Rimm, A. A. (2000). The association between hospital type and mortality and length of stay: A study of 16.9 million hospitalized Medicare beneficiaries. *Medical Care, 38,* 231.

Part II

HOW HEALTH CARE CORPORATIONS DEFEND AND PROMOTE THEIR INTERESTS

Chapter 8

COMPROMISING THE INTEGRITY OF RESEARCH

Private industry has become the major funding source for biomedical research in the U.S., even surpassing the National Institutes of Health (NIH). Almost 60% of biomedical research and development is privately funded, and two-thirds of universities have equity in industry sponsors (Bekelman, Li, Gross, 2003). The pharmaceutical industry has increased its spending on research and development more than three-times from $6.8 billion in 1990 to an estimated $23.9 billion in 2001 (PhRMA, 2002). Industry sponsored research now accounts for 70% of funding for clinical drug trials in the U.S (Bodenheimer, 2002). Biotechnology and medical device companies added another $1.6 billion to clinical research in 2001 (CenterWatch, 2001). By comparison, the NIH budget for clinical research in 2002 was $16.8 billion (NIH, 2003).

As the alliance between academic institutions and industry has strengthened over the years, clinical research has been greatly expanded and the pace of innovation accelerated. At the same time, however, the academic-industry partnership has been an uneasy alliance fraught with many challenging issues, including balancing priorities between the public good and private commercial gain, conflicts of interest of researchers and their institutions, and questions of confidentiality concerning patient privacy as well as the secrecy of research data (Kelch, 2002).

These kinds of issues are hardly new, as illustrated by the experience of Benjamin Waterhouse, one of three full-time professors at Harvard Medical School in 1799. After reading about Edward Jenner's studies in England on cowpox vaccination for the prevention of smallpox, Waterhouse proceeded to inoculate family members and 19 other children in Boston who were then exposed to smallpox. None of the children developed the disease, and he made plans to inoculate New England children for a fee on a monopoly basis. The other professors were outraged by this behavior, which was seen as self-serving and Waterhouse was finally expelled from the faculty in 1812 after years of acrimony (Blake, 1957; Beecher & Altschule, 1977; Cash & Waterhouse, 1999).

In an effort to explore how well the public interest has been served by this shift to major funding of clinical research by private industry, this chapter has four goals: (1) to examine academic-industry interrelationships as they have developed over the years; (2) to describe commercial contract research networks, largely removed from academic settings, which have been established by industry; (3) to outline various corporate practices which have led to bias and corruption of some clinical research; and (4) to give examples of the growing political influence of vested interests on biomedical research. Since research sponsored by the pharmaceutical industry, and to a lesser extent by the medical device industry, have attracted the most scrutiny and study, these areas will necessarily receive the most attention in this chapter.

THE ACADEMIC—INDUSTRY PARTNERSHIP: HOW CORRUPT IS IT?

The biomedical research communities in academic and industry settings share the common goal of advancing knowledge and therapeutic innovations in health care. Both groups need highly specialized investigators and the infrastructure to enable them to work successfully. When they come together in an economic partnership, they can each gain from the exchange of ideas, expertise, and resources to advance their common agenda. At the same time, however, each party brings different expectations, needs, and values to this partnership. Academic investigators and their institutions welcome collaboration with other investigators and the resources needed to tackle cutting-edge projects which they might otherwise not be able to undertake. Investigators based in industry likewise value the expertise and prestige of academic research settings. Beyond that, however, their expectations and needs diverge because of their respective cultures.

Investigators in universities and medical schools seek new scientific knowledge and techniques as a primary motivation. Their success is measured by such standards as the quality and number of scholarly publications in the most highly respected scientific journals, the level of support by NIH, and their advancement to tenured positions in the university. Investigators based in industry seek scientific advances which can be developed efficiently and widely marketed as a successful business venture. Their motivation is strongly influenced by financial considerations, which often include equity in their company, stock options, and royalties from the future sale of products being developed. For their employers, each one-day delay in FDA approval of a promising drug carries with it an average loss in revenue of $1.2 million (Bodenheimer, 2002). Because of these differences in the two cultures, there are many conflicts of interest which arise between them.

Conflicts of interest are especially troublesome in academic research settings. Clinician investigators may need to balance their competing responsibilities in patient care and teaching against more financially attractive research opportunities. Academic institutions must balance the attractiveness of major industry support against their responsibilities to patients and their families, the public interest, and their accrediting agencies (Moses, Braunwald, Martin, Thier, 2002). Especially in financially challenging times, as they deal with declining public and private reimbursements for patient care, they may find it difficult to turn down offers to fund research centers or other desired programs (Angell, 2000). On the industry side of the fence, investigators must serve the interests of their corporate employers' who in turn are accountable to investors (Moses, Braunwald, Martin, Thier, 2002).

After more than 30 years of large-scale federal funding for clinical research through the NIH, government priorities shifted in the late 1970s. A national slowdown of economic growth in those years, coupled with strong industrial competitors in Europe and Japan, led Congress to consider new ways to stimulate economic growth. The Bayh-Dole Act of 1980 was one piece of legislation enacted by Congress for that purpose. It was intended to accelerate innovation by encouraging academic-industry partnerships whereby new products could be brought to market faster and more efficiently. Under this Act, government subsidies were made available to university-industry cooperative ventures to more effectively translate research advances into clinical practice. It became easier for universities to own and license patents on discoveries made through publicly funded research, and provided tax breaks to industry investing more in university-based research (Bayh-Dole, 1980). By 1990, 200 U.S. universities had established technology transfer offices to identify promising discoveries that could be patented and licensed to companies. By the year 2000, the volume of these patents had increased more than tenfold resulting in over $1 billion annually in royalties and license fees (Bok, 2003; Florida, 1999).

During this period of rapid growth in academic-industry collaborative programs, many conflicts of interest involving both academic-based investigators and their institutions began to emerge. In addition to grant support, academic researchers were often given opportunities to share in patent and royalty arrangements, as well as own equity in their sponsoring companies. Many were invited to join advisory boards and speakers' bureaus for their companies, to promote their drugs at company-sponsored symposia at expensive resorts, and to be included as authors of articles ghostwritten by company staff. These financial incentives raised the possibility that researchers might undertake research projects that they otherwise would find less important; that they might shift their focus more to drug therapy and medical devices than causes and mechanisms of disease, or even that their research findings might be influenced by their financial ties (Angell, 2000). At the institutional level, as the boundaries between academic medicine and industry became blurred, medical schools could face new problems if their clinician faculty were drawn away too much from patient care and teaching, if their research proved to be compromised by commercial bias, if patient safety became threatened by lack of informed consent in research protocols, or if their own institutions were seen in any way to abuse the public trust by accepting "drug money". In addition to the kinds of potential conflicts of interest on the part of academic investigators involved in industry-sponsored research, institutional financial conflicts of interest may occur whenever key institutional decision makers (e.g., administrators, IRB members, members of other research oversight bodies) have a financial stake in the results of that research (Bok, 2003).

Since 1980, there have been so many examples of abuses by investigators and their academic institutions across the country that a rich literature base has accumulated (Bekelman, Gross, 2003; Korn, 2000; DeAngelis, Fontarosas, Flanagin, 2001; Gelijns & Thier, 2002; Emanuel & Steiner,1995). The perception of abuses, together with many documented examples in these and other reports, have led to the development of guidelines by various professional organizations and responses by government agencies in an effort to protect patient safety and the integrity of clinical research.

Several professional groups, including the Association of American Medical Colleges (AAMC, 2002) and the Association of American Universities (AAU, 2002), have developed voluntary guidelines offering guidance on financial conflicts of interest. The American Federation for Clinical Research has recommended that investigators not have any financial interest in a sponsoring company, including ownership of stock or stock options, when engaged in research on the efficacy and safety of products manufactured by that company (American Federation, 1990). In an effort to improve the safety of patients enrolled in clinical trials, a new not-for-profit Association for the Accreditation of Human Research Protection Programs (AAHRPP) was established in 2001, with the responsibility to work toward the adoption of consistent standards among research institutions (AAHRPP, 2001). Also in 2001, the International Committee of Medical Journal Editors (ICMJE) issued new, more rigorous requirements for full disclosure of the sponsor's role in the research being reported, as well as assurances that investigators are independent of the sponsor, are fully accountable for the design and conduct of the trial, have access to all of the research data, and control all editorial and publication decisions (ICMJE, 2001).

That major problems persist despite these well-intended voluntary efforts is shown by the results of a recent national study of clinical-trial agreements between medical schools and industry sponsors, which revealed that academic institutions routinely fail to adhere to ICMJE guidelines concerning trial design, access to data, and trial results. With almost 90%of medical schools participating in this study, there has been very low compliance on most counts as shown in Table 8.1. For example, none of the agreements required publication of trial results, and only 1% required access to all data for authors of reports of multicenter trials (Schulman, Seils, Timbie, Sugarman, Dame et al., 2002). Another study, reported in 2000, also gave disappointing results. Policies governing conflict of interest in clinical trials were examined in the 10 U.S. medical schools which receive the largest amount of funding from the NIH. Conflict of interest policies were found to vary widely from one institution to another in terms of financial disclosure and financial ties permitted with industry sponsors (Lo, Wolfe, Berkeley, 2000). Some academic institutions impose almost no limits on faculty members' income from consulting contracts, equity in companies, stock options, or speaking engagements (Cho, Shohara, Schissel, Rennie, 2000).

The NIH has issued general guidelines for financial conflicts of interest in human subjects research. These guidelines have set the amount above which such conflict exists at $10,000 (Drazen & Curfman, 2002; Public Health, 2002). NIH policies were relaxed in 1995, as shown in Table 8.2, in part with the intent to serve as an incentive to better recruit and retain high-level scientists at the NIH (Steinberg, 2004). A 2003 article by David Willman in the *Los Angeles Times* re-

TABLE 8.1. Compliance Scores For Coordinating-Center Agreements Between Medical Schools and Industry Sponsors of Multicenter Clinical Trials*

Item†	No.	Median Score (Interquartile Range)
Design of trial		
Agreement addresses plan for data collection and monitoring	14	83 (55–100)
Agreement addresses plan for data analysis and interpretation	13	80(20–100)
Agreement requires an independent steering or executive committee	14	3(0–50)
Agreement requires an independent data and safety monitoring board	13	1(0–50)
Access to data		
Agreement requires access to all data for authors of reports on multicenter trials	13	50(10–95)
Agreement allows use of trial data for other educational or research purposes	14	88(16–100)
Publication of results		
Agreement requires publication of trial results	13	5(0–75)
Agreement requires an independent writing or publications committee	14	6(0–23)
Agreement addresses criteria for authorship of reports on trial results	13	50(0–90)
Agreement addresses editorial control of reports on trial results	13	75 (20–100)
Agreement addresses decisions about where to submit manuscripts	13	0(0–20)
Agreement includes a commitment to publication of the results of subsequent genetic research	10	0
Other issues		
Agreement contains provision that prevents confidentiality clause from restricting investigators' publication rights	14	100 (75–100)
Agreement named as superseding document in case of conflict between agreement and protocol	10	63(20–90)
Agreement explicitly requires institution to follow protocol	13	100 (99–100)
Agreement explicitly requires sponsor to follow protocol	13	50 (1–100)‡

Source: Schulman, K. A., et al. (2002). A national survey of provisions in clinical-trial agreements between medical schools and industry sponsors. *The New England Journal of Medicine, 347,* 1337. Reprinted with permission.

*The compliance score for each item is the percentage of the institution's agreements that addressed the item.

†See the Appendix for the complete list of survey items.

‡The responses had a bimodal distribution.

TABLE 8.2. NIH Policies Regarding the Outside Activities of Employees

Before 1995	After 1995
Senior staff, including NIH director, deputy and associate directors, and institute and center directors and deputy directors, severely limited in the type of outside activities they could perform	Senior staff—with the exception of presidential appointees— no longer severely limited in the outside activities they can perform; common set of standards apply to all NIH employees
Employees limited to no more than $25,000/yr from any single source and no more than $50.000/yr from all sources combined	No dollar limit on the amount of money employees can earn from outside activities
Employees limited to a maximum of 500 hr/yr of outside activities	No limitations on the amount of time employees can devote to outside work, as long as it does not interfere with their NIH work
Employees could accept only money for performing outside activities; payment in stock or stock options was banned	Employees can accept money as well as stock and stock options for their services
All employees in a laboratory or branch were prohibited from working for an outside organization, including accepting an honorarium for speaking or lecturing, if any employee in the laboratory or branch had official dealings with the outside organization, such as through a research agreement or contract	Employees with direct official business dealings with an outside organization are prohibited from working for that organization; other employees can work for the same organization or receive compensation for speaking and lecturing

Source: Reprinted with permission from Steinbrook, R. Financial conflicts of interest and the NIH. *New England Journal of Medicine, 350,* 327–330, 2004. Copyright © 2004 Massachusetts Medical Society. All rights reserved.

ported that consulting payments were being made, often over a period of years, from tens of thousands to hundreds of thousands of dollars, and that these payments are often not publicly disclosed. Of more than 2,200 NIH employees earning over $102,168 a year, only about 6% are filing such disclosures (Willman, 2003).

New compliance guidelines were issued by the HHS Office of the Inspector General (OIG) in April 2003 with the intention of giving pharmaceutical companies a benchmark for their marketing efforts.

Although not legally binding, these guidelines list the following activities as likely to violate federal anti-kickback laws:

- "Paying physicians for lending their names to ghostwritten papers or speeches
- "Switching agreements," in which physicians are paid each time a patient's prescription is changed
- "Shadowing" arrangements, whereby drug company representatives pay to observe physicians seeing patients
- Paying doctors to listen to sales representatives market pharmaceutical products
- Compensating physicians as "consultants" for attending meetings or conferences primarily in a passive capacity
- Paying physicians for speaking about research when it is "connected directly or indirectly to a manufacturer's marketing and sales activities"
- Presentations to physicians involving meals or entertainment "if any one purpose of the arrangement is to generate business for the pharmaceutical company"
- Research contracts that originate through the sales or marketing functions or that are offered to physicians in connection with sales contracts" (Page, 2003).

In response to the developing backlash among professional groups and government agencies concerning the marketing practices of the drug industry, the Pharmaceutical Research and Manufacturers of America (PhRMA), the industry's trade group, recently put out their own voluntary guidelines to address these concerns. Not surprisingly, however, they turn out to be permissive and hardly a solution to the problem. For example, it is still "ethical" under the PhRMA code to fly 300 physicians to a resort, pay them to attend, and reimburse their costs in order to "educate and train" them to join a paid speaker's bureau to promote the company's drugs (Moynihan, 2003; PhRMA, 2003).

COMMERCIAL RESEARCH NETWORKS—CROs AND SMOs

The last 10 years have seen a rapid trend by the pharmaceutical industry to shift its drug research from academic medical centers to commercially oriented, for-profit networks. Between 1991 and 1998, the proportion of industry support for clinical drug trials at academic medical centers fell from 80% to just 40% (Getz, 1999). The industry has found that it can conduct clinical trials more quickly, more efficiently, and for less money in community settings than in academic settings. Instead of having to deal with time-consuming and complex negotiations of clinical-trial agreements with medical schools and universities, drug companies can deal with contract-research organizations (CROs) that may or may not use site-management organizations (SMOs). Compared with earlier years, many pharmaceutical companies are now well staffed with skilled investigators and their own infrastructure to manage a clinical trial from inception through completion.

An entrepreneurial marketplace has developed to facilitate clinical trials in community settings. CROs employ physician investigators, pharmacists, biostatisticians, and managers. They are prepared to develop a network of research sites, implement a trial protocol at each site, and send reports to the sponsoring company for data analyses. For smaller pharmaceutical companies, a CRO may complete the entire process under contract, including study design, data analysis, preparation of applications to the FDA, and journal articles. Among several hundred CROs across the country, the largest are Quintiles Transnational and Covance (Bodenheimer, 2002).

CROs also recruit patients for drug trials in both academic and community settings and may subcontract with SMOs, to organize community networks of physicians and patients. The entrepreneurial nature of these arrangements often leads to the lowering of research rigor. There is an inherent conflict of interest between CROs, SMOs, and sponsoring companies, with the commercial research networks entirely dependent upon the manufacturer's financial support. Critics of SMOs have called attention to inadequate training of investigators, the cost of overhead, and the poor quality of research data (Vogel, 1999; Henderson, 1999).

The most rapidly growing part of drug trials are the Phase IV post-marketing registry trials. These may have the least rigor of all, even to the point of being marketing disguised as research. Drug research firms recruit physicians and their patients to monitor the use of drugs in simple, uncontrolled trials in real-world clinical practice. Participating physicians are paid a set fee (e.g., $500 per patient) for recruiting and following appropriate patients and making reports to the sponsor. Supporters of Phase IV studies point to the value of learning more information about drug administration and patient compliance. Results may or may not be reported to the FDA. Registry trials have become common for blockbuster drugs and "vanity" drugs seeking to build a large physician and patient following. Marcia Angell, former editor of *The New England Journal of Medicine*, sums up critics' concerns about these trials in these words:

> Phase IV studies are the fastest growing components of the clinical trial enterprise and much of it amounts to bribing doctors. Essentially, doctors are paid to put their patients on the sponsor's drug. There's often no legitimate scientific purpose for the study. To a large extent, doctors buy into the fiction that they're doing "research" because it's lucrative to do so (Borfitz, 2003).

CORPORATE PRACTICES WHICH CORRUPT CLINICAL RESEARCH

We consider here four kinds of activities which corrupt industry-sponsored clinical research. Unfortunately, they are so common that they compromise the credibility of a sizable amount of research, especially in the area of drug studies.

1. Paying Consultants, Opinion Leaders, and Authors

Drug companies and prescribing physicians are joined together in a tangled web of influence that includes the kinds of interactions shown in Table 8.3 (Moynihan, 2003). The number of drug industry sales representatives has tripled over the last 10 years to about 90,000 in the U.S., about one for every five office-based physicians (Hensley, 2002). These representatives typically bring various kinds of gifts to physicians, including samples and free meals. Although physicians usually deny that these gifts influence their prescribing behavior, there is considerable evidence that they do (Wazana, 2000; Watkins, Moore, Harvey, Carthy, Robinson et al., 2003). It has been found, for example, that an increase in formulary requests for, and prescribing of, a company's drug is associated with physicians' accepting meals and expenses for travel and accommodations at sponsored educational meetings (Wazana, 2000; Leschin, 1993).

Drug companies regularly seek out academic experts as opinion leaders to promote their drugs. One study, reported in 2000, found that these arrangements include paid speaking compensation ranging from $250 to $20,000 per year; paid consultancies, usually less than $10,000 but up to $120,000 a year; paid positions on advisory

TABLE 8.3. Forms of Entanglement

- Face to face visits from drug company representatives
- Acceptance of direct gifts of equipment, travel, or accommodations
- Acceptance of indirect gifts, through sponsorship of software or travel
- Attendance at sponsored dinners and social or recreational events
- Attendance at sponsored educational events, continuing medical education workshops or seminars
- Attendance-at sponsored scientific conferences
- Ownership of stock or, equity holdings
- Conducting sponsored research
- Company funding for medical schools, academic chairs, or lecture halls
- Membership of sponsored professional societies and associations
- Advising a sponsored disease foundation or patients' group
- Involvement with or use of sponsored clinical guidelines
- Undertaking paid consultancy work for companies
- Membership on company advisory boards of "thought leaders" or "speakers' bureaus"
- Authoring "ghostwritten" scientific articles
- Medical journals' reliance on drug company advertising, company purchased reprints, and sponsored supplements

Source: Moynihan, R. (2003). Who pays for the pizza? Redefining the relationships between doctors and drug companies I: Entanglement. *British Medical Journal, 326,* 1190. Reprinted with permission of the BMJ Publishing Group.

boards, and equity holdings, typically over $10,000 and ranging up to $1 million (Boyd & Bero, 2000). An article on "the tricks of the trade" in *Pharmaceutical Marketing* asserts that the advisory process is one of the most powerful methods of influencing people (Jackson, 2001).

Drug companies aggressively market their wares at conferences of specialty associations, where the exhibit halls often resemble bazaars. Specialty organizations profit from large exhibit fees, and their journals profit further from lucrative arrangements when they publish proceedings of industry-sponsored symposia. Many clinical journals are dependent on drug advertising for their continued existence and find it difficult to reject such papers (Bero, Galbraith, Rennie, 1992; Smith, 2003). As an editor of family practice journals for 30 years, I have been approached on many occasions to publish proceedings of symposia after the fact, with no editorial role in the selection of authors (hired by industry) or their message (invariably favorable to the sponsor's drug). When confronted by the need for full peer review and disclosure of financial arrangements, they have always withdrawn their proposals.

The field of psychiatry illustrates the extent to which industry can permeate a specialty's research arm. Dr. E. Fuller Torrey, a psychiatrist and member of the Public Citizen Health Research Group for 30 years, described his observations at the July, 2001 7th World Congress of Biological Psychiatry in Berlin. Meeting officials admitted that more than one-half of the 4,000 attendees were sponsored by drug companies. In addition to business-class airline tickets and four-star hotel accommodations, honoraria for sponsored psychiatrists ranged from $2,000 to $10,000, and attendees are made fully aware that their favorable performance in a company's interests can lead to future invitations and larger honoraria. One expert who minimizes the adverse effects of Zyprexa is on a $10,000 per year retainer from Eli Lilly, while another who claims that Remeron reverses depression in suicidal patients more rapidly than other drugs receives $75,000 a year from Organon to support his laboratory (Torrey, 2002a, 2002b).

Beyond the efforts of pharmaceutical companies to bribe prescribers of their drugs, they also purchase the services of editors and authors of papers on drug therapy. Wyeth-Ayerst commissioned ghost-writers to write 10 articles promoting the combination diet drug Fen-Phen for the treatment of obesity. After the drug was withdrawn from the market in 1997 for causing heart-valve damage, it was found during litigation that adverse side effects had been minimized or even deleted by company editors (Ornstein, 1999). In 1998, tobacco companies secretly paid $156,000 to 13 scientists to write letters to influential medical journals; some of these letters were ghostwritten by tobacco-industry law firms (Hanners, 1998). Even the prestigious *New England Journal of Medicine* has found it almost impossible to find editors and authors of review articles on drug therapy issues who do not have any financial conflicts of interest with industry; their editorial policy now allows such authors up to $10,000 in the two-years before publication in payments from any one drug company (McKenzie, 2002).

2. Publishing Favorable Research Results

Another widespread practice among drug manufacturers is publication of studies with favorable findings for their drugs. This is accomplished through several strategies, including initial trial designs favoring a drug, biased analysis, "spinning" of results, misleading reports for publication, selecting journals with less rigorous peer review (especially controlled circulation journals), and suppressing the publication of unfavorable research findings.

Many drug studies are designed to compare the sponsoring company's drug against a placebo, with an insufficient dose of a competing drug, or with another drug which for other reasons, will not compare well with the sponsor's drug. For example, most trials comparing fluconazole with amphotericin B used oral amphotericin B, which is poorly absorbed in the GI tract, thereby predetermining favorable results for fluconazole (Johansen & Gotzche, 1999). In circumstances where all of the raw data are held centrally by the company, it is easy for company investigators to manipulate the data without other participating scientists being aware of such manipulations unless they have access to all of the data. It is common, especially in commercial networks, for research papers to be ghostwritten by professional writers employed by the company or writers under contract at medical communications companies. They may not be listed in a paper's authorship, while a clinical investigator (guest author) who is named has neither analyzed the data, nor written the paper (Larkin, 1999; Levy, 1996; Ghost, 1993). Under those circumstances, the ghostwriters have final say on what is submitted for publication (Rennie & Flanagin, 1994). The results of industry-sponsored research are frequently presented at symposia with little or no peer review, then submitted to journals without rigorous peer review (Bero, Galbraith, Rennie, 1992; Cho & Bero, 1996; Massie & Rothenberg, 1993).

The extent of selective bias in what is published from industry-sponsored drug research is well documented by recent studies. A 2003 report by investigators at Yale University examined the effects of financial conflicts of interest in biomedical research between 1980 and 2002. They found eight articles, which together evaluated 1,140 original studies assessing the relation between industry sponsorship and reported outcomes of research. Aggregate analysis showed that industry sponsorship was almost four times as likely (odds ratio 3.60) to lead to pro-industry conclusions than other sources of support as depicted in Figure 8.1 (Bekelman, Li, Gross, 2003). Another recent study carried out by a research team from the U.S., Canada, and Brazil looked at 30 previous studies that compared the results of industry-sponsored research with that of other sponsors. They found the same kind of systematic bias in reporting results favoring sponsor's products (odds ratio 4.05). They also found that the quality of industry-sponsored research methods were at least as good as the methods used by other sponsors of research. They conclude that publication bias (avoiding publication of unfavorable results) explains much of the difference (Lexchin, Bero, Djulbegovik, Clark, 2003).

In order to avoid the publication of unfavorable results of these studies, pharmaceutical companies have several strategies at their

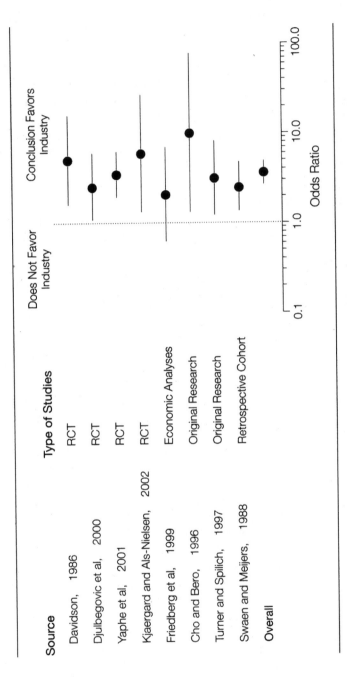

FIGURE 8.1 Relation between industry sponsorship and study outcome in original research studies. *Source:* Bekelman, J. E., et al. (2003). Scope and impact of financial conflict of interest in biomedical research. *Journal of the American Medical Association, 289,* 459. Reprinted with permission.

disposal—block or stall publication of such studies to limit threats to their drugs' market share, arrange to publish competing articles or editorials that minimize adverse findings, and stop funding of a drug trial which appears to be headed for unfavorable results. With regard to the last approach, it is estimated that 20% to 30% of clinical trials are stopped early (Pergolizzi, 2002). While there may be important reasons to abort a trial, many are stopped for "commercial" reasons, not for acknowledged scientific grounds. The latest example is the large, randomized, double-blind equivalence trials of the calcium channel blocker verapamil against less expensive standard therapies (beta-blockers and diuretics) for hypertension. The sponsoring drug company gave no explanation other than "business considerations" for stopping the trial two years early when preliminary results showed no advantage for verapamil (Psaty & Rennie, 2003; Black, et al., 2003).

3. Harass, Intimidate, and Discredit Investigators Who Conduct Unfavorable Studies

The following are just four among many examples of targeted campaigns by industry against investigators who find unfavorable results in studies of their products:

- Herbert Needleman, a pediatrician and psychiatrist, published a study in 1979 which found that children with high dentine lead levels had adverse neuropsychiatric effects, including cognitive and verbal deficits as well as increased frequency of nonadaptive classroom behavior (Needleman, 1979). An ongoing effort was carried out by the lead industry to discredit Needleman's findings by accusing him of scientific misconduct. He had to confront the administration of his university to obtain open hearings (Needleman, 1992). His accusers admitted during hearings at the University of Pittsburgh that they had no specific grounds, but that they wanted the NIH to investigate possible fraud or misconduct. In later years, Needleman's methods, data, and conclusions were confirmed by other studies, and his important work has stood the test of time (National Academy, 1993; Schwartz, 1994; Silbergeld, 1995).
- Nancy Olivieri, a researcher at the University of Toronto, found in a study funded by Apotex that deferiprone, the sponsor's drug used to treat thalassemia major, was ineffective in some

patients and caused liver toxicity in others. The company terminated the trial in 1996 and threatened legal action against Olivieri if she published the results or disclosed the risks to patients. The company invoked a confidentiality clause in the clinical trial agreement (Baird, Downie, Thompson, 2002; Thompson, Baird, Downie, 2001). Despite the concerted efforts by Apotex to suppress publication, an article was eventually published (Olivieri, et al., 1998).

- Gregory Simon, a clinician-investigator at Group Health Cooperative in Seattle, reported a controlled study in 1993 of immunological, psychological, and neuropsychological factors in multiple chemical sensitivity (MCS). The study called into question the value of immunodiagnostic tests used as evidence for disability and liability claims for MCS (Simon, Daniell, Stockbridge, Claypoole, Rosenstock, 1993). Industry representatives from immunologic-testing laboratories were joined by MCS advocacy groups and plaintiffs' attorneys in accusing Simon and his colleagues with scientific misconduct, fraud, and conspiracy. Efforts were made to revoke their licenses and investigations were carried out at three local institutions, the state medical disciplinary board, and the federal Office of Research Integrity. The investigators were completely exonerated after this expensive and stressful process, which eventually led to a local trial lawyer sponsoring a workshop promoting the tactics used in their case as a strategy to dispute unfavorable research findings (Deyo, Psaty, Simon, Wagner, Omenn, 1997).

- Betty Dong, a researcher at the University of California San Francisco, had an article already set in type for publication in the *Journal of the American Medical Association* reporting a study showing that the industry-sponsored drug Synthroid was no more effective than less expensive competing drugs. The company vetoed publication on the basis of its contract, forced withdrawal of the article, accused Dong of scientific misconduct, and began a seven-year campaign to discredit her work. This campaign included publication of another article which "reanalyzed" Dong's data without attribution to its source (Rennie, 1997). Further legal battles included a class-action suit by Synthroid users against the drug company for false advertising of Synthroid's superiority, which was finally settled out of court for $98 million. Dong's article was finally published almost seven years later, in 1997, but meanwhile the company had profited by dominating the $600-million-a-year synthetic thyroid market (Shenk, 1999).

4. Marketing Activities Masquerading as Science

We have already seen in chapter 5 a classic example of marketing disguised as science in the international effort led by Pfizer to define and treat female sexual dysfunction. A similar effort is now underway within the pharmaceutical industry to define "testosterone deficiency," and "andropause" as a silent epidemic in older men requiring widespread treatment. Unimed, the manufacturer of Andro-Gel, is currently funding ads and tests in clinics that provide services to men experiencing "low sex drive" or "low energy". Unimed is also the sole sponsor of annual "consensus conferences" on andropause; at least 9 of the 13 speakers at the 2002 conference had financial ties to Unimed. The FDA has not approved the drug for the treatment of andropause (Groopman, 2002).

The advertising industry is playing a growing role in the business of drug research, as described in a 2002 article in the *New York Times*. The three largest advertising companies have spent tens of millions of dollars to buy or invest in companies that do contract drug research. Omnicom, one of the world's largest advertising companies, paid $20 million in 1999 to become a part-owner of Scirex, one such research firm (Peterson, 2002). Here are three more examples which suggest the size and scope of pseudoscience in the drug industry:

- Although not approved for the treatment of acute pain following dental surgery, Bextra's marketers (Pharmacia and Pfizer) sponsored a small study by Scirex in Texas. "Favorable" results were found for Bextra in a small study group of younger patients, much younger than most who would likely take the drug. The paper was published by *The Journal of the American Dental Association* and Bextra's sales increased by 60% over the next three months. Marketing of drugs for unapproved uses is illegal, and the editor of the journal admitted later that he would have rejected the paper had he realized that it was not FDA-approved for that use (Groopman, 2002).
- Novartis was facing loss of market share for Ritalin, its drug for attention deficit disorder (ADD), as competitors brought longer-acting drugs to market. Without any research evidence, Novartis commissioned a medical education company owned by the global ad giant WPP, to ghostwrite a review article that would suggest theoretical efficacy of its new longer-acting version of Ritalin. That article was never published, and a disillusioned ghostwriter

resigned after 12 years' experience in medical marketing companies (Groopman, 2002).

- Neurontin is approved by the FDA only for epilepsy and the
  pain of patients with shingles. Although marketing for unapproved uses is illegal, it has been heavily marketed by its manufacturer, Warner-Lambert (acquired by Pfizer in 2000) for such
  off-label uses as bipolar disorder and restless leg syndrome. A former
  professor of neurology was paid over $300,000 for promotional
  talks between 1994 and 1997. A whistle-blower suit by a former
  company physician resulted in criminal and civil charges against
  the company. Documents that have surfaced during federal and
  state investigations revealed that Omnicom offered to write journal
  articles promoting the use of Neurontin to treat pain (Groopman,
  2002; Peterson, 2003). As we saw in chapter 5, Pfizer ended up
  paying $430 million to settle these charges (Harris, 2004).

THREATS TO SCIENCE BY THE POLITICS OF VESTED INTERESTS

When results of scientific research run counter to the interests of
industry, a powerful political backlash is often initiated by special
interest groups in an effort to discredit that research or mitigate its
effect on policy. Coalitions with misleading names are often set up to
orchestrate lobbying efforts, even to the point of attacks on funding
and regulatory agencies. The following examples illustrate the extent of these activities, which blur the boundaries between science
and policy while threatening the progress of evidence-based science:

- *Spinal-fusion surgery.* Research in the early 1990s found that spinal-fusion surgery was associated with higher costs and more
  complications than other back operations (Deyo, Cherkin, Loeser, Bigos, Ciol, 1992; Deyo, Ciol, Cherkin, Loeser, Bigos, 1993;
  Turner, Ersek, Herron, Haselkorn, Kent, 1992). These findings
  led the funding agency, the Agency for Health Care Policy and
  Research (AHCPR) to publish guidelines for managing back pain
  that favor nonsurgical approaches. The North American Spine
  Society (NASS) called the research biased, criticized the guidelines, and lobbied Congress through its front group (the Center
  for Patient Advocacy) to eliminate funding for the AHCPR. The
  FDA was also targeted in this campaign because it would not
  approve pedicle-screw devices, commonly used in spinal-fusion

procedures, beyond narrow indications. Funding for AHCPR was cut off by the House of Representatives, but was restored by the Senate at a lesser amount after industry tactics were exposed. As part of this campaign by industry, one manufacturer unsuccessfully sought a court injunction to block the AHCPR from publishing or disseminating its guidelines for treating low back pain (Deyo, Psaty, Simon, Wagner, Omenn, 1997).

- *Risks of guns.* After studies showed risks to family members of guns in the home (Taubes, 1992), coordinated attacks were launched by the National Rifle Association (NRA) and its allies against the agency which funded that research. The National Center for Injury Prevention and Control (NCIPC), part of the Centers for Disease Control and Prevention (CDC), was targeted for elimination by the NRA, which was joined by the Heritage Foundation and Doctors for Integrity in Research and Public Policy, an anti-gun control group which went so far as to call NCIPC research "incompetent and politicized research" that is "a bogus public health assault on our civil rights" (Deyo, Psaty, Simon, Wagner, Omenn, 1997; Kassirer, 1995; Suter, 1995).

- *Diesel exhaust and lung cancer.* Diesel exhaust is a potential carcinogen posing a threat to over one million U.S. workers and many more millions around the world. After conducting a feasibility epidemiologic study of diesel exhaust and lung cancer, the National Institute for Occupational Safety and Health (NIOSH) and the National Cancer Institute (NCI) initiated peer review of the study protocol in 1995. The study has been delayed for years, however, by industry lobby groups. In 1996, a coalition of mine owners and operators and other industry representatives (e.g., the Methane Awareness Resource Group) started litigation claiming that the peer review process violated the Federal Advisory Committee Act (Rosenstock & Lee, 2002; Methane Awareness Resource Group, 1996). Later delaying tactics have included calls for more peer review, access by industry to raw research data, harassment of peer reviewers, and promotion of congressional inquiries into the details of the study design. These tactics have so far successfully blocked the study (Rosenstock & Lee, 2002).

- *National Cancer Institute reversal of mammography recommendation.* In 1997, a National Cancer Institute (NCI) consensus panel concluded that scientific evidence did not support mammography screening for breast cancer for low-risk women in their 40s (NCI, 1997). That conclusion came under immediate fire from external groups with financial or emotional interests in screening. The science was repackaged and the recommendation changed to one favoring screening for women in their 40s every one to two years (Rosenstock & Lee, 2002; Fletcher, 1997).

CONCLUDING COMMENTS

Industry support and involvement is essential to research, development, and innovation in health care. This chapter, however, has revealed many examples of compromise, even corruption, of clinical research through the influence of special interests upon the scientific process. As is obvious from the widespread excesses and conflicts of interest in the interface between research and industry, more transparency and public accountability are needed. Below are some of the proposals put forward by various experts and groups to protect investigators, the integrity of research, funding agencies, and the public interest:

- Investigators must have independence to conduct and publish their own research (Bodenheimer, 2002; Angell, 2000; Deyo, Psaty, Simon, Wagner, Omenn, 1997; Relman & Angell, 2002; Sung, Crowley, Genel, Salber, Sandy, 2003).
- For profit commercial research networks should be curtailed, with strengthening of the academic-industry alliance for clinical research (Bodenheimer, 2002; Horton & Smith, 1999).
- The relationships between academic researchers, their institutions, and industry should be arm's length including more rigorous efforts to control conflicts of interest (Sung, Crowley, Genel, Salber, Sandy, 2003).
- Increased oversight is needed to eliminate conflicts of interest for those selected to serve on advisory groups to government agencies and regulatory bodies (Relman & Angell, 2002).
- The patent system should be revised, with a view toward requiring evidence of usefulness and originality of products (Relman & Angell, 2002).
- A registry should be established for all clinical trials in order to prevent publication bias (Pergolizzi, 2002; Horton & Smith, 1999; Liberati & Magrini 2003; Dickerson & Rennie, 2003).
- Budgets and staffing of the FDA and other regulatory agencies should be increased in order to strengthen the monitoring and regulatory process (Relman & Angell, 2002).

- Direct-to-consumer advertising should be banned as more marketing than educational (Relman & Angell, 2002).

REFERENCES

AAHRPP. (2001). New national accrediting entity launched, Press release. Washington, D.C. Association for the Accreditation of Human Research Protection Programs Inc. Available at *http://www.aahrpp.org/nr_05-23-01.htm*.

AAMC. (2002). Association of American Medical Colleges Task Force on Research Accountability. Report on Individual and Institutional Financial Conflict of Interest. Retrieved December 27, 2002 from *http://www.aau.edu/research/CO1.O1.pdf*.

AAU. (2002). Association of American Universities Task Force on Research Accountability. Report on Individual and Institutional Financial Conflict of Interest. Retrieved December 27, 2002 from *http://www.aau.edu/research/CO1.01.pdf*.

American Federation for Clinical Research (1990). Guidelines for avoiding conflict of interest. *Clinical Research, 38,* 239.

Angell, (2000). M. Is academic medicine for sale? *The New England Journal of Medicine, 342,* 1516.

Baird, P., Downie, J., Thompson, J., (2002). Clinical trials and industry. *Science, 297,* 2211.

Bayh-Dole Act (1980). Public Law No. 96-517, 35USC.

Beecher, H. K., & Altschule, M. D. (1977). *Medicine at Harvard: The first three hundred years.* Hanover, NH: University Press of New England.

Bekelman, J. E., Li, & Gross (2003). Scope and impact of financial conflict of interest in biomedical research. *Journal of the American Medical Association, 289,* 454.

Bero, L., Galbraith, A., Rennie, D. (1992). The publication of sponsored symposiums in medical journals. *The New England Journal of Medicine, 327,* 1135, 1992.

Black, H. R., Elliott, W. I., Grandits, G., Grambeck, P., Lucenti, T., White, W. B., et al., CONVINCE Research Group (2003). Principal results of the Controlled Onset Verapamil Investigation of Cardiovascular Endpoints (CONVINCE) trial. *Journal of the American Medical Association, 289,* 2073.

Blake, J. B. (1957). *Benjamin Waterhouse and the introduction of vaccination: A reappraisal.* Philadelphia: University of Pennsylvania Press.

Bodenheimer, T. (2002). Clinical investigators and the pharmaceutical industry. *The New England Journal of Medicine, 3342,* 1539.

Bok, D. (2003). *Universities in the marketplace: The commercialization of higher education.* Princeton and Oxford, England: Princeton University Press.

Borfitz, D. (2003, June 6). Can "Phase IV" trials work for you? *Medical Economics,* pp. 58–67.

Boyd, F., & Bero, L. (2000). Assessing faculty financial relationships with industry. *Journal of the American Medical Association, 284,* 2209, 2000.

Cash, P., & Waterhouse, B. (1999). In J. A. Garraty & M. C. Carnes (Eds.), *American national biography, Vol. 22.* New York: Oxford University Press.

CenterWatch: (2001). *An industry in evolution.* Boston, MA: Author.

Cho, M. K., & Bero, L. A. (1996). The quality of drug studies published in symposium proceedings. *Annals of Internal Medicine, 124,* 485.

Cho, M. K., Shohara, R., Schissel, A., Rennie, D. (2000). Policies on faculty conflicts of interest at U.S. universities. *Journal of the American Medical Association, 284,* 2203.

Davidson, R. A. (1986). Source of funding and outcome of clinical trials. *Journal of General Internal Medicine, 1,* 155.

DeAngelis, C. D., Fontanarosa, P. B., Flanagin, A. (2001). Reporting financial conflicts of interest and relationships between investigators and research sponsors. *Journal of the American Medical Association, 286,* 89, 2001.

Deyo, R. A., Cherkin, D. C., Loeser, J. D. Bigos, S. I., Ciol, M. A. (1992). Morbidity and mortality in association with operations on the lumbar spine: The influence of age, diagnosis, and procedure. *The Journal of Bone and Joint Surgery, 74,* 536.

Deyo, R. A., Cio, M. A., Cherkin, D. C., Loeser, J. D., Bigos, S. I. (1993). Lumbar spinal fusion: A cohort study of complications, reoperations, and resource use in the Medicare population. *Spine 18,* 1463.

Deyo, R. A., Psaty, B. M., Simon, G., Wagner, E. H. Omenn, G. S. (1997). The messenger under attack: Intimidation of researchers by special interest groups. *The New England Journal of Medicine, 336,* 1176.

Dickerson, K., & Rennie, D. (2003). Registering clinical trials. *Journal of the American Medical Association, 290,* 516.

Djulbegovic, B., Lacevic, M., Cantor, A., Fields, K. K., Bennett, C. L., Adams, J. R., Kuderer, A. M., Lyman, G. H. (2000). The uncertainty principle and industry-sponsored research. *Lancet 356,* 635.

Drazen, J. M., & Curfman, G. D. (2002). Financial associations of authors. *The New England Journal of Medicine, 346,* 1901.

Emanuel, E. J., & Steiner, D. (1995). Institutional conflict of interest. *The New England Journal of Medicine, 332,* 262, 1995.

Fletcher, S. W. (1997). Whither scientific deliberation in health policy recommendations: Alice in the wonderland of breast-cancer screening. *The New England Journal of Medicine, 336,* 1180.

Florida, R. (1999). The role of the university: Leveraging talent, not technology. *Issues in Science and Technology 15,* 67.

Gelijns, A. C., & Thier, S.O. (2002). Medical innovation and institutional interdependence: Rethinking university-industry connections. *Journal of the American Medical Association, 287,* 72.

Getz, K. A. (1999). AMCs rekindling clinical research partnerships with industry. Boston: CenterWatch, 1999.

Ghost with a chance in publishing undergrowth. (1993). *Lancet, 342,* 1498.

Groopman, J. (2002, July 29). Medical dispatch: Hormones for men. *The New Yorker,* pp. 34–38.

Hanners, D. (1998, Aug. 4). Scientists were paid to write letters. Tobacco industry sought to discredit EPA report. *St. Louis Pioneer Dispatch.*

Harris, G. Pfizer to pay $430 million over promoting drug to doctors. *New York Times,* May 14, 2004: C1.

Henderson, L. (1999). The ups and downs of SMO usage. *CenterWatch* 6(5) 1, 4–8.

Hensley, S. (2002, June 13). Side effects. As drug sales teams multiply, doctors start to tune them out. *The Wall Street Journal,* p. A1.

Horton, R., & Smith, R. (1999). Time to register randomized trials. *Lancet 354,* 1138.

ICMJE (2002). Uniform requirements for manuscripts submitted to biomedical journals: Retrieved October 1, 2002 from *http://www.icmje.org/*

Jackson, T. (2001). Are you being duped? *British Medical Journal, 322,* 1312.

Johansen, H. K., & Gotzche, P. C. (1999). Problems in the design and reporting of trials of antifungal agents encountered during meta-analysis. *Journal of the American Medical Association, 282,* 1752.

Kassirer, J. P. (1995). A partisan assault on science: The threat to the CDC. *The New England Journal of Medicine, 333,* 793.

Kelch, R. P. (2002). Maintaining the public trust in clinical research. *The New England Journal of Medicine, 346,* 285.

Kjaergard, L., & Als-Nielsen, B. ((2002). Association between competing interests and authors' conclusion: Epidemiological study of randomized clinical trials. *British Medical Journal, 325,* 249.

Korn, D. (2000). Conflicts of interest in biomedical research. *Journal of the American Medical Association, 284,* 2234.

Larkin, M. (1999). Whose article is it anyway? *Lancet 354,* 136.

National Academy of Sciences.. (1993). *Measuring lead exposures in infants, children, and other sensitive populations.* Washington, DC: Author.

Levy, D. (1996, Sept. 25). Ghostwriters a hidden resource for drug makers. *USA Today.*

Lexchin, J. (1993). Interactions between physicians and the pharmaceutical industry: What does the literature say? *Canadian Medical Association Journal, 149,* 1401.

Lexchin, J., Bero, L. A., Djulbegovic, B., Clark, O. (2003). Pharmaceutical industry sponsorship and research outcome and quality: A systematic review. *British Medical Journal, 326,* 1167.

Liberati, A., & Magrini, N. (2003). Information from drug companies and opinion leaders. *British Medical Journal, 326,* 1156.

Lo, B., Wolf, L. E. Berkeley, A. (2000). Conflict-of-interest policies for investigations in clinical trials. *The New England Journal of Medicine, 343,* 1616.

Massie, B. M., & Rothenberg, D. (1993). Publication of sponsored symposiums in medical journals. *The New England Journal of Medicine, 328,* 1196.

McKenzie, J. (2002, July). Conflict of interest. Medical journal changes policy of finding independent authors to write. ABC Evening News, June 12 and published in *Health Letter*, p. 7.

Methane Awareness Resource Group (1996). Diesel Coalition versus United States of America, filed October 23.

Moses, H. 3rd., Braunwald, E., Martin, J. B. Thier, S. O. (2002). Collaborating with industry. *The New England Journal of Medicine, 347*, 1371.

Moynihan, R. (2003). Who pays for the pizza? Redefining the relationships between doctors and drug companies, I: Entanglement. *British Medical Journal, 326*, 1189.

National Cancer Institute. (1997). Breast cancer screening for women ages 40 to 49. January 21–23, 1997, Bethesda, Maryland: National Institutes of Health Consensus Statements.

Needleman, H. L., et al. (1979). Deficits in psychologic and classroom performance of children with elevated dentine lead levels. *The New England Journal of Medicine, 300*, 689.

Needleman, H. L. (1992). Salem comes to the National Institutes of Health: Notes from inside the crucible of scientific integrity. *Pediatrics, 90*, 977.

NIH (2003). Competing and non-competing research grants, fiscal years 1992–2002. Retrieved February 12, 2003 from *http://grants.nih.gov/grants/award/research/rgmechtype9202.htm*

Olivieri, N. F., Brittenham, G. M., McClaren, C. E., Templeton, D. M., Cameron, R. G., McClellan, R. A. (1998). Long-term safety and effectiveness of iron-chelation therapy with deferiprone for thalassemia major. *The New England Journal of Medicine, 339*, 417.

Ornstein, C. (1999, May 23). Fen-phen maker accused of funding journal articles. *Dallas Morning News*, p. 1A.

Page, L. (2003). OIG warns drug makers on "suspect" relations. *Modern Physician, 7*(5), 2.

Pergolizzi, J. V. (2002). Early termination: conflicts and concerns. *Clinical Research, 2*, 4.

Peterson, M. (2002, Nov. 22). Madison Avenue plays growing role in the business of drug research. *The New York Times*, p. A1.

Peterson, M. (2003, May 30). Court papers suggest sale of drug's use. *The New York Times*, p. C1.

PhRMA. (2003). PhRMA code: On interactions with healthcare professionals. Retrieved April 28, 2003 from wwwpharmaorg/publications/policy/2002-04-19.939)

PhRMA. (2002). Pharmaceutical Research and Manufacturers of America 2002 Industry Profile. Available at *http://grants.nih.gov/grants/award/research/rgmechtype9202.htm* Accessed July 25, 2001.

Psaty, B. M., & Rennie, D. (2003). Stopping medical research to save money: A broken pact with researchers and patients. *The Journal of the American Medical Association, 289*, 2128.

Public Health (2000). 42 C.E.R. ch. 1, ¶ 50, subpart F (2000). Retrieved May 21, 2002 from *http://grants2nih.gov/grants/compliance/42_CFS_50_Subpart_F.htm*

Relman, A. S., & Angell, M. (2002, Dec. 16). America's other drug problem: How the drug industry distorts medicine and politics. *The New Republic*, pp. 27–41.

Rennie, D. M. (1997). Thyroid storm. *The Journal of the American Medical Association, 277*, 1242.

Rennie, D., & Flanagin, A. (1994). Authorship! Authorship! Guests, ghosts, grafters, and the two-sided coin. *The Journal of the American Medical Association, 271*, 469.

Rosenstock, L., & Lee, L. I. (2002). Attacks on science: The risks to evidence-based policy. *American Journal of Public Health, 92*, 14.

Schwartz, J. (1994). Low lead level exposure and children's IQ: A meta-analysis and search for a threshold. *Environmental Research, 65*, 42.

Schulman, K. A., Seils, D. M., Timbie, J. W., Sugarman, J., Dame, L. A., Weinfurt, K. P., et al., (2002). A national survey of provisions in clinical-trial agreements between medical schools and industry sponsors. *The New England Journal of Medicine, 347*, 1335.

Shenk, D. (1999, March 22). Money + sciences = ethics problems on campus. *The Nation*, pp. 11–12.

Silbergeld, E. K. (1995). Annotation: Protection of the public interest, allegations of scientific misconduct, and the Needleman case. *American Journal of Public Health, 85*, 165.

Simon, G. E., Daniell, W., Stockbridge, H., Claypoole, K., Rosenstock, L. (1993). Immunologic, psychological, and neuropsychological factors in multiple chemical sensitivity: A controlled study. *Annals of Internal Medicine, 119*, 97.

Smith, R. (2003). Medical journals and pharmaceutical companies: Uneasy bedfellows. *British Medical Journal, 326*, 1202.

Steinbrook, R. (2004). Financial conflicts of interest and the NIH. *The New England Journal of Medicine, 350*(4): 327–330.

Stelfox, H. T., Chua, G., O'Rourke, K., Detsky, A. S. (1998). Conflict of interest in the debate over calcium-channel antagonists. *The New England Journal of Medicine, 338*, 101.

Sung, N. S., Crowley, W. F. Jr., Genal, M., Solber, P., Sands, L., Sherwood, L. M., Johnson, S. B. (2003) Central challenges facing the national clinical research enterprise. *The Journal of the American Medical Association, 289*, 1278.

Suter, E. A. (1995, May 1). Internet communication concerning Doctors for Integrity in Research and Public Policy Newsletter.

Swaen, G., & Meiers, J. (1988). Influence of design characteristics on the outcome of retrospective cohort studies. *British Journal of Industrial Medicine, 45*, 624.

Taubes, G. (1992). Violence epidemiologists test the hazards of gun ownership. *Science, 258*, 213.

Thompson, J., Baird, P., Downie, J. (2001). *The Olivieri Report*. Toronto, Ontario: James Lorimer & Co Ltd.

Torry, E. F. (2002a, July 15). The going rate on shrinks: Big PhRMA and the buying of psychiatry. *American Prospect 26.*

Torry, E. F. (2002b). Big PhRMA buys psychiatry: An aura of scandal. *Health Letter, 18*(7), 1.

Turner, J. A., Ersek, M., Herron, L., Haselkorn, J., Kent, D., Ciol, M. A., Deyo, R. (1992). Patient outcomes after lumbar spinal fusions. *Journal of the American Medical Association, 268,* 907.

Turner, C., & Spilich, G. J. (1997). Research into smoking or nicotine and human cognitive performance: Does the source of funding make a difference? *Addiction, 92,* 1423.

Vogel, J. R. (1999). Maximizing the benefits of SMOs. *Applied Clinical Trials, 8*(11), 56.

Watkins, C., Moore, L., Harvey, I., Carthy, P., Robinson, E., & Brown, R. (2003). Characteristics of general practitioners who frequently see drug industry representatives: National cross sectional survey. *British Medical Journal, 326,* 1178.

Wazana, A. (2000). Physicians and the pharmaceutical industry: Is a gift ever just a gift? *Journal of the American Medical Association, 283,* 373.

Willman, D. (2003, Dec. 7). Stealth merger: drug companies and government research. *Los Angeles Times:* A1.

Yaphe, J., Edman, R., Kinishkowy, B., Herman, J. (2001). The association between funding by commercial interests and study outcome in randomized controlled drug trials. *Family Practice, 18,* 565.

Chapter 9

DISINFORMATION AND MEDIA CONTROL

Thanks to addictive doses of sympathetic governmental policies and two decades of a drive for power, a shrinking number of large media corporations now regard monopoly, oligopoly, and historic levels of profit as not only normal, but as their earned right. In the process, the usual democratic expectation for the media—diversity of ownership and ideas—has disappeared as the goal of official policy and, worse, as a daily experience of a generation of American readers and viewers.

Ben Bagdikian
Author of The Media Monopoly

We are now immersed in a period marked increasingly by corporate control of the economy, social views, and politics. In earlier chapters we have seen the growing trends toward mergers, consolidation, and oligopoly across the overall health care industry, including hospitals, insurance companies, and the pharmaceutical industry. American mass media are no exception to this pattern. A "quiet revolution" has already taken place over the last 25 years, which has led to more corporate control of the mainstream media than most Americans realize. For the first time in U.S. history, the nation's news, commentary, and entertainment media are controlled by six of the world's largest corporations, two of them foreign (Bagdikian, 2000). As will be apparent later in this chapter, this kind of control promotes the marketing agendas of corporate interests in health care while depriving Americans of objective information needed to make their own health care decisions.

This chapter has four goals: (1) to examine the extent of corporate control of the media, including print, television, radio, and the Internet; (2) to describe and illustrate various ways by which corporate interests manipulate the news and even the content of professional media; (3) to briefly discuss three important health policy issues as they have been distorted by corporate interests; and (4) to describe the current effort by a few corporations to align themselves with social responsibility.

CORPORATE CONTROL OF THE MEDIA

Six large firms dominate all American mass media. Typically, they operate across multiple industries as subsidiaries of giant corporations. Ranked in order of their annual media revenues, the top six are AOL Time Warner, Disney, Viacom (a merger of CBS and Westinghouse), News Corp, Bertelsmann, and General Electric. Rupert Murdock's News Corp is based in Australia and Bertelsmann is based in Germany (Bagdikian, 2000). The breadth of their reach is enormous. AOL Time Warner, for example, is one of the largest players in book and magazine publishing, cable television, television show production, film production, recorded music, and Internet service provision. Overall, about two dozen firms control an overwhelming proportion of American movies, television, radio, magazines, newspapers, and billboards (Bagdikian, 2002). The model in each major type of media is the same—monopoly.

Print Media

In 1946, 80% of all American newspapers were owned by individuals or independent local firms. Today, 80% are owned by corporate chains, and three corporations alone control most of the country's 11,000 magazines. The large national newspaper chains also own the more profitable television and cable channels. The five largest book publishers, in decreasing order, are Bertelsmann, AOL Time Warner, Disney, Viacom, and News Corp. As the world's third largest conglomerate, Bertelsmann holds major ownership of magazines, newspapers, television, radio, films, and online trading in 53 countries (Bagdikian, 2000).

Television

There are six television networks—Fox, United Paramount Network (also owned by Viacom), Warner Brothers, ABC, CBS, and NBC. The ten largest cable systems account for 75% of the cable market in the country. Television has become the primary medium by which large corporations influence the culture and behavior of Americans. The

100 largest corporations pay for about 75% of commercial television time and 50% of public television time. Since a half-minute of television time sells for $200,000 to $300,000, only large corporations can afford it, and it is highly profitable for the networks (Korten, 2001). Fox News, which held the franchise for Super Bowl XXXIII in 1999, charged over $53,000 per second for commercials (The New York Times, 1999). The amount of time allotted to commercials and non-program content in prime-time network shows grew from about 13 1/2 minutes per hour in 1992 to over 16 minutes in 2001 (Mink, 2002).

Radio

The Federal Communication Commission (FCC) recently permitted four giant media corporations to buy up radio stations across the country. As a result, these four corporations now control 90% of total advertising revenues (Hartmann, 2002).

Internet

Although many people assume that the Internet represents the last bastion of "free press" in our culture, even this is not the case. Anyone can establish a Web site, but it is very difficult to develop a commercially viable Web site without affiliation with or ownership by an existing media corporation. Just four corporations own the Web sites that are consistently viewed by more than 50% of Americans (Jupiter Media Matrix, 2001). Media giants have several big advantages as they colonize the Internet—they have existing digital programming, they can bring along advertisers as part of their contracts, they can publicize their Web programs through traditional media, and they have market leverage with Internet service providers, search engines and portals to get desired positioning (Bagdikian, 2002).

As a result of the increased consolidation and corporate control of the media in recent years, there has been a striking decrease in the diversity of views presented to, and genuine debate of major issues by, the public. Indeed, media power is political power, and corporate interests have put forward content that supports their interests, while avoiding content which may threaten their interests. While almost one-third of American voters hold liberal political views, according to a 1999 survey by the Roper Center for Public Opinion Research, major media news and commentary are concentrated on center-to-right politics, with comparative silence of progressive views (Roper Center, 1999). A 2000 survey by the Pew Center for People found that 61% of investigative reporters believe that corporate owners influence news decisions, with 41% of reporters able to recall specific examples of recent occasions when they had been forced to choose, change, or avoid certain news stories to meet corporate interests (Hartmann, 2002; Pew Center, 2000). The following examples illustrate important issues which have been largely suppressed or underreported by corporate media interests in recent years:

- During the 2000 presidential campaign, major television networks successfully blocked the inclusion of Green Party candidate Ralph Nader from three presidential debates, thus avoiding his discussion of corporate power and media consolidation (Bagdikian, 2002).
- Criticism of NAFTA and WTO arrangements has been quiet compared with media coverage of the claimed benefits of globalization, which serve the corporations well.
- As social programs and welfare benefits for the poor have been cut in recent years, large corporations have continued to receive tax forgiveness and payments for transferring their industries to foreign countries, with the loss of some 300,000 jobs for working people in the U.S. (*Time*, 1998; *The New York Times*, 1998).
- As Congress has proceeded to cut governmental programs, the nation's wealth has been transferred from the middle class and working poor to the most affluent so that the U.S. now has the widest gap between the rich and nonrich of any industrialized democratic country (Thurlow, 1999).

The erosion of the democratic process through corporate influences on the media led Ben Bagdikian, dean emeritus of the Graduate School of Journalism at the University of California at Berkeley and author of *The Media Monopoly*, now in its 6th edition, to this observation:

Such concentrated private power is not what the creators of the American democracy had in mind when they created the First Amendment guaranteeing free speech and free press. They could not foresee that two hundred years later, by the twenty-first century, the sacred First Amendment guaranteeing every citizen free speech would, to an appalling degree, become dependent upon the "speaker's wealth" (Bagdikian, 2000).

And further, as noted by Jeff Gates in his book *Democracy at Risk: Rescuing Main Street from Wall Street:*

> Recent changes in the rules governing this essential element of our democratic well-being ensured that access to the political arena is now "financialized"—you must pay to play. From Tom Paine's revolutionary pamphlets extolling *Common Sense*, here we are, two centuries later—with profound advances in telecommunications, yet forced to cope with a media that has morphed into a phenomenon adored by Wall Street but perilous to the open debate required for a robust democracy. Instead, democracy is fast becoming a commercial parody of itself as our airwaves are used to sell us an unsustainable lifestyle—along with mediocre political candidates—instead of exposing us to some much needed common sense. (Gates, 2000).

CORPORATE MANIPULATION OF HEALTH CARE MEDIA

There is a wide spectrum of techniques, some obvious and others less so, by which corporate interests distort health care news and reports, both for lay and professional audiences. Below are some typical examples.

Lay Public Media

1. Promotional "News" ("Infomercials")
Video news reports, through such spokesmen as Walter Cronkite, have been broadcast by local TV stations for years. More recently, that marketing strategy is being expanded to public television and the Web by hiring celebrity newscasters in an effort to buy credibility. Journalists are told that their content is educational, but in fact it is promotional material edited and approved by the PR firms. WJMK Inc., is a Florida-based firm which produces "news break" videos for drug companies, at a cost of about $15,000 each, which are then provided without charge to public television stations across the country. Disguised as news, these videos provide favorable reports of products created and funded by drug company public relations firms, and they omit mention of payments by drug manufacturers. Healthology is another firm, based in New York City, which creates videos for drug companies for distribution on the Web. Again, corporate sponsors are not disclosed, nor are the financial conflicts of interest of the speakers being interviewed, and the FDA has warned some manufacturers about statements not supported by scientific evidence (Peterson, 2003).

2. Biased News Media Coverage

Similar distortions occur regularly in newspaper and television reports, but it is less clear to what extent this is due to corporate influence or inaccurate reporting. As we saw in the last chapter, most published studies of drugs report favorable results, unfavorable results are suppressed, and commercial sponsorship of published reports is often not disclosed. It therefore comes as no surprise that coverage by the news media is frequently slanted in favor of tests or treatments. Two recent studies confirm this point. Moynihan and his colleagues studied coverage by U.S. newspapers and television networks of three drugs—pravastatin, alendronate, and aspirin. Of 207 stories, less than one-half mentioned potential harm to patients and only 30% mentioned costs. Financial ties to manufacturers were often not disclosed, as shown in Table 9.1 (Moynihan, Bero, Ross-Degnan, Henry, Lee, 2000). Those financial disclosures that were made are probably over-represented, since such ties have been found to be underreported in scientific publications (Krimsky & Rothenberg, 1998).

A second study examined the coverage by the 10 highest circulation U.S. newspapers and the three major television networks of the controversy over screening mammography for women in their 40s (Schwartz & Woloshin, 2002). As we saw in the last chapter, an NIH consensus panel concluded in January 1997 that routine screening mammography was not indicated for low-risk women in their 40s (NIH, 1997). Two months later, after intense political pressure from special interest groups, the National Cancer Institute reversed that recommendation to one favoring such screening (Fletcher, 1997). Newspaper and television coverage over the next two weeks overwhelmingly supported screening mammography for this age group (96%) while potential harms were minimized (see Figure 9.1). Advocacy groups and politicians were actively involved in this policy reversal, also pressing for insurance coverage for this procedure (Schwartz & Woloshin, 2002).

3. Other Public Relations Deceptions

Media manipulation by corporate interests through PR firms is common as they seek to increase product recognition and market share or to defuse bad publicity. Drug and biotechnology PR can be carefully scripted to promote products of questionable efficacy and safety. Many strategies are available to PR firms, including hiring consultants as product champions, funding speakers' bureaus and editorialists, organizing symposia for presentations of papers favoring products of corporate sponsors, ghostwriting journal articles, cre-

TABLE 9.1. Quantification of Benefits, Coverage of Adverse Effects and Costs, and Disclosure of Ties With Industry in Media Stories, According to Type of Medium*

Characteristic of Story	Television		Leading National Newspapers		Other Newspapers	
	$ (no./total no.)	95% CI	% (no./total no.)	95% CI	% (no./total no.)	95% CI
Did not quantify benefits	37(10/27)	19–58	36(19/53)	23–50	43(54/127)	34–52
Quantified benefits						
Only relative benefits	88(15/17)	64–98	74(25/34)	56–97	86(63/73)	76–93
Only absolute benefits	0(0/17)	0–20†	0(0/34)	0–10†	10(7/73)	4–19
Relative and absolute benefits	12(2/17)	1–36	26(9/34)	13–44	4(3/73)	1–12
Adverse effects and costs						
Adverse effects mentioned	48(13/27)	29–68	45(24/53)	32–60	48(61/127)	39–57
Costs mentioned	22(6/27)	9–42	32(17/53)	20–46	31(40/127)	24–40
Ties with industry (excluding aspirin)						
Cited expert or study	85(17/20)	62–97	89(34/39)	75–97	83(68/92)	73–90
Cited expert or study with tie‡	82(14/17)	57–96	79(27/34)	62–91	63(43/69)	51–75
Disclosed tie§	0(0/14)	0–23†	48(13/27)	13–83¶	47(20/43)	27–66¶

Source: Moynihan, R., et al. (2000). Coverage by the news media of the benefits and risks of medications. *The New England Journal of Medicine, 342,* 1648. Reprinted with permission.

*CI denotes confidence interval.

†The one-sided 97.5 percent confidence interval is given because the percentage is zero.

‡The story quoted at least one expert or study-group member with a tie, as determined by a search of the published scientific literature.

§The tie was also disclosed in the media story.

¶The 95 percent confidence intervals were adjusted for clustering by a variance-inflation factor.

Source: Reprinted with permission from Moynihan R. et al. Coverage by the news media of the benefits and risks of medications. *New England Journal of Medicine, 342,* 1648, 2000.

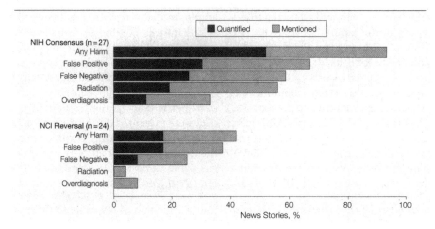

FIGURE 9.1 Proportion of news stories mentioning and quantifying specific potential risks of mammography.

Source: Schwartz, L. M., & Woloshin, S. (2002). News medical coverage of screening mammography for women ion their 40s and tamoxifen for primary prevention of breast cancer. FIGURE 2. *Journal of the American Medical Association, 287,* 3140. Adapted with permission.

ating disease awareness campaigns, and mobilizing "third party" allies to counter industry critics (Burton & Rowell, 2003a). Edelman, the largest independently owned PR firm in the world, is based in New York with an international network of offices. Excerpta Medica is another large PR firm often hired by pharmaceutical and other medical companies to help launch new products. It has even claimed responsibility for developing new medical journals to "establish a scientific base" for its clients' products (Zuckerman, 2003). Here are three examples of marketing and deceptive activities of PR firms:

- Soon after the combination diet drug fen-phen was removed from the market in 1997 due to potentially fatal damage to heart valves, the drug manufacturer commissioned "research" articles and editorials in journals claiming that the drugs were really not hazardous (Zuckerman, 2003).
- Major studies in 2001 and 2002 which revealed high complication rates and potentially life-threatening risks of breast implants were minimized in the press while a 1999 report touted by implant manufacturers and plastic surgeons claiming safety of these implants received wide press coverage (Zuckerman, 2003).

- In 2002, when the NIH stopped its eight-year trial of Prempro, Wyeth's market-leading hormone replacement therapy (HRT) drug, due to increased incidence of adverse effects, Wyeth launched a major PR counterattack. Faced with plummeting drug sales and share prices, it mobilized the Washington, D.C.-based Society for Women's Health Research (SWHR), which rebuked the NIH decision and distributed op-ed pieces and letters to newspapers across the country. Wyeth and other drug companies are represented on the group's corporate advisory board, and Wyeth sponsors its annual fundraising ball at the Washington Ritz-Carlton (Burton & Rowell, 2003b).

As editors of the quarterly *PR Watch: Public Interest Reporting on the PR/Public Affairs Industry,* John Stauber and Sheldon Rampton note how these kinds of PR campaigns place the public at a disadvantage:

> . . . ordinary citizens cannot afford the multi-million-dollar campaigns that PR firms undertake on behalf of their special interest clients, usually large corporations, business associations and governments. Raw money enables the PR industry to mobilize private detectives, attorneys, broadcast faxes, satellite feeds, sophisticated information systems and other expensive, high-tech resources to out-maneuver, overpower and outlast true citizen reformers (Stauber & Rampton, 1995).

4. "Education" of Vulnerable Groups
Two examples illustrate how corporate-sponsored "education" programs can be targeted to populations which may be more susceptible to these programs:

- Channel One is an advertiser-sponsored school television program which reaches more than 12,000 schools in the country with news and ads for candy bars, fast food, and sneakers. Schools are provided with a satellite dish and video equipment for each classroom and have to agree to show the 12 minute broadcasts on at least 90% of school days to 90% of the children, without interruption. Scholastic, Inc is a leading producer of these kinds of "curriculum" materials (Meadows, 1992; Monar, 1994).
- A 24-hour-a-day television network, Patient Channel, was recently launched by General Electric's GE Medical Systems to reach hospitalized patients. Corporate sponsors claim that these "educational" programs will empower patients with more

knowledge of diseases and treatments. Of course, there are extensive ads for sponsors' drugs, and the program is expected to reach 22 million patients and generate $20 to $40 million a year in advertising revenue (Vranica, 2002).

Professional Media

The boundaries between marketing and education/research are blurred in the professional media as well through "checkbook science," a term coined by Diane Zuckerman, president of the National Center for Policy Research for Women and Families, a nonpartisan, nonprofit think tank (Zuckerman, 2003). As we have seen earlier, corporate sponsors have many ways to hype their products through contracted communications and market research firms. Grey Healthcare Group, the world's fifth largest healthcare communications company, illustrates how this industry works. Grey provides advertising, public relations, meeting and symposium management, Web-based initiatives, and contract sales for pharmaceutical and other health care companies. Its ad for GlaxoSmith Klein's Advair Diskus asthma drug won the industry's Best Professional Ad award in 2002. Grey has established a strategic partnership with MedPanel, an online market research firm specializing in access to thought leaders. Together, according to their public trade announcement in 2002, they are "able to improve efficiency and scale on projects such as emotional insight research; branding and positioning, white paper and creative concept testing, clinical trial design research, and online Adboard momentum meetings. MedPanel prepitch studies also helped Grey achieve a 57% pitch success rate for new business (MedPanel, 2002).

Three recent studies of the content of professional literature show the extent to which it is adversely influenced by manipulation by corporate sponsors. One study compared review articles published in peer-reviewed and throwaway, controlled circulation journals which are largely supported by advertising. Not surprisingly, the more systematic and rigorous reviews in peer-reviewed journals were found to be of higher methodologic and reporting quality. Review articles in throwaway journals, especially likely to be written by authors with financial ties to corporate sponsors, were consistently rated by readers as more readable, practical, and relevant to their practices (Rochon et al., 2002). A second study examined research abstracts of presentations at scientific meetings. While they are usually preliminary and have been subjected to little peer review, they are often given extensive high profile press coverage (Schwartz, Woloshin,

Berger, 2002). This is especially true when meeting organizers issue press releases, which typically are written by press officers with little or no peer review and without disclosure of financial conflicts of interest (Woloshin & Schwartz, 2002).

SOME DISTORTED POLICY ISSUES

It is instructive to consider how the debates over two major health policy issues of our times have been influenced and distorted by media campaigns sponsored by corporate interests in defense of the present market-based system.

The Medicare Prescription Drug Benefit

The pharmaceutical industry wants, above all, to protect its pricing prerogatives and maintain its high profit margins in the U.S. market. Without price controls in the U.S., the industry generates more than 60% of its profits in this country (Siegal, 2003). The drug industry is joined by the health insurance industry as well as other health care industries in wanting to preserve and promote the market-based system. Some of the strategies orchestrated by corporate stakeholders over the last three years concerning a Medicare prescription drug benefit are described below:

- During the 2000 election campaigns, hiding behind its front group, Citizens for Better Medicare, the drug industry spent $65 million on radio and television spots. One such spot featured a concerned senior named "Flo" who was depicted as worried about the government's role in adding a prescription drug benefit to Medicare.—Flo stated"I don't want big government in my medicine cabinet" (Viason, 2002).
- In 2001 and 2002, the drug industry used another front group, United Seniors Association, as hired guns to promote its interests in the continuing debate over how a prescription drug benefit could be added under Medicare. Through radio and television "issue" ads paid for by corporate funds, government subsidies of private insurers were pushed as a strategy to increase the private sector's role and decrease the ability of Medicare to negotiate deep price discounts (Viason, 2002). This approach coincided well with the goal of many Republicans to dismantle and privatize Medicare (i.e., kill it in order to save it)!

- By the summer of 2003, as a conference committee in Congress considered how to reconcile the House and Senate bills for a prescription drug benefit, it became clear that corporate lobbying and media campaigns had been successful in avoiding price controls and discussion of the real issue—why drug prices are so high—and in gaining government subsidies supporting the private sector. This legislative victory by corporate interests took place despite the preference by most Americans over age 65 to receive their prescription drug benefit under the traditional Medicare program. For example, a national survey by the Kaiser Family Foundation released in June 2003 found that less than one-quarter of seniors preferred private health plans for a prescription drug benefit (Fong, 2003). Meanwhile, private health insurers lobbied Congress for increased payments to the private sector, warning that Medicare HMOs and PPOs cannot be relied upon, and may further exit the Medicare market, if they are underfunded (Pear, 2003).

Health Care Reform

The debate over a prescription drug benefit for Medicare beneficiaries revealed the same fault lines that exist between stakeholders in the market-based system and the public at large. As the larger debate proceeds on how to reform the health care system to increase access and quality while controlling costs, corporate-sponsored media messages perpetuate myths, spread disinformation, and avoid coverage of the basic issues.

One key issue, which is carefully avoided, is why health care costs have become unaffordable for such a large part of the population. A basic premise, put forth without evidence by private sector interests, is that *overuse* of health care is a major problem that can be controlled by giving consumers more choice and responsibility for their own health care decisions. While perhaps true for those for whom health care costs are not a problem, this premise disregards the larger role in health care inflation of the unimpeded market power of insurers, drug and medical device manufacturers, hospitals, and other suppliers of health care services (Marmor & Sullivan, 2003). It avoids discussion of the fact that health insurance costs increased 250% more than the rate of medical inflation in 2002, that for-profit HMOs take 15% to 33% of every premium dollar in overhead and profits, and that tens of millions of Americans suffer adverse consequences every day due to *underuse* of health care (Court & Flanigan, 2003).

While the overuse theory has established itself as a theoretical underpinning for cost containment among consumer-choice "reform" alternatives, market-based stakeholders nurture the myth, again without evidence, that the private sector is more efficient, gives better value (because of "competition"), and better fits the American culture than a public-based system. The rationale and evidence on both sides of this issue will be examined in chapter 12. For now, however, here are some examples of how the debate over health care reform is being shaped and slanted by the media:

- A major national awareness campaign was launched in 2002 culminating in a *Cover the Uninsured* week in March of 2003. It was funded by private foundations and corporate interests and drew broad support from the business community. Although town hall and other discussion forums were mobilized across the country to discuss alternative approaches to covering the more than 43 million Americans without health insurance, only incremental "reforms" were considered, which would leave the private sector intact without built-in cost containment. Single-payer health insurance was not on the table. Two common denominators of market-based proposals advanced by insurers for "universal health care" are that they build on the existing system and leave it to an expanded public sector to cover those who can't afford private health insurance (Court & Flanagan, 2003).
- A ballot initiative (Measure 23) to establish single-payer universal health care in Oregon was rejected in November 2002 after a disinformation campaign by a coalition of insurance companies which outspent proponents by more than 30 to 1 and blanketed the media with negative ads. An *NBC Nightly News* broadcast gave little credence to Measure 23 with biased and inaccurate reporting that repeated insurers' warnings that it could bankrupt the state while never asking how its costs would compare with the existing, more expensive system. NBC is owned by General Electric, itself heavily invested in the insurance and medical industries, but no disclosure of that conflict of interest was given (Hart & Naurecker, 2002).
- In a lengthy article on the health care proposals of the nine Democratic presidential candidates in May 2003, *The Washington Post* gave a one-sentence dismissal of Representative Dennis Kucinich's proposal for single-payer national health insurance (Goldstein & Balz, 2003).

- Canada's single-payer health care system, though costing less than one-half of the U.S. system and having better performance outcomes, is largely neglected by U.S. media, and when covered is done so in a biased and negative way. A multimedia campaign was carried out in March 2000 by Citizens for Better Medicare, a drug industry front group, urging American seniors to reject the Canadian approach to drug coverage and pricing (Marmor & Sullivan, 2000). *ABC News* and *The New York Times* called attention to Canada's current problems with overcrowding of emergency rooms without mentioning that this also has become a major problem in the U.S. Disinformation was spread about the costs of Canadian health care, its alleged inefficiency (it is much more efficient than ours), and the level of public support for it (Ackerman, 2000). In fact, the Canadian system is underfunded and does have gaps in coverage, but a recent Romanow Report has called for needed improvements in coverage and funding (Romanow, 2002). Moreover, a November 2000 poll of more than 2,500 Canadians found overwhelming support for their system (Picard, 2000).

As a result of corporate influence on the media, often below the radar screen of public awareness, a rational national debate on the costs of health care and universal health care has so far not been possible. As Marmor and Sullivan point out:

> It is almost impossible when the news media act like an echo chamber, amplifying the voices of the already heard. Well-financed interest groups have lobbyists who are paid and prodded to comment and who show up regularly in debates that journalists try to "balance." The trouble is that there are 50 industry spokespeople for every underfinanced representative of ordinary citizens. The news all too often then turns out to be what prominent figures in the medical-commercial complex claim. No wonder that Americans support the reform principles of universal coverage but express fear at most efforts to act on them. (Marmor & Sullivan, 2003).

Ralph Nader goes further, based on considerable experience with the media over the years:

> There is also a self-interest on the part of the major media conglomerates. They are after all, businesses that rely on advertising revenue and the goodwill of the surrounding business community. . . . No democracy worth its salt can rely so pervasively on the commercial media. (Nader, 2002).

CORPORATE SOCIAL RESPONSIBILITY: THE PR MASKS OF SMOKE AND MIRRORS

Recognizing increasing public concern over exorbitant CEO compensation, corporate welfare, and corporate scandals, Business for Social Responsibility was established during the 1990s. A growing number of Fortune 500 companies are joining this new national organization, including General Motors, Johnson & Johnson, Procter & Gamble, Motorola, and Reebok. Some of these companies are undertaking new socially responsive initiatives in their communities, such as offering skill development and retraining programs for their workers, and giving workers incentives to help the homeless, renovate low-income housing, or tutor in local schools (Derber, 1998). As much as this new direction is needed, there is a considerable gap between the rhetoric and image of social responsibility and actual corporate behavior, as shown by the following two examples.

Philip Morris and the Tobacco Industry

In the 1990s, tobacco companies were facing billion dollar lawsuits brought by state attorneys general for smoking-related claims. The industry agreed to a settlement, concluded in 1998, obligating it to pay about $200 billion over 25 years to the states. It also agreed to stop marketing cigarettes to children, disband the industry's think tanks and research institutes, and stop sponsoring sporting events and concerts (Center for Public Integrity, 2000; Master Settlement Agreement, 1998). The companies initially agreed to drop full-page ads in glossy magazines, such as the Marlboro Man in *Sports Illustrated* and "You've come a long way, baby" in Vogue, but a hue and cry was raised by magazine publishers as they foresaw losses in advertising revenue over $1 billion, and this concession was not included in the final agreement (Federal Document Clearing House, 1996; Mundy, 1996).

Philip Morris is now admitting in brief television news spots in the U.S. that nicotine is addictive and that smoking carries risks that can only be avoided by not smoking. The company is also running a television campaign encouraging parents to counsel their children not to smoke. However, Philip Morris has moved most of its tobacco business overseas beyond the reach of federal law and the new controls of the 1998 settlement, now dominates a global food industry to sanitize its image, and aggressively markets its tobacco products abroad (Derber, 1998). A 2003 court decision in an Illinois class-action suit imposed a $10 billion payment on the company for failing to inform consumers, even after the 1998 settlement, that its "light" cigarettes are not less harmful than its regular cigarettes (Day, 2003).

Despite the public health risk of smoking and the CDC's estimate of 440,000 annual deaths attributed to tobacco (CDC, 2002), the industry still receives millions of taxpayer dollars each year in government tax supports for tobacco. In addition, the U.S. Supreme Court recently struck down, in another of a series of cases, public health regulation of advertising as a violation of the First Amendment (Bayer, Gostin, Javitt, Brandt, 2002). Corporations since 1886 have been granted the same rights of free speech as persons (Derber, 1998). The industry still markets tobacco products in the U.S. with sophisticated marketing techniques which define target groups by their demographics as well as their attitudes, aspirations, activities, and lifestyles (Ling & Glantz, 2002).

Philip Morris joined British American Tobacco (BAT), the world's second largest tobacco corporation, and Japan Tobacco in adopting an international voluntary code for marketing known as the Global Reporting Initiative (GRI). These voluntary guidelines called for corporate reports which include information whereby customer health and safety can be protected while using tobacco products, together with accurate information about risks and outcomes of smoking. Tobacco companies were challenged by their allegiance to profits and shareholders as well as the growing clout of anti-tobacco groups in restricting tobacco advertising and promotion, especially in many Western countries. Burton and Rowell of the Center for Media & Democracy published a detailed report on the subsequent efforts by BAT to prepare its first "social responsibility report". There was much ambivalence and foot dragging along the way to its report, which was regarded as "artful PR and either cosmetic, evasive, or deceitful" by a major tobacco control advocacy group, Action on Smoking and Health. The BAT report omitted information on adverse effects of smoking, and disregarded many of the indicators called for in the GRI guidelines (Burton & Rowell, 2002). Meanwhile, Philip Morris, which makes about 80% of the cigarettes smoked in the Czech Republic accounting for 20% of deaths there each year, responded to local complaints that it was saddling the country with large health care costs by issuing a report which calculated that the country was actually *saving* money due to early mortality (PNHP, 2002).

General Electric

General Electric, the largest corporation in the world, has a wingspan almost as broad as the U.S. government. Its interests include manufacturing of locomotives, jet engines, industrial turbines, robotics, and medical diagnostic equipment, while its activities also include stock brokering, banking, and financial services. It is also a media giant, with broadcast and cable television operations like NBC, CNBC, MSNBC and Bravo. As an active member of the Business Roundtable, which orchestrates the political agenda of Fortune 500 companies, it is a Republican institution that sponsors the right-wing TV talk show, the *McLaughlin Group*. It has been active in many socially responsive activities, including helping with early childhood education and initiatives to help the poor and disadvantaged minorities (Greider, 1992; Elliott, 2003). It can boast a long succession of technological advances from Edison's invention of the light bulb to medical imaging equipment.

Concerned about growing anti-corporate public opinion in the U.S. and negative publicity about the retirement benefits of its former CEO, Jack Welch, General Electric has recently launched a $100 million public relations campaign to burnish its image. It has changed its corporate slogan from "We bring good things to life" to "Imagination at work," and the airwaves are now filled with dramatic illustrations of its innovative advances over the years. The intent of the campaign is to promote its spirit of innovation and downplay its enormous scale (Elliott, 2003). Yet there are problems behind the public façade that the corporation keeps away from public view. GE has opposed any examination of its business operations by its network program, *NBC News*, as described in a book by a former NBC correspondent, who alleges that GE degraded and censored the news to favor its corporate interests (Kent, 1997; Kent, 1998). Over the 11-year period ending in 1992, it shed more than one-quarter of its U.S. workforce while more than tripling its net income (Naisbitt, 1994). Together with other large U.S. corporations, GE has developed a large, contract workforce beyond our borders. These workers are often paid less than two dollars a day, without benefits, in countries with no legal or union protections (Derber, 1998). Corporations in a global economy can readily make profits at the expense of social needs by avoiding public accountability in their host countries. William Greider sums up the political prowess of today's global corporations in these words:

> Given its girth and skill and other attributes, a politically active corporation like General Electric acts like a modern version of the "political machine," with some of the same qualities of the old political machines that used to dominate American cities (Greider, 1992).

CONCLUDING COMMENTS

The struggle goes on as to how best to reconcile corporate self-interest with the public interest, more challenging than ever in our new global economy. Corporations still hold the upper hand, with liberal government subsidies and tax breaks, friendly regulatory agencies, First Amendment rights as persons, dominance over the media, and the lack of effective campaign finance reform. There is a growing counterforce in defense of the public interest, however, as reflected by national and local media watch groups (e.g., Fairness & Accuracy in Reporting), organizations such as Public Citizen, People for Better Television, and the Center for Digital Democracy, as well as the public outcry by over 1 million Americans over a June 2003 decision by the FCC to relax the rules of media ownership, which led the Senate Commerce Committee to override that decision (Bagdikian, 2002; Marciniak & Dreazen, 2003). For now, one has to conclude that more corporate accountability is needed, voluntary guidelines have not been effective, and more government oversight and regulation will be required in order to provide Americans with objective and accurate information with which to make their own health care decisions. For that to happen, the money culture of government will have to be reined in through campaign finance reform—which leads us to the next chapter.

REFERENCES

Ackerman S. (2002, May/June). U.S. media favor radical health reform—for Canada. *ABC, New York Times* distort problems of single-payer system. EXTRA! p. 7.

The New York Times (1999, Jan. 28) Advertising money flows. p. C1.

Bagdikian, B. (2002a). *The Media Monopoly,* Boston: Beacon Press.

Bagdikian, B. (2002). In: R. W. McChesney, & J. Nichols, *Our Media, Not Theirs: The Democratic Struggle Against Corporate Media.* New York: Steven Stories Press.

Bayer, R., Gostin, L. O., Javitt, G H., & Brandt., A. (2002). Tobacco advertising in the United States: A proposal for a constitutionally acceptable form of regulation. *Journal of the American Medical Association, 287,* 2990.

Burton, B., & Rowell, A. (2002). British American Tobacco's socially responsive smoke screen. *PR Watch,* p. 6.

Burton, B., & Rowell, A. (2003). Disease mongering. *PR Watch, 10*(1) 1.

Burton, B., & Rowell, A. (2003b). From patient activism to astroturf marketing. *PR Watch* l0 (1), 5.

Centers for Disease Control and Prevention (CDC). (2002). Annual smoking attributable mortality, years of potential life lost and economic costs— United States 1995–1999. *Morbidity and Mortality Weekly Report, 51,* 300.

Center for Public Integrity. (2000). Off the Record: What Media Corporations Don't Tell You About Their Legislative Agendas. Washington, D.C. 41.

Corporate welfare. (1998, Nov. 9). *Time,* p. 34.

Corporate welfare. (1998, Dec. 8). *New York Times,* p. C27.

Court, K., & Flanagan, J. (2003, Mar. 18). Insurance "reform"? Consider the source. *The Wall Street Journal.* Day, S. (2003, Mar. 22). Philip Morris is convicted of fraud in marketing. *The New York Times,* p. A8.

Derber, C. (1998). *Corporation nation: How corporations are taking over our lives, and what we can do about it.* New York: St. Martin's Griffin.

Elliott, S. (2003, Jan. 16). G.E. to spend $100 million promoting itself as innovative. *The New York Times,* p. C1.

EXTRA. (1997, July/August). Fairness and accuracy in reporting. p. 24.

Fletcher, S. W. (1997). Whither scientific deliberation in health policy recommendations: Alice in the wonderland of breast-cancer screening. *The New England Journal of Medicine, 336,* 1180.

Fong, T. (2003, June 23). Medicare. Public dismay for private plan. *Modern Healthcare,* p. 9.

Document ClearingHouse Political Transcripts. (1996). Freedom to Advertise. Coalition news conference, August 23.

Gates, J. (2000). *Democracy at Risk: Rescuing Main Street from Wall Street.* Cambridge: Perseus Publishing. Goldstein, A., & Balz, D. (2003, May 26). Universal health care gets boost. Democratic rivals push new plans. *The Washington Post,* p. A1.

Greider, W. (1992). *Who Will Tell the people? The betrayal of American democracy.* New York: Simon & Schuster.

Hart, P., & Naurecker, J. (2002, Dec.). NBC slams universal health care. EXTRA! December, p. 4.

Hartmann, T. (2002). *Unequal Protection: The Rise of Corporate Dominance and the Theft of Human Rights.* New York: Rodale.

Jupiter Media Matrix (2001). Research company, 2001 report. Available at www.jmm.com

Kent, A. (1998, June 8). Breaking down the barriers. *Nation,* p. 29.

Kent, A. (1997). Risk and redemption: Surviving the network news wars. Tortola, British Virgin Islands: Interstellar.

Korten, D. C. (2001). *When corporations rule the world.* San Francisco: Kumarian Press & Berritt-Koehler Publishers.

Krimsky, S., & Rothenberg, L. S. (1998). Financial interest and its disclosure in scientific publications. *Journal of the American Medical Association, 280,* 225. Ling, P. M., & Glantz, S. A. (2002). Using tobacco-industry marketing research to design more effective tobacco-control campaigns. *Journal of the American Medical Association, 287,* 2983.

Marciniak, S., & Dreazen, Y. J. (2003, June 20). Senate panel votes to override FCC on recent ruling. *The Wall Street Journal,* p. A4.

Marmor, T., & Sullivan, K. (2000, July/august). Canada's burning! Media myths about universal health coverage. *Washington Monthly*, p. 15.

Marmor, T., & Sullivan, K. (2003, Feb. 12). Who's shaping the debate on health care reform? *The Hartford Courant.*

Master Settlement Agreement between Settling State Officials and Participating Manufacturers. (1998, November 23). p. 19. Available at *www.naag.org/tobac/index.html*

Meadows, D. (1992, oct. 3). Corporate-Run Schools Are a Threat to Our Way of Life. *Valley News*, p. 22.

MedPanel (2002). Announcement. Retrieved on May 1, 2002 from Erin. *Sheehan@medplanel.com*

Mink,, E. (2002, Nov. 4). What ad slump? *Time Inside Business*, pp. A17–18.

Monar, A. (1994). *Corporations in the classroom. Co-op American Quarterly 19*, Winter.

Moynihan, R., Bero, L., Ross-Degman, P., Henry, B., Lee, K., Watkins, J., et al. (2000). Coverage by the news media of the benefits and risks of medications. *The New England Journal of Medicine, 342*, 1645.

Mundy, A. (1996, oct. 14). Magazine pages will burn: A new federal plan to limit tobacco ads leaves many publishers under a cloud of uncertainty. *Mediaweek.*

Nader, R. (2002). *Crashing the party: Taking on the corporate government in an age of surrender.* New York: St. Martin's Griffin.

Naisbitt, J. (1994). *Global Paradox.* New York: William Morrow.

National Institutes of Health (NIH) (1997). Breast Cancer Screening in Women Ages 40–49. NIH Consensus Statement No. 103. U.S. Dept. of Health and Human Services, Bethesda, Maryland.

Pear, R. (2003, July 1). Private health insurers begin lobbying for changes in Medicare drug legislation. *The New York Times*, p. A20.

Peterson, M. (2003, May 7). A respected face but is it an ad or news? *The New York Times*, p. C1.

Pew Center for the People and the Press (2000). Available at *http://people-press.org*

Picard, A. (2000, Nov. 27). Health care not so bad. Survey. *The Toronto Globe and Mail.*

PNHP (2002). Data Update. *PNHP Newsletter*, p. 7.

The Wall Street Journal (2001). *PNHP Newsletter*, January 2002, p. 7. Report, July 16, 2001.

Rochon, P. A., Bero, L. A. Bay, A. M., Gold, J. L. Dergal, J. M. Binne, M. A., et al., (2002). Comparison of review articles published in peer-reviewed and throwaway journals. *Journal of the American Medical Association, 287*, 2853.

Romanow, R. (2002). Building on Values: The Future of Health Care in Canada. Final report of the Commission on the Future of Health Care in Canada. Retrieved November 28, 2002 from *www.finalreport.healthcarecommission.ca.*

Roper Center for Public Opinion Research (1999). News reporting and commentary. Question ID: USMS. 99 Feb R20.022. EXTRA! July/August p. 24.

Schwartz, L. M., Woloshin, S., Baczek, L. (2002). Media coverage of scientific meetings: Too much, too soon? *Journal of the American Medical Association, 287,* 2859. Schwartz, L. M., & Woloshin, S. (2002). News media coverage of screening mammography for women in their 40s and tamoxifen for primary prevention of breast cancer. *Journal of the American Medical Association, 287,* 3136.

Siegel, M. (2003, June 22). This doesn't have to be the price we pay. *Washingtonpost.com* p. B02.

Stauber, J., & Rampton, S. *Toxic sludge Is good for you: Lies, damm lies, and the public relations industry.* Monroe, ME: Common Courage Press.

Thurlow, L. (1999). *Building Wealth.* New York: Harper Business.

Viason, J. (2002). Rx drug industry spent millions on sham issue ads to influence drug benefit debate. *Public Citizen News, 22*(5), 1, 15.

Vranica, S. (2002, Sept. 26). Patient channel to blast ads at bedridden. *The Wall Street Journal,* p. B1.

Woloshin, S., & Schwartz, L. M. (2002). Translating research into news. Press releases *Journal of the American Medical Association, 287,* 2856.

Zuckerman, D. (2003). Hype in health reporting: "Checkbook science" buys distortion of medical news. *International Journal of Health Services, 33*(2), 383.

Chapter 10

LOBBYING THE GOVERNMENT

The culture of money dominates Washington as never before; money now rivals or even exceeds power as the preeminent goal. It affects the issues raised and their outcome; it has changed employment patterns in Washington; it has transformed politics; and it has subverted values. It has led good people to do things that are morally questionable, if not reprehensible. It has cut a deep gash, if not inflicted a mortal wound, in the concept of public service.

—*Elizabeth Drew*
Journalist and Political Analyst

Money not only determines who is elected, it determines who runs for office. Ultimately, it determines what government accomplishes—or fails to accomplish. Congress, except in unusual moments, will listen to the 900,000 Americans who give $200 or more to their campaigns ahead of the 259,600,000 who don't. Real reform of democracy, reform as radical as those of the Progressive era and deep enough to get government moving again, must begin by completely breaking the connection between money and politics.

— *Bill Bradley, U.S. Senator*

The last two chapters have described two ways by which corporate interests in health care advance their agendas, often without regard for the public interest. Lobbying of government at both state and federal levels is a third way. Corporate influence is extremely effective in this area as well, particularly in the money culture surrounding the activities of government alluded to in the above quotes (Drew, 1999; Phillips, 2002).

This chapter has four goals: (1) to give a brief overview of the corporate media as "the fourth branch of government," (2) to describe and illustrate lobbying activities at federal and state levels; (3) to discuss the impact of corporate lobbying efforts on the democratic process; and (4) to consider whether recent campaign finance reform legislation can be expected to redress some of the problems prevailing in the money culture of politics today.

CORPORATE MEDIA AS "THE FOURTH BRANCH OF GOVERNMENT"

Beyond its powerful role in shaping popular opinion, the press plays a large role in influencing legislation, and has been called by many the "fourth branch of government" for good reason. As a result, corporate interests which control the media often trump the public interest in health care. This has become even more true since the 1980s, when the media corporations achieved control of the national airwaves. They successfully lobbied for the airways and channels to be sold to the highest bidders at frequency auctions. As deregulation moved into the 1990s, the corporate media lobbied hard for the 1996 Telecommunications Act, which removed the consumer and diversity protections established in the earlier 1934 Act (Hartmann, 2002). The giant media conglomerates such as General Electric, AOL Time Warner, Disney, and the News Corporation all have their own lobbying machines, which collectively are considered by Alan Murray of the *Wall Street Journal* to be the most powerful lobby in Washington (Murray, 1997). From 1996 to 2000, the 50 largest media companies spent over $111 million to lobby Congress and the executive branch of government, fighting against any restrictions on tobacco advertising or any effort to give political candidates free air time during election campaigns (Center for Public Integrity, 2000).

Campaign revenues have become very lucrative for the media corporations. The average campaign for the U.S. Senate now costs candidates $6 million, win or lose. That means that a senator must take in an average of $20,000 a day during his or her six-year term to prepare for the next election. During the 1998 House and Senate campaigns, the media corporations were paid over $1 billion for ads by parties, politicians, and interest groups. This is *seven times* the amount generated in the 1978 campaigns before deregulation of the media (Hartmann, 2002).

Several common approaches used by large lobbying initiatives are illustrated by the following examples.

The Corporate Media

One favored strategy often used by media and communications lobbies is to bring local station managers to Washington, D.C. to meet with members of Congress. Station managers thereby control television appearances of politicians in their home districts. In order to develop closer relationships with legislators, the National Association of Broadcasters (NAB) has even recruited the spouses of members of Congress to give televised public service announcements (McChesney, 2002).

Astroturfing and Coalition-Building

"Astroturf" lobbying is a covert advertising practice whereby a public relations campaign creates the illusion of "grass" in a phony "grassroots" lobbying effort. Typically, a PR firm will contact community groups to request signatures on a petition that has misleading information about its source and no disclosure of its funding (Barry, 2002). The lobbying campaign by the health insurance industry, which played a key role in killing the Clinton Health Plan in 1994, provides a good example of how effective such a campaign can be. The Coalition for Health Insurance Choices was created and funded by the Health Insurance Association of America (HIAA) with additional funding from the National Federation of Independent Business (NFIB). Blair Childs, a PR leader for that campaign with previous experience with the American Tort Reform Association, described the Coalition's strategies in these words: "Forming coalitions is a way to provide cover for your interest. We needed cover because we were going to be painted as the bad guy. You also get strength in numbers. Some have lobby strength, some have grassroots strength, and some have good spokespersons . . . Start with the natural, strongest allies, sit around a table and build up . . . to give your coalition a positive image" (Childs, 1994). Additional lobbying clout was provided by the Independent Insurance Agents of America (IIAA), which mobilized almost 140,000 insurance agents across the country against the proposal (Stauber & Rampton, 1995; Lewis, 1998).

Another common ploy of PR-orchestrated lobbying campaigns is the use of front groups with misleading names. As not-for-profit, tax-exempt organizations, they are not required to disclose their funding sources (Lewis, 1998). Crass commercial self-interest is often disguised by names that create the illusion of public interest, such as Citizens for Better Medicare (the drug industry front group to oppose a prescription drug benefit under Medicare with accompanying price controls), and the Coordinated Care Coalition (the HMO industry's front group aimed at improving the image of for-profit HMOs).

Think Tanks

Another important strategy to influence public policy and shape popular opinion is through the work of think tanks. Many have been established in the U.S. since the 1970s, are well-funded by corporate interests, and have as their goal to conduct and disseminate "policy research." They vary along the political spectrum, but most are conservative. Three of the major think tanks that represent the neoconservative movement are the American Economics Institute for Public Policy Research, the Heritage Foundation, and the Business Roundtable. The latter comprises the CEOs of about 200 of the country's largest corporations, representing about one-half the GNP of the U.S. and more than the GNP of any other country in the world except for the United States. (McQuaid, 1981). Although the Roundtable cultivates an image of statesmanlike-moderation, it promotes its sponsors' political agenda through commissioned studies, position papers, op-ed pieces, editorials, television commentaries, and news releases (Green & Buchsbaum, 1980).

Revolving Door

Many legislators, at both federal and state levels, become paid lobbyists when they leave office, often without any time lapse from their departure. This can be one of the most effective ways to lobby for special interest agendas—hire government insiders with recent experience in the legislative process. In 1997, for example, three former Senate majority leaders (Republicans Howard Baker Jr., and Robert Dole, and Democrat George Mitchell) became lobbyists for the tobacco industry. A study by the Center for Public Integrity in the mid-1990s found that about 15% of senior Senate and House aides left to become registered lobbyists, many with senior staff experience on such key committees as Commerce, Finance, and Ways and Means (Lewis, 1998). Former Surgeon General C. Everett Koop, though he had taken a principled stand against the tobacco industry while in office, lobbied members of Congress after leaving office in support of a drug company without disclosing that his own nonprofit organization, the Koop Foundation, had received a $1 million grant earlier that year from that same drug company (Noble, 1999).

LOBBYING OF GOVERNMENT AT THE FEDERAL AND STATE LEVELS

Lobbying of the government at all levels has become an industry of its own, as will become clear in this brief overview. In state capitals across the country, for example, there were 36,959 companies, business associations, and other interest groups registered to lobby state legislators in 2000, about five lobbying interests per lawmaker. The number of lobbyists, of course, is measured by hundreds of thousands. As documented by analyses carried out by the Center for Public Integrity, the involvement of lobbying interests goes far beyond lobbying per se, even to the point of writing legislation. Legislators in many states are part-time, have limited staffs, and are overwhelmed by the volume of detail contained in the many bills upon which they will vote. Lobbyists with expertise, time, and strong interpersonal skills are often welcomed by harried legislators as aides or consultants who help draft legislation and work it through the approval process. Lobbyists often play an additional role as conduits for campaign contributions, especially in states without limits. Many larger business interests carry out ongoing lobbying activities at federal and state levels. What they can't accomplish in Washington, D.C. can perhaps be achieved by targeted lobbying efforts at the state level (Renzulli & Center for Public Integrity, 2002).

Federal Level

As of 2002, there were more than 20,000 registered lobbyists in Washington, D.C., or about 38 for every member of Congress; of these, 138 were former members of Congress (Hartmann, 2002, p.158). Almost all of the Fortune 500 companies maintain public relations offices in Washington, D.C. Many participate actively in front organizations, which provide political cover for their own agendas. For example, the Business Roundtable created a front organization USA* NAFTA that enrolled about 2,300 U.S. corporations and associations as members. It was intended to show broad support for free trade, but all of its state captains were corporate members of the Roundtable, which actively promoted the view that NAFTA would provide Americans with high-paying jobs and stop immigration from Mexico (Anderson, Cavenaugh, Gross, 1993).

Several additional examples of lobbying activities by health care groups at the national level.

- *Health insurance.* Proposed legislation by the National Federation of Independent Business (NFIB) and other business allies would free association health plans (AHPs) from state regulations and place them under lighter federal oversight. It is being opposed by the Blue Cross-Blue Shield Association, as well as state regulators, consumer, and labor groups. Both sides have formed coalitions that hold receptions and seminars for Capitol

Hill staffers and provide patch-through phone lines connecting constituents with their legislators. Proponents claim that AHPs make health insurance more affordable for smaller employers and their employees, while critics see further cherry-picking of the market without assurances of adequate coverage. If enacted into law, annual sales of AHPs could total more than $100 million for bare-bones policies which benefit the insurance industry more than the beneficiaries (Hamburger, 2003).

In another instance, the two largest insurance trade groups, the American Association of Health Plans (AAHP) and the Health Insurance Association of America (HIAA) agreed to merge in September 2003. They spent over $9 million in 2002 lobbying for a larger role for private insurers in the Medicare prescription drug legislation being debated in Congress, as well as for increased payments to private Medicare HMOs (Gerber, 2003).

- *Dietary Supplements.* As we saw in chapter 7 the dietary supplement industry is an enormous, highly profitable, and mostly unregulated industry. Many of these products act as drugs and carry significant health risks, including death. A strong ongoing lobby effort has been conducted by the industry and its supporters to avoid more regulation or accountability. According to the Center for Responsive Politics, dietary supplement manufacturers gave more than $3.3 million to Democrats and Republicans alike during the last two election cycles. Senator Orrin Hatch (R-Utah) co-authored the 1994 Dietary Supplement Health and Education Act (DSHEA), which deregulated the industry. Many of these companies are based in Utah, which describes itself as "the Silicon Valley of the supplements industry" (Neubauer, Pasternak, Cooper, 2003). The industry has donated almost $137,000 to Senator Hatch's campaigns over the last 10 years, and spent nearly $2 million in lobbying fees to firms that employ his son Scott. Although ephedra has been linked to over 100 deaths and its largest manufacturer, Metabolife, has been under investigation for lying to the FDA about safety complaints, the FDA, with Hatch's support, still refused to ban ephedra until the end of 2003 (Vinson, 2003).
- *Pharmaceuticals Industry.* According to federal lobbying disclosure records the drug industry hired 675 lobbyists from 138 different firms in 2002, or almost seven for every U.S. Senator. This army of lobbyists includes 26 former members of Congress, and 51% have revolving-door connections between their K Street offices and the federal government. The industry has

spent almost $650 million on political influence since 1997, including lobbying, hiring academics, funding nonprofits, and issue ads. Brand-name drug manufacturers outspent generic manufacturers by more than 20 times and hired seven times as many lobbyists (Public Citizen, 2003a). The industry's main efforts were directed toward avoiding price controls under any prescription drug benefit enacted under Medicare, and toward protecting its patent rights. As the conference committee in Congress worked through the summer of 2003 to reconcile the House and Senate bills for a Medicare prescription drug benefit, other health care industry lobbyists pressed for attachment of their own pet interests to the legislation. These ranged from coverage for self-injected drugs, improved reimbursement of radium implants for prostate cancer, and accelerated coverage decisions by Medicare for medical devices, to coverage of chiropractic services under Medicare (McGinley & Lueck, 2003). By the time the Medicare bill passed in November 2003, the health care industry (including HMOs and the drug industry) had contributed about $8 million to President George W. Bush and another $3 million to six key legislators on both sides of the aisle involved in its passage, or more than $15,000 per day and $1,896 per hour since 2000 (Schlesinger & Hamburger, 2003).

Interests in each health care industry often unite behind an issue being promoted, but on many issues these interests are split among themselves. Examples of divisive issues include brand-name vs. generic drug manufacturers, large employers vs small employers concerning health insurance, and general hospitals vs. specialty hospitals. These splits don't reduce lobbying efforts; instead, they make them more complex.

On some occasions, special interest provisions are attached to legislation and proceed to passage without committee review or debate. A classic example is the anonymous inclusion in the Homeland Security Bill of 2002 of a provision, that would prevent lawsuits by families claiming that a mercury-based vaccine caused autism in their children. No legislator claimed responsibility for this provision. A furor arose among these parents and several moderate Senate Republicans, which led Congress to repeal the legislation in January 2003, but a Republican-led effort several months later sought to attach a similar provision to a bill being considered concerning research on a SARS vaccine (Firestone, 2003; Stolberg, 2003). Another good example of a "mystery amendment" is a 46-word provision attached to a House bill in the dead of night which would have granted $50 billion in tax breaks to the tobacco industry.

The bill was passed the next day with most House members unaware of its inclusion. Again, nobody claimed responsibility for it. The Senate later voted it out after *Time's* Margaret Carlson exposed that it had been written by Haley Barbour, tobacco lobbyist and former chairman of the Republican National Committee (Chen, 1997).

State Level

Much of the action in government now takes place in the state capitals across the country, especially during this period of "new federalism" launched by President Ronald Reagan in the 1980s and which shifted power to the states. Since 1998, over 100,000 laws have been passed by state legislators. Some industries such as insurance are largely controlled at the state level. In 1945 Congress passed the McCarran-Ferguson Act, which ceded most insurance regulation to the states. The insurance industry outnumbers all other lobbying interests at the state level (Renzulli & Center for Public Integrity, 2002).

Only nine states have full-time legislatures. Most state legislators work part-time, earn modest salaries in their legislator roles, and have other jobs on the side. The most common occupation, by far, is the legal profession. Most state legislatures impose few, if any, restrictions on legislators' outside income. According to the Center for Public Integrity, seven states have weak or no disclosure laws, and legislators can hide their private financial interests from the public in about half of the states. Revolving door shifts from legislator to lobbyist are pervasive, and conflicts of interest are extremely common (Renzulli & Center for Public Integrity 2002). In North Carolina, for example, 60% of state legislators sit on committees whose decisions directly affect their private income (Editorial, 2003).

There were more than 3,000 health care-related companies and organizations registered to lobby in statehouses in 1999, each lobbying for favorable laws and regulations. The nursing home industry fought against increased regulations even as their safety violations became more prevalent. The health insurance industry lobbied against managed-care reforms, while groups of health care professionals battled to protect their own roles against competitors, (e.g,, ophthalmologists opposing the right of optometrists to perform laser eye surgery Renzulli & Center for Public Integrity, 2002, p. 150).

Several examples of recent hard-fought issues at the state level are described below:

- *For-profit HMOs.* During the November 2000 election campaign, HMOs spent $34 million in Massachusetts to successfully defeat, by a narrow margin, a statewide single-payer plan (PNHP, 2001). In Virginia, HMOs spent lavishly and lobbied hard to defeat, also by a slim margin, patients' rights legislation that would have allowed patients to sue their HMOs. At the time, 26 Virginia legislators had ties to the insurance industry (Renzulli & Center for Public Integrity, 2002, pp. 94–95).

• *Pharmaceutical industry.* As we saw in chapter 6 Maine introduced legislation in 2000 to require price discounts for drugs under its Medicaid program. After its passage, PhRMA fought that bill all the way to the U.S. Supreme Court. Faced by exploding costs of prescription drugs in their own Medicaid programs, 19 other states attempted to pass similar legislation in 2001. All were battled to a standstill by drug industry lobbyists (Renzulli & Center for Public Integrity, 2002) In Massachusetts, PhRMA spent seven times as much on lobbying in 2002 as in 1998, in successful efforts to block bulk discounts on drugs as well as bills mandating disclosure of spending on drug promotion and gifts from companies to physicians (Dember, 2003).

• *Health insurance industry.* In California, with premium rate increases for health insurance in the 20% to 40% range for small employers and individuals, a 2003 bill to require state approval for such insurance rate increases is stalled in committee due to heavy lobbying by the industry. Blue Cross of California, now for-profit and the state's largest health insurer, claims that required state approval for premium increases could "put insurers at risk of insolvency or force them to pad their increase requests to keep up with rising health care costs" (Lawrence, 2003). In Oregon, Regence Blue Cross-Blue Shield (Regence BCBS) of Oregon lobbied strongly against Measure 23, Oregon's 2002 attempt to achieve universal coverage, contending that the market can meet the state's health care needs better than a single-payer program. A year later, Regence BCBS announced that it would phase out its commercial HMO offering in Oregon by the end of 2004, forcing 130,000 individuals to change plans (Moody, 2003).

THE CORPORATE MONEY CULTURE AS A THREAT TO DEMOCRACY

The political rhetoric of our times, carried nearly to the point of patriotic fervor, that holds that free trade and markets in a global economy are an effective way to advance democracy. In truth, they are fundamentally antidemocratic. In a true political democracy, each person has one vote, while in the marketplace, each dollar is a vote. Markets are, therefore, biased in favor of the affluent and against the less affluent. As markets become freer and more global, it follows that governance increasingly passes from national governments to global corporations (Korten, 2001).

The U.S. is fully committed to the global market, and governance has largely shifted to corporate interests. Corporate governance takes place through a mix of strategic alliances, contracting networks, and interlocking board directorships that link almost all Fortune 500 corporations with each other (Drew, 1999, p. 18). It also occurs through coordinated advocacy efforts of the Business Roundtable, which includes the heads of 42 of the 50 largest U.S. industrial corporations, 9 of the 11 largest U.S. utilities, 7 of the 8 largest U.S. commercial banks, 7 of the 8 largest U.S. transportation companies, 7 of the 10 largest U.S. insurance companies, and 5 of the 7 largest U.S. retailers. The Roundtable campaigned strongly for NAFTA, and actively pursues the bottom-line interests of its members quite aside from the usual legislative process. Their interests are further served by the granting of "fast track" authority by Congress to the President for trade negotiations like those of the General Agreement on Tariffs and Trade (GATT). Once a trade agreement is reached, Congress can only vote once to approve or reject the entire package, without any opportunity to amend or reject particular sections (Greider, 1992).

For-profit public relations firms and business-sponsored policy institutes provide another vehicle for corporate advocacy and image-building campaigns. In what Greider has termed "democracy for hire," these firms produce opinion polls, op-ed pieces, press releases, and policy-oriented papers aimed at the public as well as legislators (Greider, 1992, p. 35). In the U.S., there are now some 170,000 public relations employees serving the interests of paying clients compared with only about 40,000 news reporters. More than one-third of the news content in a typical U.S. newspaper is based on public relations press releases, story memos, and suggestions submitted by PR firms (Korten, 2001, p 148). Meanwhile, ownership of much of the media by our largest corporations further serves the interests of corporate America under the umbrella of managed news. Ralph Nader has this to say about corporate governance:

> Big corporations are out of control, in large part, because they control government and its responsibility to defend the people. The financial

scandals exposed the utter failure of the various expected private watch-dogs or gatekeepers of accounting firms, corporate law firms, invest-ment bankers, major credit rating agencies, and stockbrokers, all of whom receive direct compensation or large fees for not watchdogging the CEOs and their rubber-stamp boards of directors. (Nader, 2002)

Corporations have exerted major influence over the electoral and legislative process through their large contributions to the political parties and their candidates. Over the last 10 years, the drug industry has spent more than $1 billion to influence the public policy process in Washington, DC with over 600 lobbyists working its issues on Capitol Hill. (Lewis and the Center for Public Integrity, 2004). In the 1996 election cycle, 96% of Americans made no direct contributions to a politician or political party and less than one quarter of 1% gave more than $200, while each of the top 500 U.S. corporations gave more than $500,000 to both Republicans and Democrats during the preceding 10 years (Hartmann, 2002, p. 222). This has led Senator John McCain to describe our campaign finance system as "an elabo-rate influence-peddling scheme by which both parties conspire to stay in office by selling the country to the highest bidder" (Phillips, 2002, p. 325).

As a result of these changes, a large part of the U.S. population has been turned off and has withdrawn from the political process. Over the last 40 years, there has been a 25% decline in voting and a 50% drop in activities in political campaigns. Only about one-half of eligi-ble voters vote in presidential elections, while one-third turn out for congressional elections (Green, 2002). Table 10.1 shows the level of public concern about campaign contributions and the unethical or illegal behavior of politicians (Phillips, 2002, p. 328).

WHERE IS CAMPAIGN FINANCE REFORM HEADED?

After seven years of increasing public calls for campaign finance re-form, the McCain-Feingold Bipartisan Campaign Reform Act of 2002 (BCRA) was passed and became effective on November 6, 2002. As the most significant reform since the 1970s, it has these major provi-sions:

Soft money donations to the national parties are banned; state and local parties may collect contributions as large as $10,000, but these funds may not be used for broadcast ads for federal candidates.

TABLE 10.1. Public Concern About Unethical or Illegal Behavior by Officeholders Obligated to Campaign Contributors

- Percentage of the public that thinks politicians often do special favors for people and groups who give them campaign contributions: 8076 (*ABC News*, March 2001)
- Percentage who think this is not a problem: 11%
- Percentage who think those special favors tend to be unethical: 74%
- Percentage who think these special favors tend to be illegal: 46%
- Percentage of candidates for statewide office who report spending at least one out of every four of their waking hours raising money for their campaigns: 55% (*Campaigns and Elections* survey, April 2001)
- Percentage who report spending more than half their time raising money: 23%
- Percentage of the public that thinks unlimited contributions to political parties (soft money) should be banned: 66% (Reuters/Zogby Poll, March 2001)

Source: Public Campaign, Washington, D.C.

Outside groups (corporations, unions, and nonprofits) are barred from using soft money to air ads that clearly identify a candidate within thirty days of a primary or within sixty days of the general election. Anyone or any group may still air such ads before these deadlines but (a) can't coordinate the ads with candidates, (b) must use only hard money, and (c) must comply with reporting and disclosure rules.

The limits on hard money contributions from individuals are increased to $2000 per election (or a total of $4000 for primary and general elections combined). Individuals may make up to $95,000 in total contributions per two-year election cycle. (Green, 2002, p. 81).

Opposition to the BCRA was fast and furious. Eighty-four groups filed complaints against the U.S. Department of Justice (DOJ) and the Federal Elections Commission (FEC) challenging the constitutionality of the new law. These groups ranged across the political spectrum, including the Republican National Committee, the California Democratic Party, the AFL-CIO, the NRA, and the ACLU. One court case, McConnell vs. FEC, consolidates 11 separate lawsuits filed by the 84 plaintiffs (Holman & Morrison, 2003). A special three-judge panel upheld most of BCRA's provisions by a 2 to 1 margin in a complex set of rulings over 1,600 pages long. The case has been sent to the U.S. Supreme Court, which was expected to hold hearings the case in late 2003 at the earliest. The Supreme Court rejected limits on campaign spending in 1976 on the basis of the First Amendment and restriction of free speech, and court watchers anticipate that this will be a central concern this time around (Greenhouse, 2003; Lewis & Oppel, 2003).

In the aftermath of the passage of the BCRA and as its legal standing remains uncertain, the financial needs of the political parties and their candidates for office are still high. Other creative approaches to raise funds are now being taken. Four public interest advocacy groups—Public Citizen, Common Cause, Democracy 21, and the Center for Responsive Politics—have charged that the parties are now establishing nonprofit organizations, with lax reporting requirements as conduits to evade the new law. They have called for more rigorous reporting and disclosure requirements (Public Citizen, 2003b). Another major concern is the acknowledged weakness of the FEC as a watchdog over campaign finance laws. The FEC was created by Congress in 1974 with six commissioners, three Republican and three Democrat. It has often been deadlocked along partisan lines and has been called by many "a watchdog without a bite" (Project FEC, 2002). As to the future of campaign finance reform, Scott Harshbarger, president of Common Cause, makes this observation: "McCain-Feingold is only an incremental step. If this becomes the final step, we have failed" (Holman & Morrison, 2003, p. 83).

Meanwhile, as the contentious issue of campaign finance reform winds its way through the court system, the Bush-Cheney re-election campaign proceeds in high gear to make a mockery of any commitment to such reforms. By November of 2003, when he was claiming that his campaign hadn't yet started, President Bush's "Dash for Cash" tour had already passed the $100 million mark, largely through bundled $2,000 contributions of corporate interests, and was well on its way to its $200 million goal. According to Frank Clemente, director of Public Citizen's Congress Watch, which monitors campaign contributions through WhiteHouseForSale.org, "Bush has already accomplished his mission of destroying the presidential public financing system" (Public Citizen, 2003c).

CONCLUDING COMMENTS

From the foregoing, it is clear that the money culture of government, especially as manipulated by large corporate special interests, remains a major obstacle to issues such as health care reform. In a 1994 report, *Well-Healed: Inside Lobbying for Health Care Reform*, the Center for Public

Integrity drew this conclusion which still appears to be true 10 years later:

> For 200 years of America's democratic experiment, factions or interest groups were natural and inherent to our society and representative government was the objective arbiter between competing, rival groups. In recent years, however, and especially in the current health care reform debate, we have seen that some factions are so strong they overwhelm the decisionmaking process. (Center for Public Integrity, 1994)

REFERENCES

Anderson, S., Cavenaugh, J., Gross, S. (1993). NAFTA's Corporate Cadre: An Analysis of the USA NAFTA State Captains. Institute for Policy Studies, Washington, D.C.

Barry, P. (200). Drug industry spends huge sums guarding prices. *AARP Bulletin*, 43(5): 3–15.

Center for Public Integrity. (1994). Well-Healed: Inside Lobbying for Health Care Reform. Washington, D.C.

Center for Public Integrity. (2000). Off the Record: What Media Corporations Don't Tell You About Their Legislative Agendas. Washington, D.C.

Chen, E. (1997, Sept. 11). $50 billion tobacco tax break rejected by senate. *Los Angeles Times*, p. 1.

Childs, B. (1994, Dec. 9). Shaping Public Opinion: If You Don't Do It, Somebody Else Will Conference address. *Chicago*, Illinois.

Dember, A. (2003, May 16). Drug firms boost their lobbying in state. *Boston Globe*, p. A1.

Drew, E. (1999). *The corruption of American politics: What went wrong and why.* New York: The Overlook Press. Editorial. (2003, April 14) Conflicts of interest have no boundaries. *The Honolulu Advertiser.* April 14, p. A8.

Editorial. Conflicts of interest have no boundaries. *The Honolulu Advertiser*, April 14, 2003, pA8.

Firestone, D. (2003, Jan. 13). G. O. P. leaders promise repeal of provisions hidden in bill. *The New York Times*, p. A9.

Gerber, M. S. (2003, Sept. 23). Insurance trade groups okay merger: AAHP and HIAA consolidate Hill lobbying efforts. *The Hill.*

Green, M., & Buchsbaum, A. (1980). The corporate lobbies: Political profiles of the business roundtable and the chamber of commerce. Washington, DC: Public Citizen Gale Research.

Green, M. (2002). *Selling out: How big corporate money buys elections, runs through legislation, and betrays our democracy.* New York: Regan Books.

Greenhouse, L. (2003, May 3). An assessment: 1,638 pages, but little weight in Supreme Court. *The New York Times*, p. A14.

Greider, W. (1992). *Who will tell the people: The betrayal of American democracy.* New York: Simon & Schuster.

Hamburger, T. (2003, May 28). Trade group poses health plan. *The Wall Street Journal,* p. A4.

Hartmann, T. (2002). *Unequal protection: The rise of corporate dominance and the theft of human rights.* Emmanus, PA: Rodale Press.

Holman, C., & Morrison, A. (2003, Jan/Feb). All rise—campaign finance reform fight shifts to courts. *Public Citizen News, 23*(1), 1.

Korten, D. C. (2001). *When corporations rule the world.* San Francisco: Berrett-Koehler Publishers.

Lawrence, S. (2003, May 14). Bids to regulate health insurance rate hikes stalls. *Contra Costa Times.*

Lewis, C., & the Center for Public Integrity. (1998). *The buying of the Congress: How special interests have stolen your right to life, liberty and the Pursuit of Happiness.* New York: Avon Books.

Lewis, C., & The Center for Public Integrity. *The Buying of the President 2004: Who's really bankrolling Bush and his democratic challengers—and what they expect in return.* New York; Harper-Collins Publishers, Inc., 2004: pp. 104–105.

Lewis, N. A., & Oppel, R. A., Jr. (2003, May 3). U.S. Court issues discordant ruling on campaign law. *The New York Times,* p. A1.

McChesney, R. W., & Nichols J. (2002). *Our media, not theirs: The democratic struggle against corporate media.* New York: Seven Stories Press, p. 78.

McGinley, L., & Lueck, S. (2003, July 14). Medicare bill: Prescription for politics. *The Wall Street Journal,* p. A4.

McQuaid, K. (1981, May/June). The Roundtable. *Getting Results in Washington,* p. 114.

Moody, R. J., (2003, Sept. 29). Regence decides to exit HMO field in Oregon. *The Business Journal of Portland.*

Murray, A. (1997, Sept. 29). Broadcasters get a pass on campaign reform. *The Wall Street Journal,* p. A1.

Nader, R. (2002). *Crashing the party: Taking on the corporate government in an age of surrender.* New York: St. Martin's Griffin.

Neubauer, C., Pasternak, J., Cooper, R. T. (2003, Mar. 5). Senator, his son get boosts from makers of ephedra. *Los Angeles Times,* March 5.

Noble, B. N. (1999), Sept. 4). Hailed as a surgeon general, Koop criticized on Web ethics. *The New York Times.*

Phillips, K. (2002). *Wealth and democracy: A political history of the American rich* (p. 435). New York: Broadway Books.

Physicians for a National Health Plan (PNHP (2001, May). Data update. PNHP Newsletter.

Project FEC. (2002, April). No Bark, No Bite, No Point. The Case for Closing the Federal Election Commission and Establishing a New System for Enforcing the Nation's Campaign Finance Laws. Available at *www.democracy21.org*

Public Citizen (2003a, June 23). Press Release. Drug industry employs 675

Washington lobbyists, many with revolving-door connections, new report finds. Washington, D.C.

Public Citizen (2003b, Feb. 4). Press Release. Non-profit organizations are becoming the new conduit for soft money and cloaked electioneering activities. Washington, D.C.

Public Citizen (2003c, Nov. 13). Press Release. Mission half-accomplished: Bush's "Dash for Cash Tour" to top $100 million after two Florida fund-raisers today. Washington, D.C.

Renzulli, D., & Center for Public Integrity. (2002. *Capitol offenders: How private interests govern our states (pp. 158–159).* Washington, DC: Center for Public Integrity.

Schlesinger, J. M., & Hamburger, T. (2003, Nov. 25). Democrats take on business as campaign weapon. Medicare will be a double-edged sword. *The Wall Street Journal*, p. A4.

Stauber, J., & Rampton, S. (1995). *Toxic sludge is good for you: Lies, damm lies and the public relations industry.* Monroe, ME: Common Courage Press.

Stolberg, S. G. (2003, April 9). Republicans press for bill to shield vaccine makers from suits. *The New York Times*, p. A8.

Vinson, J. (2003, May/June). FDA hides behind Sen. Hatch's dietary supplement law, refuses to ban ephedra. *Public Citizen News, 23(3),*

Chapter 11

CO-OPTING THE REGULATORS

> Market mechanisms are essential to modern societies. However,
> for the market to serve the public good, business must recognize
> and accept the essential roles of government and civil society in
> maintaining the conditions on which the economic and social
> efficiency of markets depends, even though this may reduce cor-
> porate profits, limit the freedom of corporate action, and increase
> the prices of some consumer goods.
> —*David C. Korten, Economist and Author of*
> When Corporations Rule the World

The matter of corporate influence on government regulators is closely
related to lobbying practices discussed in the last chapter. Corporate
interests typically lobby government for less regulation, or in some instances, for *more* regulation designed to better serve their own interests
and put their competitors at a disadvantage. As Korten implies above,
the tail should not be wagging the dog. (Korten, 2001). This chapter has
four goals: (1) to present a brief historical overview of the politics of
deregulation, using the FDA as an example; (2) to describe ways in
which the FDA is regularly manipulated by the industry it is expected to
regulate; (3) to look at how health insurance regulators are influenced
by the insurance industry at the state level; and (4) to consider the extent
to which the court system supports the regulatory process in health care.

REGULATORY POLITICS

The regulatory power of the federal government, while potentially a
countervailing force to corporate excesses, also helps corporations to
prosper in ways not readily apparent to the public. We have a system of
"corporate welfare" involving some $300 billion a year in subsidies and
tax breaks, and this alliance between government and our largest corpo-

rations has led to U.S. economic dominance in the new global economy (Derber, 1998). Within this alliance, large corporations are skilled at designing and manipulating governmental regulatory programs to suit their needs. Monsanto, a pioneer in genetically altered crops, provides a case in point. It started lobbying the government for regulation in 1986, even before genetically modified foods were brought to market. Monsanto successfully obtained the regulations it desired from the EPA, the USDA and the FDA, which allowed manufacturers to avoid labeling and to determine on their own the risks and need for testing of genetically modified foods (Eichenwald, 2001). Beyond their major role in determining government regulations, corporations play an ongoing dominant role in governmental policy through lobbying, campaign contributions, and a revolving door of leadership between government, its regulatory agencies, and corporate management.

Free trade and globalization have become the centerpiece of U.S. economic policy over the last 20 years, and deregulation across industries has accompanied this policy. The U.S. played a leading role in the creation of the World Trade Organization (WTO), world banking institutions, and international trade agreements. WTO governance is largely a process of closed-door negotiations, which in many instances supersede the laws or regulations of any given country. As a result of these trends, more than one-half of the 100 largest "economies" in the world today are corporations, not countries (Hartmann, 2002). Nine of the 12 largest publicly-held health care corporations in the world are American (The Wall Street Journal, 2002).

Deregulation and the FDA

Concerns for the importance of regulating drugs in the public interest date back almost 100 years. Passage of the Pure Food and Drug Act in 1906 later led to creation of the FDA as the regulatory agency for enforcing the provisions of the Act. The FDA's first head, Harvey Wiley, recognized in 1930 the challenge in regulating the food and drug industries: "There is a distinct tendency to put regulations and rules for the enforcement of the law into the hands of the industries engaged in food and drug activities. I consider this one of the most pernicious threats to pure food and drugs" (Lewis & The Center for Public Integrity, 1998, p. 144). Table 11.1 lists the chronology of some of the major federal legislation which has been enacted over the years to modify the FDA's responsibilities and activities. Much of this legislation in recent years has included corporate friendly provisions which have weakened the FDA's purview and enforcement authority.

TABLE 11.1. Major Legislation Concerning the FDA

1906	Pure Food and Drug Act passed including a goal to ensure the safety of drugs (Lewis, 1998)
1938	Food, Drug and Consumer Act passed which required drugs to be shown safe before marketing (Ramsey et al, 1998)
1962	Kefauver-Harris amendment required that drugs be demonstrated by well-controlled studies to be safe and effective for intended uses (Lewis, 1998)
1976	Passage of Medical Device Amendments, which established an oversight and regulatory role of the FDA for medical devices; it divided medical devices into three risk categories and required premarket notification only for high-risk devices without rigorous methods of clinical evaluation (Ramsey et al, 1998)
1992	Passage of Prescription Drug User Fee Act in an effort to increase FDA's funding and decrease the time lag in review of drug applications (Lewis et al, 1998)
1994	Dietary Supplement Health and Education Act enacted, authorizing regulation of manufacturing practices, liberalizing labeling and marketing, and minimizing requirements for review of dietary supplements by the FDA (Barrett, 2003)
1997	Passage of the Food and Drug Administration Modernization Act, which reauthorized user fees, exempted more low-risk medical devices from premarket notification requirements, authorized manufacturers of drugs and devices to disseminate information about off-label users, and established a pilot program for third- party (private sector) review of device pre-market notifications (Merrill, 1999)
2002	Medical Device legislation passed whereby manufacturers partially fund safety reviews and are authorized to hire private contractors to inspect manufacturing facilities and review some devices for approval (Public Citizen, 2002)

The FDA is often in the "hot seat" trying to balance the needs of the public interest against pressures from industry and from Congress. "User fees" (payments by drug companies to the FDA toward the costs of the regulatory process for their drugs) now account for slightly more than one-half of the FDAs budget for review of marketing applications (Public Citizen Health Research Group, 2002). Congress is under heavy lobbying pressure from an industry that helps to support politicians' re-election campaigns. Two examples of the dynamics between these groups reveal the extent to which the FDA can be held captive by political forces:

- In 1996, Republican legislators in both the House and Senate launched a campaign to "reform" the FDA. Although unsuccessful that year, with the strong support of industry, Congress passed the FDA Modernization Act the next year, which gave industry more leeway in several respects. Drug companies could send physicians information on untested uses of drugs, and only one instead of two clinical trials were required for approval of a new drug, while manufacturers of dietary supplements could make health claims for their products without FDA approval. The legislation passed through both houses of Congress by wide margins. That the public interest was not well served by this legislation is illustrated by the adverse experience with off-label use of drugs to treat arrhythmias several years previously. After encainide and flecainide had been shown to suppress 90% of the complex ventricular arrhythmias in patients who suffered heart attacks, they were prescribed more widely for off-label uses for more benign arrhythmias until they were shown in a clinical trial to cause twice the mortality compared with placebo therapy (Echt, et al., 1991; Deyo, 1998). An estimated 40% of drugs prescribed in the U.S. are used for off-label purposes, without FDA approval, and there are over 5,000 off-label uses now listed in the AMA *Drug Evaluations.* Hazards to the public are therefore substantial through off-label use of drugs that are beyond the FDA's reach, while industry avoids the costs and delays involved in seeking new FDA approvals (Lewis & The Center for Public Integrity, 1998, p 153).

- In 2002, Congress quietly tacked on an amendment renewing the ten-year old user fees for the FDA to an unstoppable larger bill on bioterrorism. Legislators removed themselves from the renewal negotiations, encouraging representatives from the FDA and the drug companies to meet in closed-door sessions. With the strong support of industry, the amendment passed without a hearing, debate, or vote in any Congressional committee. Although concerns about the user fee program were raised by three Democrats in a House Subcommittee, Congress made no effort to carefully review its record, which was not good. In exchange for industry funds which allowed the FDA to increase its reviewer staff by 77%, industry gained a 20% increase in the approval rates of new drug applications and a faster review process. However, the percentage of new drugs approved between 1997 and 2000 which were withdrawn from the market for safety reasons increased more than threefold compared with the period from 1993 to 1996. Not one of the 13 dangerous drugs withdrawn over the last 10 years met a medical need not already being met by other drugs. Although touted as a "reform" by the Administration, many in Congress, and industry, the renewal amendment put added pressure on the FDA by industry for faster approvals and further tied the hands of the FDA in important ways. For example, user fee funds cannot be used to monitor the safety of any drug submitted for review before October 2002 or to assess unanticipated safety concerns which arise after marketing begins for new drugs. In addition, the FDA still does not have the authority to levy civil penalties for violations of its regulations, to subpoena industry records to investigate industry wrongdoing, or to require mandatory drug recalls not undertaken voluntarily by manufacturers (Sigelman, 2002).

The Faustian bargain struck between industry and the FDA, cemented in place by Congressional approval of continued user fees, builds obvious conflicts of interest into the regulatory process. To a considerable extent, the FDA is held hostage by the industry it is chartered to regulate. User fees now fund about one-half of the costs of the FDA's review of marketing applications (Pear, 2002). Pressures from industry for rapid approval of new drugs have led to a "sweatshop" environment within the FDA, with rapid turnover of staff and increasing barriers to scientific debate of adverse effects of drugs under review. A 1998 survey by Public Citizen of FDA physician reviewers found that they had opposed the approval of 27 drugs approved during the previous three years. A 2002 report from the General Accounting Office (GAO), an investigative branch of Congress, revealed occasions when physicians were precluded from presenting adverse drug information at FDA Advisory Committee meetings and even received harassing phone calls from industry (General Accounting Office, 2002). Moreover, as the costs of prescription drugs keep soaring and become less affordable for millions of Americans, the FDA continues to refuse to consider drug costs or their cost effectiveness as legitimate criteria within the review and approval process. Instead, recognizing that addition of these criteria would be furiously opposed by industry, the new head of the FDA pursues a goal of making the review process shorter and more efficient for both drugs and medical devices as a way to reduce the costs of their development (Abboud & McGinley, 2003).

MANIPULATION OF FEDERAL REGULATORS BY INDUSTRY

Outlined below are several examples of ways in which the FDA appears to be held captive by the industry it seeks to regulate in the public interest:

- *Misleading advertising.* Direct-to-consumer advertising (DTCA) has increased by almost 150% since 1997, when FDA regulations or such advertising were relaxed. As a marketing strategy, DTCA is very effective. The GAO estimates that over 8 million people each year request and purchase prescriptions for specific drugs they hear or see advertised. Many of these ads are inaccurate or misleading, most often overstating the benefits and downplaying the risks of drugs being promoted. Yet the FDA's regulatory effectiveness is hampered by shortage of staff, the lack of authority to impose penalties on violators, and delays in sending regulatory letters created by recent requirement for legal review of all such letters. In instances where ads have violated FDA standards, regulatory letters may be delayed by as much as 11 weeks, often allowing misleading ads to complete their cycle, and some companies continue to violate ad requirements, without penalties, even after receiving multiple regulatory letters from the FDA (Gahart, Duhamel, Dievler, Price, 2003). Although there is no evidence that the accuracy of DTCA has improved since 1997, by 2003 the FDA stopped only 24 misleading ads, an 85% drop since 1998 (Public Citizen Health Research Group, 2004).
- *Advertising for unapproved uses.* Video news releases (VNRs) are entire news stories, written, filmed and produced by public relations firms and sent by Internet or satellite feed to television stations around the world. By 1991, 4,000 such releases were being produced each year. They are presented to the public as breakthrough news announcements implying a third party, without disclosure of their drug company source, thereby circumventing the FDA requirements for such advertising. The FDA has no formal guidelines for VNR's, which are in wide use by drug manufacturers, including for unapproved uses of drugs being advertised (Bosik, 1991; Foley, 1993).
- *Fighting against worrisome but necessary labels.* Tylenol® is taken in one form or another by almost 50 million Americans every week, with annual sales in the billions. It also accounts for more than 100,000 calls a year to poison control centers, 56,000 emergency room visits, and 26,000 hospitalizations. Tylenol is contained in many combination over-the-counter products, overdosing is common, and drug overdoses lead to 450 deaths a year in the U.S. In 2002, FDA staff wanted to reduce the public's access to Tylenol by considering such approaches as reducing maximal dosage, limiting manufacturers' flexibility in combination products, and requiring more safety warnings on

labels. Confidential documents obtained by an investigative reporter, however, revealed how these approaches were avoided in FDA Advisory Committee discussions for fear of offending Johnson & Johnson, the manufacturer of Tylenol and the third largest health care corporation in the world. Discussion of the positive experience in the United Kingdom with safety controls of Tylenol were ruled out of order by senior FDA managers and only minimal labeling changes were made (Moynihan, 2002; (Public Citizen Health Research Group, 2002).

- *Underreporting of adverse drug effects.* One half of approved drugs are later found to have serious adverse effects not detected before FDA approval (General Accounting Office, 1990), and adverse drug effects that do not stem from human error account for 1.5 million hospitalizations and more than 100,000 deaths each year in the U.S. (Lazarou, Pomeranz, Corey, 1998). Despite this alarming public hazard, the FDA estimates that only about 10% of adverse drug effects are ever reported (Wolfe, 2003). In fact, it has recently been calculated that the probability of a drug being found to have a life-threatening risk or being withdrawn from the market over a 25-year period is 20% (Lasser, Allen, Woolhandler, Himmelstein, Wolfe et al., 2002). Yet, drug companies regularly underreport adverse drug effects to the FDA, as already shown by the examples in chapter 5 of Baycol and Regulin.

- *Delaying or failing to complete required Phase IV studies.* Phase IV post-marketing drug surveillance studies are often required by the FDA as a condition for approval, and they can provide essential information about the safety and effectiveness of new drugs. Once drugs are on the market, however, drug companies often drag their feet in completing these required studies. By 2002, little more than one-third of 2,400 Phase IV studies were completed and submitted to the FDA. Although the FDA has the authority in some cases to withdraw approval if Phase IV studies are not done, it has never done so (Adams, 2003). It is therefore obvious that monitoring of Phase IV studies has been relaxed significantly.

- *Withholding information about unfavorable studies.* As we saw in Chapter 6, ephedra is a commonly used drug which, as a "dietary supplement," is partly shielded from some FDA regulatory procedures. The burden of proof of its lack of safety falls on the FDA. A study was carried out by manufacturers in the late 1990s and was touted by industry as confirming the safety and effectiveness of ephedra for weight loss. But industry sponsors and researchers withheld information about the study until recently when an agreement was reached to have a panel of three scientists review the methods and assess the conclusions of the study. All three scientists criticized the study as flawed for such reasons as being too small to be valid, and for minimizing increases in heart rate and blood pressure among study participants (Drew & Fessenden, 2003). Yet industry lobbyists and some supporters in Congress continued to battle against an FDA ban on the drug linked to thousands of reports of strokes, cardiac arrhythmias, and other acute problems, including more than 100 deaths (Pear & Grady, 2003).

- *Using a "home brew" strategy to avoid the need for FDA approval.* Diagnostic tests that are marketed to hospitals, commercial laboratories, and physicians' offices, must go through the FDA approval process. One way to bypass approval requirements, now increasingly used by some manufacturers, is to market the basic ingredients of such tests, which are then put together by users, hence the term "home brew". An advisory committee to HHS recommended in 2000 that the FDA should regulate some genetic tests, including home brew tests. The FDA is now considering extending the regulatory umbrella to all high-risk diagnostic tests, which of course the testing industry opposes for time and cost reasons (Pollack, 2003a).

- *Lobbying for faster approvals.* Industry has complained for many years about the time lags in the FDA approval process. Now that industry is paying one-half of the costs of this process through user fees, it is even more insistent in its demands for rapid reviews. A 2003 report by the HHS's Inspector General revealed new concerns that the integrity of the review process is now threatened by inadequate time, excess workload for reviewers, and too much political influence on the process (Frieden, 2003). That the threshold for approval has been lowered is suggested by the May, 2003 approval of Iressa, Astra Zeneca's new cancer drug, which was approved for the treatment of lung cancer despite the findings that it shrank tumor size in only 10% of patients in one small study, that tumors begin growing again in one-half of those patients after seven months, that it failed to prolong life when combined with chemotherapy in larger studies, and that it is linked to 246 deaths in Japan. Astra Zeneca executives anticipate that annual sales could reach $1 billion (Pollack, 2003b).

- *Inadequate notification of patients after drug recall.* Recalls of drugs are voluntary on the part of their manufacturers, and it is they who control the pace and scope of patient notification when drugs are recalled. Recalled drugs may or may not be removed from retail pharmacies, and companies are often reluctant to fund widespread notification efforts. There are no federal regulations in place for the notification process. In one follow-up study carried out by researchers at Cook County Hospital in Chicago after Baycol was recalled, only 20% had heard of the recall, more than one-half of patients continued to take the drug, and 40% of these patients had physical symptoms of muscle damage. Public Citizen's Health Research Group has noted that drug companies pay out only a small fraction of their profits for a given drug to losses through litigation, and calls for expanded authority of the FDA to include mandatory drug recalls, more rigorous patient notification requirements, and civil monetary penalties for violations by drug companies (Wolfe, 2002).

- *Lobbying against imports of less expensive drugs.* Congress passed legislation in 2000, signed into law by President Clinton, which would allow imports of less expensive prescription drugs if it could be certified by HHS that such imports would be safe. Since then, under heavy lobbying pressure from industry, no Administration has assured such safety. A similar bill was passed by the House with strong bipartisan support in July 2003, sponsored by Representative Jo Ann Emerson (R-Mo) and Representative Gil Gutnecht (R-Minn). This proposal would establish a system for consumers, pharmacists, and wholesalers to import FDA-approved drugs from FDA-approved facilities in Canada and Europe. A provision was also included to assure counterfeit-resistant packaging (Stolberg, 2003a). Despite strong public demand for cost containment of prescription drugs, the growing volume of purchases of Canadian drugs by Americans, the lack of documented safety of these drugs (Davey, 2003), and restrictions against lobbying by governmental agencies, FDA officials have personally lobbied hard in Congress against this bill as the drug industry continues to press its claims that such imports impose a risk to the public and that price controls in the U.S. would jeopardize research and development of new drugs (Stolberg, 2003b).

THE HEALTH INSURANCE INDUSTRY AND STATE REGULATORS

As we saw in the last chapter the insurance industry is largely regulated at the state level where the industry maintains a formidable lobbying effort to promote its own interests. Within the health care arena, state insurance agencies regulate health insurance practices for about one-third of people in an average state. Medicare, Medicaid, Veterans Administration coverage, and other federal plans are exempt from state regulation, as are self-funded plans, which are exempted under the Employee Retirement Income Security Act (ERISA) (Iglehart, 1997).

In 1999, more than 2,200 insurance-related companies and organizations had lobbyists deployed in the states (Renzulli & The Center for Public Integrity, 2002). Many state regulatory agencies are understaffed and vulnerable to influence by industry. In Indiana, for example, there are only three consumer consultants and no investigators in a state commission receiving more than 5,000 complaints each year. The *Indianapolis Star* has published an editorial stating that "the conflicts of interest are so pervasive that the industry is actually regulating the regulators, rather than vice versa" (Renzulli & The Center for Public Integrity, 2002, p. 107).

Hundreds of laws and regulations are enacted every year in statehouses across the country, which control insurance practices across a broad spectrum of issues. A 2000 50-state survey of insurance commissions on health insurance or managed care requested information on the following areas:

- Prescription drug coverage and regulation of annual limits, caps, and copays
- Coverage of off-label drug use and for specific terminal conditions, such as cancer, AIDS, and HIV
- Right to use restricted formularies
- Coverage of medically necessary treatments associated with AIDS and HIV
- Consumers' ability to sue their insurer or health plan for denial of care or refusal to cover all medically necessary prescriptions
- Coverage of routine costs associated with experimental prescriptions and treatments (Bolin, Buchanan, Smith, 2002).

Not surprisingly, the survey found a regulatory maze, with wide variability in regulations from one state to another, and with many states providing few consumer protections. For example, 39 states do not require private health insurers to offer prescription drug coverage, lifetime dollar limits are allowed in most states, and none of the states require managed care organizations to provide all necessary medications to beneficiaries with terminal illness such as AIDS (Bolin, Buchanan, Smith, 2002).

HEALTH CARE REGULATIONS AND THE COURTS

On most issues related to health care, the court system comes down on the side of corporate interests. This has been true for over 100 years, since a landmark case before the U.S. Supreme Court in 1886 accorded corporations the rights of persons, including freedom of speech (to lobby their interests), protection from searches, Fifth Amendment protections, and coverage by due process and antidiscrimination laws (Derber, 1998, pp. 129–131). As "legal persons," corporations have been granted special freedoms to pursue their interests, and also have advantages over private citizens. They can live forever, can live in many places at the same time (including overseas), and can change at will or even sell themselves to foreign owners. Furthermore, when corporations are prosecuted for crimes, they can claim that they are "artificial legal entities," not personally accountable for alleged misdeeds (Greider, 1992). These protections have led to some surprising alliances through corporation friendly interpretations of the First Amendment by the courts. Between 1988 and 1996, for example, the ACLU and its branches secretly received over $1 million in donations from the tobacco industry to fund ACLU committees in their efforts to protect "smokers' rights" and to support the rights of tobacco companies to advertise their products (Mintz, 1998).

Although the FDA has won 94 federal court cases since 1990, it has lost 23 such cases during that period. Table 11.2 lists some important

TABLE 11.2. Some Important Losses by FDA in Federal Courts

Date	Outcome
1999	Appeals court says the FDA improperly rejected health claims by dietary supplement makers
2000	Court challenge by a conservative foundation opens the door to drug companies mailing out medical articles on unapproved ("off-label") uses of their drugs
2000	Supreme Court rejects attempts to regulate tobacco: "It is plain that Congress has not given the FDA the authority that it seeks"
2002	Supreme Court strikes down rules barring pharmacies from advertising special "compounded" drug mixtures
2002	Judge says FDA rule requiring some drugs to be tested on children "usurps" Congress

Source: Adams, C. (2002). FDA isn't holding up in court. *The Wall Street Journal,* November 19, p. A4.

examples of these losses, which have tended to undermine and limit the agency's regulatory authority (Adams, 2002).

Despite the conservative leanings of many courts concerning health care, there are some areas where the courts have sided with consumer interests. An important example is the 5-4 decision by the U.S. Supreme Court in June, 2002 (*Rush Prudential HMO, Inc.* vs. *Moran*), which upheld an Illinois state law requiring binding independent external review when an HMO disagrees with a patient's physician over questions of medical necessity (Lueck, Greenberger, Rundle, 2002). Over 40 states have established independent review boards to adjudicate disputes between HMOs, physicians, and their patients over coverage of procedures and treatments. Many cases of this kind have been overturned through appeal mechanisms across the country (Mariner, 2002).

CONCLUDING COMMENTS

The four chapters in Part II provide abundant evidence that serious health care reform is needed because corporate self-interest, in many cases, trumps the public interest, and existing approaches to regulating the health care industry is failing at both federal and state levels. Stronger regulation is urgently needed that is independent of co-option by corporate self-interest. Given the pervasive money culture in politics today, it is now time to shift gears into Part III, where we will ask whether serious health care reform is possible and assess the advantages and disadvantages of alternative approaches.

REFERENCES

Abboud, L., & McGinley, L. (2003, April 16). FDA chief embarks on novel mission: Cut drug costs. *The Wall Street Journal*, p. A4.

Adams, C. (2002, Nov. 19). FDA isn't holding up in court. *The Wall Street Journal*, p. A4.

Adams, C. (2003, Jan. 28). Test data for some drugs are long overdue at the FDA. *The Wall Street Journal*, p. B1.

Barrett, S. (2003). How the Dietary Supplement Health and Education Act of 1998 weakened the FDA. Retrieved May 13, from *www.quackwatch.org/02 ConsumerProtection,dshea.html* Bolin, J. N., Buchanan, R. J., Smith, S. R. (2002). State regulation of private health insurance: prescription drug benefits, experimental treatments, and consumer protection. *American Journal of Managed Care, 8.*

Bolin, J. N., Buchanan, R. J., & Smith, S. R., (2002). State regulation of private health insurance: prescription drug benefits, experimental treatments, and consumer protection. *American Journal of Managed Care, 8,* 977.

Bosik, D. (1991, April). TV Stations Desire Health, Medical VNRs the Most. O'Dwyer PR Services Report, p. 12.

Davey, M. (2003, Oct. 27). Illinois seeks permission to buy drugs in Canada; Governor cites study on safety and savings. *The New York Times,* p. A11.

Derber, C. (1998). *Corporation nation: How corporations are taking over our lives and what we can do about it* (p. 65). New York: St. Martin's Press.

Deyo, R. A. (1998). Using outcomes to improve quality of research and quality of care. *Journal of American Board of Family Practice 11,* 465.

Drew, C., & Fessenden, F. (2003, July 23). Expert panel finds flaws in diet pill safety study. *The New York Times,* p. A14.

Echt, D. E., Liebson, P. R., Mitchell, L. B., Peters, R. W., Obias-Manno, D., Barker, A. H., Areneberg, D., Baker, A., Friedman, L., Green, H. L. (1991). Mortality and morbidity in patients receiving encainide, flecainide, or placebo: The cardiac arrhythmia suppression trial. *The New England Journal of Medicine, 324,* 781.

Eichenwald, K. (2001, Jan. 25). Redesigning Nature: Hard Lessons Learned. *The New York Times.*

Foley, K. E. (1993, April). Ethics and Sigma are in 'VNR Cartel.' O'Dwyer's PR Services Report, April, p. 13.

Frieden, J. (2003). Inspector General faults FDA drug review process. *Family Practice News, 33,* 53.

Gahart, M. T., Duhamel, L. M., Dievler, A,. Price, R. (2003, Feb. 26). Examining the FDA's oversight of direct-to-consumer advertising. *Health Affairs,* February 26, W3, 120.

General Accounting Office. (1990). *FDA drug review: Postapproval risks, 1976–85.* GAO/PMD-90-15. Washington, DC: Author.

General Accounting Office. (2002). GAO report backs link between drug user fees and higher rate of drug withdrawals. *Health Letter 18,* 11.

The Wall Street Journal (2002, Oct. 14). Global Giants: Amid Market Pain, U.S. companies Hold Greater Sway. p. R10.

Greider, W. (1992). *Who will tell the people: The betrayal of American democracy* (p. 349). New York: Simon & Schuster.

Hartmann, T. (2002). *Unequal protection: The rise of corporate dominance and the theft of human rights* (p. 37). Emmaus, PA: Rodale Press.

Iglehart, J. K. (1997). State regulation of managed care: Interview with NAIC President Joseph Musser. *Health Affairs (Millwood) 16,* 36.

Korten, D. C. (2001). *When corporations rule the world (p. 98).* San Francisco: Berrett-Koehler Publishers.

Lasser, K. E., Allen, P. D., Woolhandler, S. J., Himmelstein, D. U., Wolfe, S. M., Bor, D. H. (2002). Timing of new black box warnings and withdrawals for prescription medications. *Journal of the American Medical Association 287,* 2215.

Lazarou, J., Pomeranz, B. H., Corey, P. N. (1998). Incidence of adverse drug reactions in hospitalized patients: A meta-analysis of prospective studies. *Journal of the American Medical Association, 279,* 1200.

Lewis, C., & The Center for Public Integrity. (1998). *The buying of the congress: How special interests have stolen your right to life, liberty and the pursuit of happiness* (p. 142). New York: Avon Books.

Lueck, S., Greenberger, R, Rundle, R. (2002, June 25). Court backs patient appeals in battle over HMO coverage. *The Wall Street Journal.*

Mariner, W. K. (2002). Independent external review of health maintenance organizations' medical necessity decisions. *The New England Journal of Medicine, 347,* 2178.

Merrill, R. A. (1999). Modernizing the FDA: An incremental revolution. *Health Affairs (Millwood) 18,* 96.

Mintz, M. (1998, Spring). The ACLU and the tobacco companies. *Nieman Reports,* p. 66.

Moynihan, J. (2002). FDA fails to reduce accessibility of paracetamol despite 450 deaths a year. *British Medical Journal, 325,* 678.

Pear, R. (2002, Dec. 12). FDA seeks quicker approval of new drugs. *The New York Times,* p. A16.

Pear, R., & Grady, D. (2003, March 1). Government moves to curtail use of diet supplement. *The New York Times,* p. A1.

Pollack, A. (2003a, July 18). FDA asks if a genetic test is sold without approval. *The New York Times,* p. C2.

Pollack, A. (2003b, May 6). Drug's approval hints at flexibility in FDA process. *The New York Times,* p. C1.

Public Citizen (2002, Oct. 18). Public Citizen decries conflict of interest created by new law regulating safety of medical devices. Press release. Washington, D.C.

Public Citizen Health Research Group. (2002). Unsafe drugs: Congressional silence is deadly (Part 2). *Health Letter, 8*(11): 1.

Public Citizen Health Research Group. (2002). FDA caves in to industry, fails to adequately address acetaminophen (Tylenol) overdoses. *Worst Pills, Best Pills 8,* 87.

Public Citizen Health Research Group (2004). Overselling Donepezil (Aricept) and exploiting patients with Alzheimers disease: Why isn't the FDA stopping these ads? *Health Letter, 20*(3), 1.

Ramsey, S. D., Luce, B. R., Deyo, R., Franklin, G. (1998). The limited state of technology assessment for medical devices: Facing the issues. *American Journal of Managed Care, 4,* 188.

Renzulli, D., & The Center for Public Integrity. (2003). *Capitol offenders: How private interests govern our states.* Washington, D.C.: Center for Public Integrity.

Sigelman, D. (2002). Unsafe drugs: Congressional silence is deadly. *Public Citizen Research Group Health Letter, 18,* 1.

Stolberg, S. G. (2003a, July 26). House passes drug measures, but faces fight with Senate. *The New York Times,* p. A11.

Stolberg, S. G. (2003b, July 25). FDA officials press legislators to oppose bill in importing less expensive drugs. *The New York Times,* p. A18.

Wolfe, S. M. (2002). Drug safety withdrawals: Who is responsible for notifying patients? *Pharmacoepidemiology Drug Safety 11,* 641.

Wolfe, S. M. (2003). Remedies needed to address the pathology in reporting adverse reactions and Food and Drug Administration use of reports. *Journal of General Internal Medicine, 18,* 72.

Part III

IS REFORM POSSIBLE?

Chapter 12

PRIVATIZATION vs. THE PUBLIC UTILITY MODEL OF HEALTH CARE

We're either going to have a health care system where people who live in this country are welcome, or we're not. If we're not, then let's just say, "Okay, we're *not* going to be a first-rate health care system," instead of clinging to this fantasy that as long as you can beg for services or work the system, you can get care. The unreliability of such an approach is appalling. It is also a wrong assumption that all the uninsured are perfectly willing to be treated as charity cases. Someone who lived on my block was too proud to go to an emergency room, because he couldn't pay. He died of pneumonia.

—Emily Friedman
Ethicist and Health Policy Analyst

In this and the next two chapters we will consider whether, and to what extent, any real reform is possible for the U.S. health care system. In past years, it has been a given that we start with the existing system and ask what incremental changes can address its problems. As we have seen in earlier chapters, however, incremental reforms have consistently failed to resolve the problems of access, costs, quality, and performance. With the system now collapsing around us and ever more obviously unsustainable without major change, we therefore need to revisit these fundamental, interrelated, and still mostly unanswered questions:

- Is health care a basic human need and right, or is it just another commodity for sale on the open market?
- Should health care be provided on a for-profit or not-for-profit basis?
- Should health care delivery be based on a market system or on a public utility model?
- Whom should the health care system serve primarily, the patient or the stakeholders in providing care?

• If the private market is to retain its central role in U.S. health care, can its excesses be regulated in the public interest?

These questions, underscored by Emily Friedman above (Brown, 1999), underpin the national debate over any effort to reform our health care system. To the extent that they remain unanswered, they will render effective reform unlikely. This chapter is concerned with the first three of these questions. Since Part II has already cast serious doubt upon the degree to which the excesses of corporate self-interest can be regulated, the stakes associated with these questions are raised even higher.

This chapter has four goals: (1) to briefly revisit the issue of health care as a right or commodity for sale; (2) to compare the track record of privatized corporate health care against its claims of greater efficiency and value; (3) to consider the extent to which public-private partnerships can address system problems; and (4) to briefly describe an alternative approach to health care delivery within a not-for-profit, public utility model of care.

HEALTH CARE: ANOTHER COMMODITY OR A HUMAN RIGHT?

We have already touched on this question in chapter 1 including the views of the Institute of Medicine and the U.S. Supreme Court favoring the "human right" position, and further qualified by the thoughtful observations of the ethicist, Larry Churchill. While all other industrialized Western countries have built their health care systems around one or another form of social health insurance with universal coverage, the U.S. remains locked in a long unresolved debate about health care as an entitlement versus a commodity for sale on the open market. Princeton's health economist Uwe Reinhardt brings sharp focus to this issue with this pointed question: "As a matter of national policy, and to the extent that a nation's health system can make it possible, should the child of a poor American family have the same chance of avoiding preventable illness or of being cured from a given illness as does the child of a rich American family?" (Reinhardt, 1997). Opponents of a system of national health insurance base their opposition on a libertarian view and their preference for a limited role of government. As a result, the observation by Reinhardt below accurately describes the current health care marketplace with its plethora of increasingly unaffordable private sector programs and a beleaguered, underfunded public "safety net."

As a matter of conscious national policy, the United States always has and still does openly countenance the practice of rationing health care for millions of American children by their parents' ability to procure health insurance for the family or, if the family is uninsured, by their parents' willingness and ability to pay for health care out of their own pocket, or if the family is unable to pay, by the parents' willingness and ability to procure charity care in their role as health care beggars (Reinhardt, 1997).

With the shift toward more conservative government in the U.S. since 1980, and the current environment of fiscal deficits at both federal and state levels, gains made in the 1960s to assure access to health care for the poor and elderly are now under attack. In his excellent 2003 book, *The Political Life of Medicare,* Jonathan Oberlander documents that a bipartisan consensus supporting Medicare as a universal government program was maintained from 1965 to 1994. Medicare politics changed as this consensus unravelled after the 1994 congressional elections, when the ideological debate over Medicare reverted to that of the 1950s and 1960s. The opponents of Medicare in 1965 had proposed that, instead of operating a single-payer health insurance plan, the government should subsidize beneficiaries so that they could purchase private health insurance. Since the late 1990s Medicare politics have come full circle, with conservative legislators pushing for increased privatization and dismantling of traditional Medicare as an entitlement program (Oberlander, 2003).

In his book *The Social Transformation of American Medicine,* Paul Starr saw all of this coming more than 20 years ago. His assessment then describes today's chaotic health care landscape quite well:

The rise of a corporate ethos in medical care is already one of the most significant consequences of the changing structure of medical care. It is likely to aggravate inequalities in access to health care. Profit-making enterprises are not interested in treating those who cannot pay. The voluntary hospital may not treat the poor the same as the rich, but they do treat them and often treat them well. A system in which corporate enterprises play a larger part is likely to be more segmented and more stratified. With cutbacks in public financing coming at the same time, the two-class system in medical care is likely to become only more conspicuous. (Starr, 1982)

PRIVATIZATION: CLAIMS VS. TRACK RECORD

The continued drumbeat by proponents of the market-based health care system maintains that this approach provides greater efficiency and choice to patients. As we have seen in Part I, however, the well-documented track record of corporate, for-profit health care has a demonstrated track record quite the opposite—higher costs, lower quality, and less value compared with not-for-profit care. Whether one looks at investor-owned hospitals, HMOs, dialysis centers, nursing homes, or mental health companies, the results are the same—the only increase in efficiency is in separating the more lucrative parts of the market from the less lucrative. Table 12.1 summarizes evidence across the health care industry which documents that investor-owned care is more expensive and of lesser quality than not-for-profit care.

TABLE 12.1. Investor-Owned Care: Comparative Examples vs. Not-For-Profit Care

Hospitals	Costs 3–13% higher, with higher overhead, fewer nurses and death rates 6 to 7% higher (Chen, Radford, Wang, Marciniak, Krumholz, 1999; Hartz, Krakauer, Kuhn, Young, Jacobsen et al., 1989; Kovner & Gergen, 1998; Silverman, Skinner, Fisher, 1999; Woolhandler & Himmelstein, 1997; Yuan, Cooper, Einstadter, Cebul, Rimm, 2000)
HMOs	Higher overhead (25 to 33% for some of the largest HMOs), worse scores on 14 of 14 quality indicators reported to the National Committee for Quality Assurance (Himmelstein, Woolhandler, Hellander, Wolfe,1999; HMO honor roll, 1997; Kuttner, 1999)
Dialysis centers	Death rates 30% higher, with 26% less use of transplants (Devereaux, Schunemann, Ravindran, Bhandari, Garg et al., 2002; Garg, Frick, Diener-Wiest, Power, 1999)
Nursing homes	Lower staffing levels and worse quality of care; 30% committed violations which caused death or life-threatening harm to patients (Harrington, Woolhandler, Mullen, Carillo, Himmelstein, 2001)
Mental health centers	Medicare expelled 80 programs after investigations found that 91% of claims were fraudulent (Wrich, 1998), for-profit behavioral health companies impose restrictive barriers and limits to care (eg, premature discharge from hospitals without adequate outpatient care) (Munoz, 2002)

Source: Adapted with permission from the American Board of Family Practice, Lexington, Ky: In J. P. Geyman. The corporate transformation of medicine and its impact on costs and access to care. *Journal of the American Board of Family Practice,* 16(5):559.

As we saw in chapter 1, HMOs, nursing homes, home care agencies, and dialysis centers are predominantly for-profit and investor-owned. This dominance of the market continues as their prices soar unabated. According to Hewitt Health Resource, for example, average HMO premiums had increases of 21% and 17% in 2002 and 2003, respectively, and are expected to increase by another 18% in 2004 (Bennett, 2003). HMOs are increasing their profits, as they raise their premiums, by reducing benefits and increasing cost sharing with patients. They are marketing a broader range of products, including "more affordable" plans with reduced benefits that are tailored to medium and lower-income individuals. An analyst with the Carlyle Group, a New York investment firm, describes this business success in these terms: "Now there is a broad [range] of products and prices. There is a price point for everyone" (Kazel, 2003).

As escalating health care costs continue out of control, fraud runs rampant across the health care industry, especially in investor-owned corporations, as illustrated by these examples:

- HCA and Tenet, the two largest investor-owned hospital chains in the country, recently paid the government $631 million and $54 million, respectively, to settle charges of fraudulent overbilling (Bowe & Chaffin, 2003); although Tenet has been scandalized recently for its multiple aggressive and dishonest marketing and accounting practices, its CEO received $116 million in total compensation in fiscal 2002 (McLaughlin, 2003).
- Within the drug industry, TAP Pharmaceuticals Products Inc. paid $875 million in 2001 in civil and criminal penalties and pleaded guilty to a charge of conspiring with physicians to bill government insurers for free samples of its drug for prostate cancer (Callahan, 2003).
- Within the medical device industry, Guidant admitted that it failed to report malfunctions of its device for abdominal aortic aneurisms and the injuries and deaths which occurred as a result, paying $92 million in 2003 to settle those charges (Callahan, 2003).

The National Health Care Anti-Fraud Association, a nonpartisan group of insurers, self-insured companies, and government investigators, estimates that fraud accounts for 3% of the nation's health care spending each year (about $50 billion in 2003) (Callahan, 2003).

As a single-payer public insurance program since 1965, Medicare has been far more efficient than private health insurers, both in controlling overall health care costs and in administrative overhead. Figure 12.1 shows that Medicare has been more successful than private health insurers over the last 30 years in constraining its per-enrollee cost growth for personal health care. This capability in cost control has been largely attributed to Medicare's ability to aggressively price for the services it covers (Boccuti & Moon, 2003). It has done so while providing universal coverage for all individuals 65 years of age or older and still maintaining higher levels of patient satisfaction across income groups of both sick and healthy beneficiaries (see Figure 4.2) (Boccuti & Moon, 2003). Medicare is administered with an overhead of about 3% compared with overhead costs five to nine times higher for private insurers (PNHP, 2002). Indeed, Medicare could be even more efficiently administered were coverage decisions not decentralized to almost 50 local private contractors across the country that process individual claims for payment. Because of a political compromise when Medicare was enacted in 1965, private contractors were empowered to determine whether claims are a covered benefit, and if so, whether the service is "reasonable and necessary". Most Medicare coverage decisions are therefore made at the local level (Foote, 2003). Since there is considerable variation from one area of the country to another in local medical review policies (LMRPs, 9,000 of which were posted in 2001) the Medicare Payment Advisory Commission (MedPAC) has recently recommended that this local process of policy and regulation be eliminated in order to reduce Medicare's current complexity, inconsistency, and uncertainty" (MedPac, 2001). As expected, this issue has touched off an intense debate on both sides of the issue. Organized medicine has called for uniform national standards for coverage decisions (Aston, 2002), while the medical device industry, concerned about possible delays in coverage decisions made nationally on an all or none basis, supports the current local process (AdvaMed, 2001).

As we saw in chapter 4, the private health insurance industry, mostly for-profit, is bloated with middlemen, bureaucracy, and high administrative overhead. Fragmentation, inefficiency, and waste are unavoidable with over 1,200 private health insurers offering many thousands of different policies. One study of 2,000 patients in one city found that they were covered by 189 different plans with 755 different policies (Grembowski, Diehr, Novak, Roussel, Martin, 2000). A 2003 study found that health care administrative costs total at least $294 billion each year in the U.S. (31% of annual national health care expenditures), or $1,059 per capita compared with only $309 per capita across the border in Canada (see Table 12.2). Administrative and

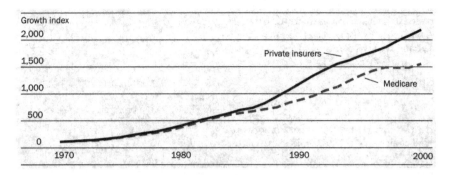

FIGURE 12.1 Cumulative growth in per enrollee payments for personal health care, Medicare, and private insurers, 1970–2000.

Source: Boccuti, C., & Moon, M. (2003). Comparing Medicare and private insurers: Growth rates in spending over three decades. *Health Affairs (Millwood), 22,* 230. Reprinted with permission.

clerical personnel now account for 27% of the U.S. health care work force. Table 12.3 shows that employees of private health insurers in the U.S. vastly outnumber their counterparts in the Canadian single-payer system (Woolhandler, Campbell, Himmelstein, 2003a). These inefficiencies, however, do not constrain profits of private health insurers in this country, which averaged 25% in 2001 (Terry, 2003). These profits are achieved by lowering the "medical loss" ratio, restricting benefits, increasing cost-sharing with enrollees, and avoiding sicker patients.

TABLE 12.2. Costs of Health Care Administration in the United States and Canada, 1999

| | Spending Per Capita (U.S. $) | |
Cost Category	United States	Canada
Insurance overhead	259	47
Employers' costs to manage health benefits	57	8
Hospital administration	315	103
Nursing home administration	62	29
Administrative costs of practitioners	324	107
Home care administration	42	13
TOTAL	1,059	307

Source: Woolhandler, S., et al. (2003a). Costs of health care administration in the United States and Canada. *The New England Journal of Medicine, 349,* 771.

TABLE 12.3. Number of Enrollees and Employees of Major U.S. Private Health Insurers and Canadian Provincial Health Plans, 2001

Plan Name	No. of Enrollees†	No. of Employees	No. of Employees/ 10,000 Employees
U.S. Plans:			
Aetna	17.170,0W	35,7W	20.9
Anthem	7,983.000	14,800	18.9
Cigna	14.300.OW	44,6W	31.2
Humana	6,435,8W	14.500	22.5
Mid Atlantic Medical Services	1.932,400	2.571	14.0
Oxford	1.490,600	3,400	22.8
Pacificare	3,388,100	8,200	24–2
United Healthcare	8,S40,000	30,000	35.1
WellPoint	10,146,945	13,900	13.7
Canadian Plans:			
Saskatchewan Health	1.021,288	145	1.4
Ontario Health Insurance Plan	11,742,672	1,433‡	1.2

*Data are from the Annual Reports filed with the Securities and Exchange Commission, the Government of Saskatchewan and the Government of Ontario.

†Numbers include administrative-services-only contracts as well as Medicare. Medicaid, and commercial enrollees; numbers exclude recipients of pharmacy-benefit management, life, dental, other specialty. and nonhealth insurance products.

‡The estimate is based on wage and salary expenses and on the assumption that the average annual wage is $38,250.

Source: Reprinted with permission from Woolhandler, S., Cambell, T., & Himmelstein, D. U. (2003a). Costs of health care administration in the United States and Canada. *The New England Journal of Medicine, 349,* 768.

Privatization of Medicare is being promoted by its many advocates despite the largely negative experience with Medicare+Choice HMOs in recent years. About one-third of seniors enrolled in these plans were dropped between 1999 and 2003 as many providers found the market for such plans less than lucrative (Bodenheimer, 2003). After a $1 billion increase in Medicare reimbursement in 2001, only a few such programs increased benefits or re-entered the market, and more than 800,000 Medicare enrollees lost coverage (Medicare minus choice, 2002; Waldholz, 2002). In a recent pilot program for Medicare PPOs, fewer than 1 million Medicare patients signed up for that option in 23 states even 3 months after its launch (Japsen, 2003).

Despite this experience, market proponents are still promoting Medicare PPOs as a strategy to "save Medicare." There are now about

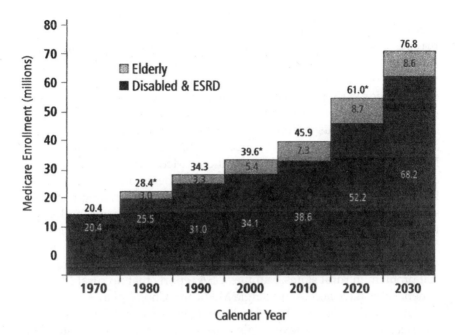

FIGURE 12.2 Number of Medicare beneficiaries: the number of people Medicare serves will nearly double by 2030.

Source: Physicians for a National Health Program (2002). Retrieved from *www.pnhp.org* Reprinted with permission.

40 million Medicare beneficiaries and their number is expected to nearly double by 2030 (see Figure 12.2). Faced with this demographic reality, conservative politicians and market advocates are hoping to dismantle the social contract of traditional Medicare as an entitlement program and shift it to a federally subsidized, privatized model requiring increased cost sharing with patients. This battle underlies the ongoing political debate over a Medicare prescription drug benefit.

The Federal Employees Health Benefits Program (FEHBP) is the largest employer-sponsored health benefits program in the United States today, covering more than 8 million federal employees, retirees, and their dependents. The FEHBP, "the health plan that members of Congress have," is being touted as a model for "reform," despite the fact that its premiums are increasing by double-digits each year and that private plans have consistently failed to control health care costs. A 2003 study by the Commonwealth Fund found that average out-of-pocket spending for Medicare+Choice enrollees in poor health more than doubled between 1999 and 2003 from $2,211 to $5,305 (Commonwealth Fund, 2003). In addition to being less efficient than the traditional Medicare fee-for-service program, private plans pay physicians and hospitals about 15% more than Medicare reimbursement rates, according to a study by the Medicare Payment Advisory Commission involving health plans of over 31 million people (Pear, 2003a). Private Medicare plans exit the market unless they receive sufficient reimbursement from the government to compensate for this difference and to maintain their profitability.

A recent report by Public Citizen found that the government paid Medicare HMOs 13% more than traditional Medicare costs between 1998 and 2000 (Public Citizen, 2002). In addition to being more expensive and less efficient than traditional Medicare, they end up limiting choice for seniors. A 2003 study by Public Citizen found, for example, that less than one-half of the Medicare general physicians in 20 counties of 5 states were in the Blue Cross-Blue Shield plan, the private plan with the most Medicare physicians (Wolfe, 2003). Restrictions in choice are a special problem in rural states. Families USA reports that no rural Medicare beneficiaries have access to a single Medicare+Choice plan if they live in any of the following 19 states: Alaska, Arkansas, Connecticut, Delaware, Georgia, Kansas, Kentucky, Maine, Maryland, Mississippi, Montana, Nebraska, New Hampshire, North Dakota, South Carolina, South Dakota, Utah, Vermont, or Wyoming (Armstrong, 2003).

Increased cost sharing which occurs in private plans inevitably leads to decreased access to care, lower utilization of services, and impaired clinical outcomes, especially for lower income, fragile or disabled elderly patients. Patricia Neuman, Vice President and Director of the Henry J. Kaiser Family Foundation's Medicare Policy Project, called attention in recent testimony before Congress to the "triple jeopardy" of seniors faced with increased cost sharing:

> Those with low incomes are more likely to be without any form of supplemental insurance that covers Medicare's cost-sharing requirements; since those with low incomes also tend to be in poorer health and need more medical services, Medicare's cost-sharing requirements will account for a greater portion of their limited income if they use the necessary additional services; and if they do not use the additional services they need, their health is likely to suffer as a result. (Neuman, 2003).

PUBLIC—PRIVATE PARTNERSHIPS: ARE THEY REALLY A REFORM OPTION?

As our market-based health care system steams full-speed ahead, leaving an increasing part of the population behind, many call for new kinds of public-private partnerships. The concept has an attractive ring to it, even if it is not clear what it means. For such a potentially important subject, the literature is relatively sparse, and the concept is variously and often vaguely described.

At the international level, public-private partnerships have been growing in recent years, and often involve collaboration between the public and private sectors for such purposes as stimulating product development and expanded availability of vaccines for infectious disease in the developing world. There have been a number of successful initiatives around the world using this approach, such as agreements made by some drug companies to provide drugs at low cost to underdeveloped countries besieged by the AIDS pandemic (Reich, 2002), but it has also been recognized that public-private partnerships are not appropriate in such areas as public health policy making and regulatory approval, where the for-profit motive of the private sector biases the collaboration (Widdus, 2001).

Closer to home, there are many ongoing public-private partnership projects, especially at the community level, involving foundations, associations, nonprofit organizations, Federal and state agencies, provider groups, and members of the business community. Most of these projects are focused on improving access to care for underserved and vulnerable populations, and in many cases are conducted as Medicaid demonstration projects (Models That Work Campaign, 2003). The Institute of Medicine has recently proposed five major initiatives for targeted demonstration projects as a foundation for reform of the health care system: (1) information technology development, (2) expanded health insurance coverage, (3) malpractice reform, (4) chronic disease management, and (5) primary care enhancement. Each strategic initiative would require an investment of government funds and involve some degree of collaboration between the public and private sectors. For example, demonstration projects targeted to expand health insurance coverage would likely involve use of tax credits or expansion of public programs such as Medicaid and SCHIP (Institute of Medicine, 2002).

Although the concept of closer collaboration between the public and private sectors sounds appealing, the critical word requiring closer scrutiny is the term "partnership". These examples are clearly not partnerships in the public interest, although they meet the profit mission of private sector participants:

- Medicaid HMOs in New Jersey have become efficient in tracking down low-income families without telephones, enrolling them, and then rejecting 17 to 30% of their claims for hospital care (Freudenheim, 2003).

- Medicare HMOs have dropped 2.4 million elderly patients in the last five years, complaining of inadequate federal payments, already 13% more than for the traditional fee-for-service Medicare program (Freudenheim, 2003; Public Citizen, 2002); while receiving higher reimbursement than fee-for-service Medicare and abandoning more costly markets, Medicare+Choice plans increased their earnings by 118% in 2002 (Rose, 2004).
- A joint venture between almost 400,000 Medicaid recipients in Massachusetts for mental health care from two of the country's largest for-profit behavioral health companies ended up bringing millions of dollars to these companies even as their systems of care collapsed; many covered children were left stranded unnecessarily in locked wards of psychiatric hospitals without arrangements for outpatient followup as the companies collected capitation dollars without accountability (Wolfe, 2001).
- Discount cards now being offered by some pharmaceutical companies to some low-income patients, while helpful to those patients, are not in the long term public interest to the extent that they provide the industry with political and public relations cover as they fight against price controls, importation of drugs from Canada, cost-effectiveness comparisons of "me-too" drugs, or any relaxation of their assumed rights.

While there are many examples of well-motivated and successful collaborations between the public and private sectors in the U.S., one can find little evidence that real partnerships, with built-in public accountability, will provide much opportunity for health care reform. At best, these collaborations can help some communities in some parts of the country. At worst, these collaborations give a false impression of progress toward reform while preserving the interests of stakeholders in a failing system.

TOWARD A PUBLIC UTILITY MODEL OF HEALTH CARE

The foregoing shows how distorted traditional values of public service in health care have become in the largely deregulated health care marketplace. The problem is not so much the predictable behavior of the for-profit enterprise as the system itself, which creates and maintains incentives for business to thrive at the expense of patient care. As Kuttner, with long experience as a health care analyst, has pointed out, the problem is also not so simple as distinguishing for-profits from not-for-profits, since market pressures drive some not-for-profits to adopt some of the practices of for-profit organizations in order to survive (Kuttner, 1998).

If the Darwinian marketplace undermines our health care system, even to the point of its not being sustainable in the long run, and if public-private partnerships do not hold the key to reform, what then are our options to rebuild a sustainable and humane health care system? To answer that question, we need to decide what kind of system we want. As is well documented in earlier chapters, the Wall Street model of health care gives us:

- a large and still growing part of the population which is either uninsured or underinsured, with increasingly restricted health benefits (Institute of Medicine, 2003; Pear, 2003b)
- millions of people crowding our emergency rooms with urgent and emergent problems, many of which could have been prevented with earlier care, and if they are uninsured, being charged the highest rates often without adequate follow-up care (Derlet, 2002; Ornstein, 2002; Weber & Ornstein, 2003)
- uncontrolled health care costs which, together with increased cost-sharing with patients, renders even basic health care services unaffordable for many millions of Americans (Kaiser, 2002a, Kaiser, 2002b)
- soaring costs of prescription drugs such that many patients with multiple chronic diseases can afford to fill only some of their prescriptions, and consequently reduce the doses or frequency because of costs (Taylor & Leitman, 2001)
- of the estimated 200,000 uninsured patients with newly diagnosed cancer each year, a recent study of their health expenditures on diagnosis and treatment was only 57% compared with insured patients with cancer; outcomes were not studied, but can only be expected to be considerably worse (Thorpe & Howard, 2003)

An alternative model, as will be described in more detail in the next chapter, would change our method of financing health care from its present maze of private-public approaches to a system of universal social insurance. Single-payer coverage, whether on a state by state or national basis, would trade in our uncontrolled administrative costs, waste, and profits for a sustainable system of universal coverage which could provide universal access to all medically necessary health care services while building in more quality controls and fiscal accountability (Woolhandler, Himmelstein, Angell, Young and the Physicians Working Group for Single-Payer National Health Insurance, 2003b). The basic structural flaw in our present system of for-profit, private health insurance is that this coverage is most expensive and least accessible for those patients who need it most—the sickest people with the lowest disposable income. As observed by Sara Rosenbaum, chairman of the Department of Health Policy at the George Washington University School of Public Health and Health Services, "from both an operational and economic perspective, it is simply a policy nonstarter for this group to rely on a market that does not want them and that will (logically, from a business perspective) attempt to block entry and retention through risk avoidance and pricing techniques" (Rosenbaum, 2003).

The Institute of Medicine's Committee on Quality of Health Care in America issued a landmark report in 2001 calling for 10 new directions to improve and transform our health care system (Institute of Medicine, 2001). Although the Committee's recommendations are important and laudable, its report pays little attention to the main barrier to implementing its recommendations—the transformation from a service to a business that has already occurred in health care (Relman, 2001). In response to that report, Gordon Schiff and Quentin Young have noted that you can't cross the quality chasm in U.S. health care in two jumps. They make a persuasive case that the proposed reforms will be ineffective unless accompanied by a public system of universal coverage. Table 12.4 presents their analysis comparing, for each IOM recommendation, the inhibitors/barriers in today's market-based system with facilitators /motivators in a public system of universal coverage (Schiff & Young, 2001).

It is the premise of this book that the single most important element of health care reform is changing our financing system to a public, single-payer model. The private sector could still do well in such a system, with stabilized reimbursement to health care facilities, reasonable reimbursement to health care providers, and fair return on investment to other industries such as the pharmaceutical and medical device industries. Administrative simplification and bulk purchasing of drugs and other products for large population groups, could extend health care to the whole population, increase the level of social justice within our system, and provide new opportunities to improve quality of care and system performance (Himmelstein & Woolhandler, 2003).

TABLE 12.4. Friction vs. Traction: Barriers and Facilitators to IOM's 10 "New Rules" to Transform Health Care

New rules to improve care, adapted from IOM report	Inhibitors/barriers in current market-oriented system	Facilitators/motivators in a public, universal system
Care based on continuous healing relationships 24-7 access/responsiveness Minimize unneeded face-to-face visits	Disruptions in continuity, e.g., resulting from annual employer bids for best deal, monthly Medicaid eligibility changes, S-CHIP enrollment, contingent on fluctuating eligibility (Forrest & Starfield, 1998; Starfield, 2002) Barriers to access (including financial) fuel cycle of anxiety, more demand, more barriers, and so on.	Stable funding, with no requirement to switch providers for reasons other than patient choice Public accountability for access/conveniences Public health approach to decrease unnecessary encounters Fewer incentives for wasteful encounters
Customization based on patient needs Patient values drive variations	Emphasis on brands and branding for product differentiation, giving illusion of marketplace choices, often without independent, comparative evidence on which to base decisions New technology promoted/favored over more careful fine-tuning of skills, processes, interactions	Research and improvement efforts facilitated, e.g., research with Medicare database for prostatic hypertrophy shared decision-making paradigm (Lu-Yao, McLerran, Wasson, Wennberg, 1993) Mobility and portability to achieve best-fit relationships; trusting environment would enable healthier transactions (Davis, Collins, Schoen, Morris, 1995)
Patient as source of control	One dollar, one vote: profit-driven institutions cater to rich and well-insured, and neglect others Locus of decision-making shifted away from primary care relationships and local communities to distant corporate headquarters	More democratic local control of direction of resources and system Ultimate accountability is to patient/public, not stock owners
Shared knowledge Free flow of information	Protection of proprietary information Inhibitions on public release of negative information or suppression of research studies to protect corporate image or profits (Angell & Relman, 2001) Modes of reimbursement and the decision-making process itself concealed	Favors open source information/systems Nonproprietary approach to information, e.g., PubMed; journals such as *British Medical Journal* free on Web Traditions of right to information, epidemiologic reporting, availability of claims data

continued

TABLE 12.4. *(continued)*

New rules to improve care, adapted from IOM report	Inhibitors/barriers in current market-oriented system	Facilitators/motivators in a public, universal system
	Ad hoc purchasing of computer software/systems fragments information	Information sharing facilitated by public standards for confidentiality, storage, and release
Evidence based decision-making	Primary data often withheld or transformed into proprietary data	Independent consensus evaluative review processes and forums (NIH Consensus Conferences, professional society recommendations, AHRQ guidelines)
	Marketing and promotion encourages one-sided education and stimulates excess demand (Avorn, Chen, Hartley, 1982; Wilkes, Doblin, Shapiro, 1992)	
		Better insulated from market biases
	Information flow and practice conditioned by market considerations such as pressures to quickly reap returns on drug research investments	
Safety as a system property	Temptation for profit motivation to compromise staffing and safety standards (Stapleton, 2001)	Public safety as historic goal of public service and agencies, e.g., EPA, FAA, OSHA, NHTSA
	Short-term rewards from stretching and stressing staff more lucrative than long-term improvement/investment	Leading role of not-for-profits and government sector in current safety movement (AHRQ, CMS, USP, VA hospitals)
Need for transparency	Numerous incentives and mechanisms to conceal (noted above)	Public sector by definition is public, with oversight from citizens, volunteer groups, and publicly elected officials.
		Decision-making points and processes identifiable
Anticipate needs	Needs of profit-making dominate and shape planning and policy	The essence of public health practice, which is steeped in principles of epidemiology, outcomes research, health planning, workforce training, and resource allocation
	Fragmentation of community as obstacle to population-based practice (Ibrahim, Savitz, Carey, Wagner, 2001)	
		Some positive experience attempting to constrain excessive/imbalanced capital allocation
Waste continuously decreased	Massive unmeasured private sector waste buried in accounting systems that	An ongoing challenge

TABLE 12.4. *(continued)*

New rules to improve care, adapted from IOM report	Inhibitors/barriers in current market-oriented system	Facilitators/motivators in a public, universal system
	measure only selected costs, e.g., staffing costs, and externalizing others such as environmental impacts	
	Administrative/marketing waste (Woolhandler, Campbell, Himmelstein, 2003a)	
	Unconscionable executive rewards	
	Frills contrasted to frugality of public sector	
Cooperation	Enshrines competitiveness and selfishness as desired engines of improvement, as if all progress depends on humans being acquisitive, individualistic, and aggressive, and on the strong displacing the weak (Kohn, 1999)	Based on and encourages a non-market, more cooperative, value system (Korten, 1999; Waitkzin, 2001) Better balance of collective and individual needs; orientation around collective progress, group and cooperative caring endeavor, and public service

AHRC	Agency for Healthcare Research and Quality
CMS	Centers for Medicare and Medicaid Services (formerly the Health Care Financing Administration)
EPA	Environmental Protection Agency
FAA	Federal Aviation Administration
IOM	Institute of Medicine
NHTSA	National Highway Traffic Safety Administration
NIH	National Institutes of Health
OSHA	Occupational Safety and Health Administration
S-CHIP	State Children's Insurance Program
USP	United States Pharmacopoeia
VA	Veterans Administration

Source: Reprinted with permission from Schiff, G. D. & Young Q. D. (2001). You can't leap a chasm in two jumps: The Institute of Medicine Health Care Quality Report. *Public Health Reports, 116,* 56.

Simplifying the financing system could by itself, in large measure, replace the market ethics and values of the present system with a public service ethic which had a long tradition in precorporate health care. Moving toward a public utility model, profiteering in health care would be regulated by public control while universal coverage, cost-efficiency, and affordability of health care are extended to the entire population (Flanagan & Smith, 2003). If U.S. health policy moves in this direction, the country will be joining all other industrialized Western countries with some form of social health insurance. Many of these countries have better performing health care systems that perform better than the U.S system. (Starfield, 1998; 2000; World Health Report, 2000), and we already know that we can afford such a system by changes in the allocation of today's health care expenditures (Himmelstein & Woolhandler, 2003; Woolhandler, Himmelstein, Angell, Young and Physicians Working Group for Single-Payer National Health Insurance, 2003b).

CONCLUDING COMMENTS

This chapter has provided evidence and a rationale that our basic questions at the outset need to be answered in favor of health care as a basic human need and right, and of the advantages of converting health care delivery to a not-for-profit, public utility model. It seems obvious that the health care system should meet the needs of the public first, not of the stakeholders in our failing system. It is remarkable how our country, as advanced and successful as it is in so many ways, has embraced philosophies and structures for its health care system based on unproven and untested concepts. Thus, the theoretical advantages of managed competition have produced today's chaotic and unfair system, while proponents of Medicare privatization through PPOs disregard evidence of the widespread failure of Medicare HMOs in the open marketplace. A major reason for the lack of an evidence-based approach to health policy, of course, is the political power and influence of the stakeholders in the present system. That leads us to the next chapter where we will consider the politics operating for and against the major options for health care reform.

REFERENCES

Adva Med. (2001). Testimony for the Record by the Advanced Medical Technology Association [AdvaMed] before the House Ways and Means Subcommittee on Health, "Hearing on H.R. 2768, the Medicare Regulatory and Contracting Reform Act of 2001" Retrieved May 5, 2003 from *www.advamed.org/publicdocs/testimony-hr2768.html*

Angell, M., & Relman, A.S. (2001, June 20). Prescription for profit. *The Washington Post*, p. A27.

Armstrong, J. (2003, July 15). Washington Watch: Medicare+Choice not an option for rural seniors. *Physicians' Financial News, 21*(9), 13.

Aston, G. (2002, April 20). Doctors Urge National Standards for Medicare Carriers. *American Medical News*, p. 3.

Avorn, J., Chen, M., Hartley, R. (1982). Scientific versus commercial sources of influence on the prescribing behavior of physicians. *American Journal of Medicine 73*, 4.

Bennett, J. (2003, June 24). HMO rates are expected to rise 18%. *San Francisco Chronicle.*

Boccuti, C., & Moon, M. (2003). Comparing Medicare and private insurers: Growth rates in spending over three decades. *Health Affairs (Millwood) 22*, 230.

Bodenheimer, T. (2003, June). The dismal failure of Medicare privatization. Senior Action Network. San Francisco, California, p. 1.

Bowe, C., & Chaffin, J. (2003, Aug. 13). Convictions for U.S. healthcare fraud up by 22%. *Financial Times,* Retrieved from *www.ft.com/healthcare*

Brown, C. (1999). Ethics, policy and practice: interview with Emily Friedman. *Image: Journal of Nursing Scholarship, 31*, 260.

Callahan, P. (2003, Aug. 18). Health industry sees a surge in fraud fines. *The Wall Street Journal*, p. B1.

Chen, J., Radford, M.J., Wong, Y. Marciniak, T. A., Krumholz, H. M. (1999). Do "America's Best Hospitals" perform better for acute myocardial infarction? *The New England Journal of Medicine, 340*, 286.

Commonwealth Fund. (2003, Aug. 11). Press release. New York

Davis, K., Collins, K. S., Schoen, C., Morris, C. (1995). Choice matters: Enrollees' views of their health plans. *Health Affairs (Millwood), 14*(2), 99.

Derlet, R. A. (2002). Trends in the use and capacity of California's emergency departments, 1990–1999. *Annals of Emergency Medicine, 39*, 430.

Devereaux, P. J., Schunemann, H. I., Ravindran, N., Bhandari, M. Garg, A. X., Choi, P. T. (2002). Comparison of mortality between private for-profit and private not-for-profit hemodialysis centers: A systematic review and meta-analysis. *Journal of the American Medical Association, 288*, 2449.

Flanagan, J., & Smith, F. (2003, Jan. 2). Public utility model of health care reform. *San Francisco Chronicle,* Available at *http://www.pnhp.org/news/2003/january/publicutility_model.pnp*

Foote, S. B. (2003). Focus on locus: Evolution of Medicare's local coverage policy. *Health Affairs (Millwood), 22*, 137.

Forrest, C. B., & Starfield, B. (1998). Entry into primary care and continuity: The effects of access. *American Journal of Public Health, 88*, 1330.

Freudenheim, M. (2003, Feb. 19). Some concerns thrive on Medicaid patients. *The New York Times*, p. C1.

Garg, R. P., Frick, K. D., Diener-West, M., Power, N. R. (1999). Effect of the ownership of dialysis facilities on patients' survival and referral for transplantation. *The New England Journal of Medicine, 341*, 1653.

Grembowski, D. E., Diehr, P., Novak, L. C., Roussel, A. E., Martin, D. P., Patrick, D. L. et al. Measuring the "managedness" and covered benefits of health plans. *Health Services Research, 35*, 707, 2000.

Harrington, C., Woolhandler, S., Mullan, J., Carillo, H., Himmelstein, D. U. Does investor-ownership of nursing homes compromise the quality of care? *American Journal of Public Health, 91*(9), 1, 2001.

Hartz, A. J., Krakauer, H., Kuhn, E. M., Young, M., Jacobsen, S. I., Gay, G. Muenz, L., Katzoff, M., Bailey, R. C., Rimm, A. A. Hospital characteristics and mortality rates. *The New England Journal of Medicine, 321,* 1720, 1989.

Himmelstein, D. U., Woolhandler, S., Hellander, I., Wolfe, S. M. (1999). Quality of care in investor-owned vs not-for-profit HMOs. *Journal of the American Medical Association, 282,* 159, 1999.

Himmelstein, D. U., & Woolhandler, S. (2003). National health insurance or incremental reform: aim high, or at our feet? *American Journal of Public Health, 93*(1), 31.

HMO honor roll. *U.S. News & World Report,* p. 62.

Ibrahim, M. A., Savitz, L. A., Carey, T. S., Wagner, E. H. (2001). Population-based health principles in medical and public health practice. *Journal of Public Health Management Practice, 7*(3), 75.

Institute of Medicine. Committee on Quality of Health Care in America. (2001). *Crossing the Quality Chasm: A New Health System for the 21st Century.* Washington: National Academy Press.

Institute of Medicine. (2002, Nov. 19). Press Release. Bold initiatives aim to solve key health care problems. Demonstration projects lay foundation for statewide reform. Institute of Medicine. National Academies of Science, Washington, D.C.

Institute of Medicine. Committee on the Consequences of Uninsurance. (2003). A Shared Destiny: Community Effects of Uninsurance. Washington, D.C.: Institute of Medicine, The National Academy Press, p. 182.

Japsen, B. (2003, Mar. 23).Seniors spurning pilot Medicare PPO effort. *Chicago Tribune.*

Kaiser Commission on Medicaid and the Uninsured. (2002a, Feb.) Health Insurance Coverage in America: 2000 Data Update, p. 9.

Kaiser Family Foundation (2002b, Fall). Survey, June 5, reported in the PNHP Newsletter, Fall.

Kazel, R. (2003, Aug. 25). Insurers post robust profits for the second quarter. *American Medical News.*

Kohn, A. (1999). *Punished by rewards.* Boston: Houghton Mifflin.

Korten, D. C. (1999). *The post corporate world.* West Hartford, CT and San Francisco, CA: Kumarian Press & Berrett-Koehler.

Kovner, C., & Gergen, P. J. (1998). Nurse staffing levels and adverse events following surgery in U.S. hospitals. Image: *Journal of Nursing Scholarship, 30,* 315.

Kuttner, R. (1999). The American health care system: Wall Street and health care. *The New England Journal of Medicine, 340,* 664.

Kuttner, R. (1998). Must good HMOs go bad? First of two parts: The commercialism of prepaid group health care. *The New England Journal of Medicine, 338,* 1558.

Lu-Yao, G. L., McLerran, D., Wasson, J., Wenneberg, J. E. (1993). An assessment of radical prostatectomy: Time trends, geographic variation and outcomes. *Journal of the American Medical Association, 269,* 2633.

McLaughlin, N. (2003, Aug. 4). Plenty of money: Healthcare industry bestows some outrageous, some sane pay packages. *Modern Healthcare,* p. 7.

MedPac. (2001, Dec.). Reducing Medicare Complexity and Regulatory Burden. Washington, DC: Author.

Models That Work Campaign. (2003, Aug. 18). Bureau of Primary Health Care. Bethesda, Maryland: available at *http://bphc.hrsa.gov/programs/MTWProgramInfo.htm*

Munoz, R. (2002, May 22). How health care insurers avoid treating mental illness. *San Diego Union Tribune.*

Neuman, P. (2003). Testimony to the Committee on Ways and Means Subcommittee on Health, U.S. House of Representatives, Washington, D.C. (2003, May 1). Available at *http://waysandmeans.house.gov/hearings.asp?formmode=view&id+338*

Oberlander, J. (2003). *The Political Life of Medicare.* Chicago: University of Chicago Press.

Ornstein, C. (2002, April 3). Bill could aid uninsured patients. *Los Angeles Times,* p. B1.

Pear, R. (2003a, May 6). Critics say proposal for Medicare and private health plans could increase costs. *The New York Times.*

Pear, R. (2003b, May 13). New study finds 60 million uninsured during a year. *The New York Times,* p. A20.

PNHP (2002). Slide set prepared by Physicians for a National Health Program, Chicago, Illinois. Available at *www.pnhp.org*

Public Citizen (2002). Medicare Privatization: The Case Against Relying on the HMOs and Private Insurers to Offer Prescription Drug Coverage. Available at *www.citizen.org/congress/reform/rx_benefits/drug_benefit/articles.cfm?ID-8298* Accessed October 2, 2003.

Reich, M. R. (Ed.). (2002). *Public-private partnerships for public health.* Cambridge: Harvard University Press.

Reinhardt, U. E. (1997). Wanted: A clearly articulated social ethic for American health care. *Journal of the American Medical Association, 278,* 1446.

Relman, A. S. (2001). The Institute of Medicine report on the quality of health care: *Crossing the quality chasm: A new health system for the 21st century. The New England Journal of Medicine, 345,* 702.

Rose, J. R. (2004, Feb. 6). Focus on practice. HMO coffers overflow. *Medical Economics,* p. 19.

Rosenbaum, S. (2003). Why Entitlements Matter. *Health Affairs (Millwood),* 22(5), 257.

Schiff, G. D., & Young, Q. D. (2001, Sept./Oct.). You can't leap a chasm in two jumps. The Institute of medicine health care quality report. *Public Health Reports, 116,* 53.

Silverman, E. M., Skinner, J. S., & Fisher, E. S. (1999). The association between for-profit hospital ownership and increased Medicare spending. *The New England Journal of Medicine, 341,* 420.

Stapleton, S. (2001, June 18). Where's the nurse? *American Medical News,* 50.

Starfield, B. (2002). Evaluating the state Children's Health Insurance Program: Critical considerations. *Annual Review of Public Health, 21,* 569.

Starfield, B. (1998). *Primary care, balancing health needs, services, and technology.* New York: University Press.

Starfield, B. (2000). Is U.S. health care really the best in the world? *Journal of the American Medical Association, 284,* 483.

Starr, P. (1982). *The social transformation of American medicine* (p. 448). New York: Basic Books.

Taylor, H., & Leitman, R., (Eds.) (2001). Out-of-pocket costs are a substantial barrier to prescription drug compliance. *Health Care News, 1*(32),

Terry, T. (2003, Jan. 10). Where has all the money gone? *Medical Economics,* p. 72.

Thorpe, K. E., & Howard, D. (2003, Jan./June). Health insurance and spending among cancer patients. *Health Affairs Web exclusive,* W3, 189-97.

Waitkzin, H. (2001). *At the front lines of medicine: How the health care system alienates doctors and mistreats patients and what we can do about it.* Landham, MD, Rowman & Littlefield.

Waldholz, M. (2002, Oct. 3). Prescriptions. Medicare seniors face confusion as HMOs bail out of program. *The Wall Street Journal,* p. D4.

Weber, T., & Ornstein, C. (2003, April 23). County USC doctors say delays fatal. *Los Angeles Times.*

Widdus, R. (2001). Public-private partnerships for health: Their main targets, their diversity, and their future directions. *Bulletin of the World Health Organization, 79,* 713.

Wilkes, M. S., Doblin, B. H., Shapiro, M. F. (1992). Pharmaceutical advertisements in leading medical journals: Experts' assessments. *Annals of Internal Medicine, 116,* 912.

Wolfe, S. M. (2003). Bush Administration plan to privatize Medicare would limit seniors' choice of doctors. *Health Letter, 19,* 1.

Wolfe, S. M. (2001). Unhealthy partnership: How Massachusetts and its managed care contractor shortchange troubled children. *Public Citizen Health Research Group Health Letter, 17*(2), 1.

Woolhander, S., & Himmelstein, D. U. (1997). Costs of care and administration at for-profit and other hospitals in the United States. *The New England Journal of Medicine, 336,* 769.

Woolhandler, S., Campbell, T., Himmelstein, D. U. (2003a). Costs of health care administration in the United States and Canada. *The New England Journal of Medicine, 349,* 768.

Woolhandler, S., Himmelstein, D. U., Angell, M., Young, Q. D., and the Physicians Working Group for Single-Payer National Health Insurance (2003b). Proposal of the Physicians' Working Group for Single-Payer National Health Insurance. *Journal of the American Medical Association, 290,* 798.

World Health Organization (2000). Report Available at http://www.who.int/whr/2000en/report.htm

Wrich, J. (1998). *Brief summary of audit findings of managed behavioral health services.* Chicago: J. Wrich & Associates.

Yuan, Z., Cooper, G. S., Einstadter, D., Cebul, R. D., Rimm, A. (2000). The association between hospital type and mortality and length of stay: A study of 16.9 million hospitalized Medicare beneficiaries. *Medical Care, 38,* 231, 2000.

Chapter 13

POLITICS AND OPTIONS FOR HEALTH CARE REFORM

Health care administration in America is a Tower of Babel that reaches to the moon, built over decades specifically to cope with a "system" designed by historic accident, regulatory redundancy, and ever more ingenious entrepreneurial ambitions. The recurring impulse among everyone who tries to simplify and clarify the U.S. health care system is to dream up a business scheme that ultimately complicates and obfuscates it further. The result of every attempt at reform is the creation of more jobs.

—*J.D. Kleinke*
Health Care Analyst and Information Technology CEO

The health care system makes patients feel powerless, and it makes many of those who work within it feel exactly the same way. But until we change the infrastructure and the corporate culture of health care, until the fiefdoms and the turfs and the lust for money and the competition and the power positions are broken down, until teamwork replaces individual arrogance and patients replace power mongers as the focus of the system, innocent people will continue to be terrified, humiliated, injured and killed unnecessarily—not because of any individual wrongdoing, but because the system does not and cannot serve them well.

—*Emily Friedman*

The above two observations, from two vantage points by two health care analysts with long experience studying the U.S. health care system (Kleinke, 2001; Friedman, 2003), pinpoint different challenges which have frustrated all past attempts to reform the "sick elephant" which is our failing health care system. With the exception of Medicare and Medicaid, enacted as part of the Great Society legislation in 1965, all attempts to reform the system over the last 60 years have consisted of relatively minor, incremental changes around the edges of an increasingly complex and incoherent "system". Politics and ideology have trumped rationality and evidence along the way as one-seventh of the world's largest economy is handed from one untested organizational and financing concept to another. As an example, "managed competition," touted by many economists over the last 25 years as the basis for market solutions to health care, though now largely discredited as an organizing principle, is still being proposed by one of its architects, Alain Enthoven, in the form of another untested concept—"employer-created exchanges" The idea here is that employers offer their employees a wide selection of carriers and plan designs from which they can make their own individual choices of plans and delivery systems. (Enthoven, 2003).

This chapter undertakes four goals: (1) to consider ways in which the politics of health policy in the U.S. differ from other Western industrialized countries; (2) to describe three basic approaches to health care reform, including their advantages and, disadvantages, and the supporting evidence; (3) to discuss the political dynamics of the debate among these options; and (4) to summarize surveys of public opinion concerning the health care system.

WHY ARE HEALTH CARE POLITICS SO DIFFERENT IN THE U.S.?

The trend in many European countries during the late 1800s and early 1900s was to establish one or another form of social health insurance covering their whole populations (Starr, 1982). By the end of the 20th Century, all other Western industrialized nations, including South Africa, had such a program. The U.S., as the only exception in the industrialized world to this trend, has resisted five attempts since 1912 to enact a national plan for health insurance. How can we explain such a difference in health care politics, especially since many other parts of our society have drawn liberally from European culture?

Bruce Vladeck, Professor of Health Policy and Geriatrics at Mount Sinai Medical Center in New York, has carefully considered this question and offers us ten explanations, each one of which is significant in its own right:

Historical-cultural
1. Americans have more negative attitudes toward government than people in most other countries.
2. Population is more independent and individualistic.

3. Absence of a well-developed working class as most Americans identify themselves with the middle class.
4. Many low-income Americans own some property, thereby furthering their self-identification with the middle class.
5. Persistent racial cleavage working against a widespread, cohesive political movement.

Political-structural

1. Difficulty in redistribution of resources from affluent to middle and lower-income people due to division of powers between executive, congressional, and judicial branches of government.
2. Social diversity and political heterogeneity without religious, ethnic, or class identity upon which to build a national political movement.
3. Relatively weak political parties.
4. Increased influence of money in politics in the absence of strong political parties.
5. Relatively little differences between the political parties which end up in the middle ground on health policy. (Vladeck, 2003).

Vicente Navarro, professor of Health Policy and Management at Johns Hopkins University and editor-in-chief of the *International Journal of Health Services,* makes a persuasive case that the power and influence of the labor movement is the single most important factor in establishing national health insurance in any country (Navarro, 1989, 2003). Since only about 13% of the U.S. workforce is now unionized (Snider, 2002), that source of political power is much less than in other industrialized societies.

MAJOR OPTIONS FOR HEALTH CARE REFORM

As political pressure has mounted in recent years to address the growing ranks of uninsured and underinsured Americans who face increasing unaffordability of health care, three major alternatives emerge from a plethora of proposals to reform the system. Although discussion of these proposals tends to revert quickly to technical details, the three basic options involve:

1. building on the employer-based insurance system, including various strategies for *employer mandates* by which employers are required to offer health insurance to their employees

2. phasing out the employer-based system and moving into a consumer choice model, including strategies to promote an *individual mandate,* whereby all citizens will be required to purchase
   health insurance
3. replacing the private insurance industry with a national (or
   state-by state) system of public financing of social health insurance

All three options preserve a private system for delivery of health
care. The first two options make incremental changes in the existing
system and rely on expansion of public programs such as Medicare,
Medicaid, and S-CHIP to cover those who cannot afford private coverage and care. Admittedly, there is some overlap between the first
two alternatives, with some similar strategies to help employers provide, or individuals purchase, health insurance, but these three remain the basic alternatives for reform.

Building on Employer-Based Health Insurance

As we saw in chapter 4, employer-based health insurance took root
in the U.S. during the 1930s and grew rapidly during and after World
War II. Tax policy exempting employers and individuals from the
cost of health insurance has supported this policy since that time.
Today, these exemptions account for over 9% (more than $130 billion)
of annual health care expenditures in the U.S. As a result, despite the
common misperceptions that our system is mostly privately financed,
it is best described as "public money, private control," with 60% of
total health care expenditures, including the subsidies and public
employee health benefits, funded by public tax financing (Woolhandler & Himmelstein, 2002a).

The concept of an employer mandate was a core element in President Nixon's "play or pay" proposal put forward in the early 1970s
which, if enacted, would have required employers to either offer
health care coverage to their employees or pay a tax that would
finance their coverage from an insurance pool that would also cover
the unemployed (Kuttner, 1997). The State of Hawaii has had a 30–
year experience with an employer mandate system. Most recently,
faced with one in five of its residents uninsured, California passed an
employer mandate plan in September 2003. Starting in 2006, employers with 200 or more workers will be required to subsidize health
care for individuals and families, or pay into a new state fund to
cover the uninsured. In 2007, companies with 50 to 200 employees
must cover their employees, but not their dependents. Later on,
employers with 20 to 50 employees will be required to provide health

care coverage, but only if the state provides for tax credits to enable that coverage. This bill was supported by Democrats, opposed by Republicans, and passed by a vote along party lines. Backers included organized labor, many physicians, and patient advocacy groups. The Chamber of Commerce and business groups strongly opposed the measure, planning court challenges and some threatening to downsize or move their businesses out of state (Freudenheim, 2003).

While proponents of employer mandates claim that the employer-based health insurance system, now over 60 years old, is a solid rock upon which to build, there are many problems with it as documented by this kind of evidence:

- Faced with unabated increases in health insurance premiums, many employers are dropping coverage of their employees, restricting benefits, or opting for defined contribution arrangements (as opposed to defined benefits), which shift more costs to employees and will progressively fall below the full costs of insurance coverage for their employees (Appleby, 2002; Taylor, 2002)
- According to the Bureau of Labor Statistics of the U.S. Department of Labor, the proportion of employees covered by employer-sponsored health insurance dropped from 63% in 1992–1993 to only 45% in 2003; defined benefit plans cover a smaller proportion of employees today, as defined contribution plans have grown (Bureau of Labor Statistics, 2003)
- Workers who lose their jobs, or change jobs to work for an employer not offering health insurance benefits, often find coverage on the individual market unaffordable, while only one-fourth of workers who lose their jobs can afford to continue their coverage through COBRA (the Consolidated Omnibus Budget Reconciliation Act of 1985) (Commonwealth Fund, 2002)
- Many lower-income workers cannot afford health insurance even if offered by their employers (Gabel, Pickreign, Whitmore, Schoen, 2001)
- With an increasingly unstable workforce in this country, only about one-half of employed men or women now claim to have held their job for more than 10 years (Tejada, 2002)
- Many small employers are exempt from employer mandates, while a growing part of the U.S. workforce works part-time, often in two or more jobs, without employer-based coverage (Institute for the Future, 2000)
- The present tax subsidies for employment-based health insur-

ance have many inequities which disproportionately favor the affluent (e.g., the tax subsidy is worth one-third of the premium for families with annual incomes over $200,000, but only 10% of the premium for families making less than $10,000 a year (Synthesis Project, 2003)

- California's new employer mandate will, at best, cover only about one in seven of the uninsured (Freudenheim, 2003)
- Hawaii's experiment with its employer mandate, while initially dropping the uninsured rate below 5%, has ultimately failed due to the lack of effective cost controls—and after three consecutive years of 10 to 28% premium increases, the ranks of the uninsured are again increasing; health care premiums in 2002 increased 250 times faster than medical inflation (DePiero & Kilo, 2000)

Shifting Toward Consumer-Choice Model

This approach is being strongly promoted by the Administration, Republicans in Congress, and business interests as a means of shifting more responsibility to consumers in choosing their own care and, theoretically, helping to control health care costs. This approach may be combined with an *individual mandate* to require individuals to purchase their own health insurance, assisted by government subsidies if their incomes are below a specified amount. The consumer-choice model is based on several assumptions—that there is a free market in health care, that consumers can be well-informed about an adequate number of choices, and that they will spend their own money more prudently than other people's money (DePiero & Kilo, 2000). Increasingly, "consumer driven" plans are being marketed by health insurers which enable consumers to choose providers and health plans, and even customize their own benefit packages. They assume more financial risk as they do so, and the least expensive plans necessarily provide the least benefits (Gabel, Lo Sasso, Rice, 2002).

Within the consumer-choice model, three commonly proposed strategies illustrate how this approach will play out:

1. *Tax credits and premium support subsidies.* Proponents claim that these can enable many uninsured to purchase health insurance. President Bush has proposed a tax credit of $1,000 per individual ($2,000 per family). However, average annual HMO premiums are now over $6,000, and this approach also runs the risk that employers may drop

TABLE 13.1. What's Wrong with Tax Subsidies and Vouchers?

- Taxes go to wasteful private insurers, overhead >13%
- Amounts too low for good coverage, especially for the sick
- High costs for little coverage—much of subsidy replaces employer-paid coverage
- Encourages shift from employer-based to individual policies with overhead of 35% or more
- Costs continue to rise (e.g., FEHBP)
- Many are unable to purchase wisely—e.g., frail elders, severely ill, poor literacy

Source: Woolhandler, S., & Himmelstein, D. U. (2002). Vouchers by another name: Defined contribution and premium support plans. *PNHP Newsletter,* *January 19.*

coverage for employees who are eligible for tax credits. Moreover, a study reported in 2000 showed that tax subsidies would buy little new coverage, with a $13 billion annual subsidy covering only 4 million (less than 10%) of the uninsured (Gruber & Levitt, 2000). Table 13.1 summarizes the problems with this approach when vouchers are used to buy health insurance (Angell, 2001; Woolhandler & Himmelstein, 2002b).

2. Medical Savings Accounts (MSAs). Advocates of this approach to personal responsibility for purchasing of health care services argue that individuals will think twice before spending their own money. MSAs allow individuals to put money aside in tax-free accounts in order to pay their health care bills out of pocket; if unused in any one year, the remainder accumulates without being taxed.

While potentially attractive to younger and healthier individuals, MSAs nevertheless have a number of problems. They often fall far short of covering health care bills for many with acute and chronic disorders, and remove any opportunity for individuals to leverage down the costs of health care services, as may be accomplished by employers. Table 13.2 lists other major problems with MSAs, which render them ineffective as a reform strategy (PNHP, 2002).

3. Federal Employees Health Benefits Program (FEHBP) as a model. Many legislators in both parties are looking to the FEHBP as a model for offering consumers choice among private health plans. It covers all federal employees—over 8 million people, including 2.2 million active workers, 1.8 million retirees, and 4.2 million dependents (Pear, 2003b), and offers more than 200 plans nationwide (Lee, 2003). Critics

TABLE 13.2. Problems With Medical Savings Accounts (MSAs)

- Sickest 10% of Americans use 72% of care, MSAs cannot lower these catastrophic costs
- The 15% of people who get no care would get premium "refunds," removing their cross-subsidy for the sick, but not lowering use or cost
- Discourages prevention
- Complex to administer—insurers have to keep track of all out-of-pocket payments
- Congressional Budget Office projects that MSAs would increase Medicare costs by $2 billion

Source: Physicians for a National Health Program (2002). Available at www.pnhp.org

of this model, however, point to its inability to constrain rising insurance premiums much better than other parts of the market. According to Janice Lachance, former director of the Office of Personnel Management, FEHBP's costs increased by 50% between 1997 and 2002 (PNHP, 2002); its premiums are still expected to increase by another 10.6% in 2004 (Lee, 2003).

Aside from the above problems involved with each of these three strategies, and their lack of cost controls, there are other concerns with the consumer-choice model:

- As we saw in chapter 1, there is no competitive open market in health care (Evans, 1997)
- More than one-third of the U.S. population lives in smaller markets where their range of choices is limited (Kronick, Goodman, Weinberg, Wagner, 1993)
- The consumer choice model is a boon to the private insurance industry; without adequate controls against shrewd underwriting, increased risk segmentation and adverse selection will occur, thereby increasing the cost of insurance for the sick and chronically ill (Fuchs, 2002)
- As private insurers promote plans with lower benefits and higher deductibles and copayments, this increased cost-sharing with patients, especially in lower income groups, can be expected to result in decreased utilization of necessary care and, therefore, worse outcomes (Rasell, 1995; Tamblyn, 2001), with most of the cost savings reverting to the health plans themselves (Joyce, Escarce, Solomon, Goldman, 2002)

- An AARP survey of seniors has found that few had enough knowledge to make informed choices among health plans (Hibbard, Jewett, Engelmann, Tusler, 1998)

Publicly-Financed Social Health Insurance

This approach is based on the premise that the best way to improve the health of individuals and the population, as well as the performance of the health care system itself, is by assuring that everyone has insurance coverage for necessary health care services. It is also based on the philosophy that health care is a social service which should be distributed on the basis of need, not just another commodity available to those best able to pay. Further, it fosters the notion that health care, as an essential human need, should be delivered largely on a not-for-profit basis. The paradox of today's market-based system is that the business model generates maximal profits by avoiding the sick.

As is well documented in earlier chapters, the Wall Street model of corporate health care has shifted a large amount of our health care resources from patient care to administration and largely profits a bloated private sector bureaucracy. Many examples of increased cost, poorer outcomes, and less value were summarized in the last chapter for investor-owned industries compared with their not-for-profit counterparts.

Over the last 30 years, all incremental efforts to achieve full coverage of the uninsured have failed. As a result, many millions of Americans go without basic health care services each year, with increased rates of preventable morbidity and death. The Institute of Medicine's Committee on the Consequences of Uninsurance has calculated the impact of uninsurance in its 2003 report *Hidden Costs, Value Lost: Uninsurance in America*, as illustrated in Figure 13.1 (Institute of Medicine, 2003).

What would a system of social health insurance look like, whether administered nationally or initially on a state by state basis? It can best be understood as "Medicare for All," an expanded and improved version of traditional Medicare. All citizens would have an insurance card providing access to all necessary medical services, including preventive services, long-term care, mental health and dental services, and prescription drugs. Patients would have free choice of hospitals, physicians, and other providers. Unnecessary or ineffective services, as determined by boards of medical experts and community representatives, would not be covered. Copayments and deductibles

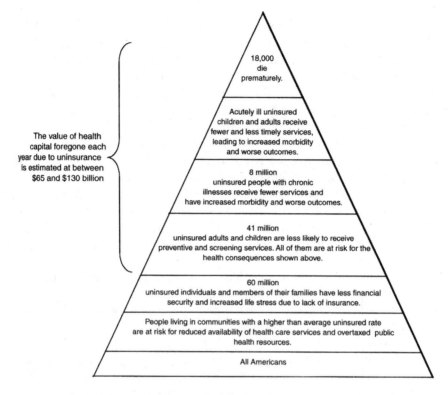

FIGURE 13.1 Consequences of uninsurance.

Source: Institute of Medicine (2003). *Hidden costs, value lost: Uninsurance in America.* Washington, DC: National Academy Press. Reprinted with permission.

would be eliminated, together with private insurance duplicating necessary health care services. A single-source, tax-financed public insurer would be established in each state, and would be federally mandated but locally controlled. Public funds now flowing through private insurers would be used to fund universal coverage. For-profit facilities and providers would be converted over a 10 to 15-year transition period to not-for-profit status. Hospitals and other facilities would operate under a global budget negotiated each year. Physicians and other providers could choose between fee-for-service, salaried practice in institutions on global budgets, or salaried practice in group practices or HMOs receiving capitation payments. As a single-payer system, administrative savings would fully offset the costs of covering all of the uninsured as well as giving full coverage of prescription drugs for all Americans. More specifics can be found in the 2003 Proposal of the Physicians' Working Group for Single-Payer National Health Insurance, endorsed by more than 12,000 U.S. physicians representing all specialties (Woolhandler, Himmelstein, Angell, Young and Physicians Working Group for Single-Payer National Health Insurance, 2003a). Appendix 1 provides a two-page summary of the United States National Health Insurance Act, H.R. 676, as introduced into the House of Representatives in 2003.

In contrast to the inability of incremental changes in either employer-based insurance or the consumer choice model to achieve universal coverage, a publicly financed system of universal coverage would do so while putting in place more effective cost controls than any of the market-based approaches. That this is the only effective way to achieve affordable universal coverage and not just wishful thinking is grounded on this kind of evidence:

- Based upon 1999 data, a 2003 report found that U.S. health care costs could be cut by $209 billion each year if reduced to the administrative costs of the single-payer Canadian system (Woolhandler, Campbell, Himmelstein, 2003b)
- A follow-up study by Harvard researchers and Public Citizen's Health Research Group updated these findings to 2003 spending as estimated by the Office of the Actuary, National Center for Health Statistics; based on these estimates, $286 billion could be saved in 2003, $6,940 for each of the 41 million uninsured Americans, considerably more than would be needed to provide them with comprehensive coverage. Appendix 2 lists the potential savings, state-by state under national health insurance (NHI) (Himmelstein, Woodlhandler, Wolfe, 2003)
- According to analysis by the Institute of Medicine Committee on the Consequences of Uninsurance, the annualized cost of diminished health and shorter life spans of Americans without health insurance is between $65 and $130 billion for each year of health insurance foregone; the Committee further estimates that the value of uncompensated health care services to the uninsured is about $35 billion a year (Institute of Medicine, 2003)
- Experience has shown that tax credits and vouchers can never work as approaches to effectively cover the uninsured (Gruber & Levitt, 2000; Angell, 2001)
- While covering all Americans, independent projections by several government agencies and private sector analysts have concluded that single-payer national health insurance would *not* increase total health care costs (Brand, Ford, Sager, Socolar, 1998;

CBO, 1993; GAO, 1991; Kahn, Bodenheimer, Grumbach, Lingpappa, Farey, 2002; Sheils & Haught, 2000; Smith, 2001)
- Many countries with national health insurance have effectively
  controlled health care costs without the use of copayments or
  deductibles (Woolhandler, Himmelstein, Angell, Young and Physicians Working Group for Single-Payer National Health Insurance, 2003a)
- Alex Preker, a leading health economist at the World Bank, has
  concluded that universal health care results in cost containment,
  not explosion of costs (Preker, 1998)
- Taiwan is the latest of advanced world economies to adopt national health insurance; since it was established in 1995 with a
  comprehensive benefit package, Taiwan's health care spending
  has not exceeded historical trends, and the program enjoys a
  public satisfaction level of about 70%, one of the highest for a
  public program in the country (Lu & Hsiao, 2003)

POLITICS OF THE HEALTH CARE DEBATE: DENIAL, MISINFORMATION, AND OBFUSCATION

As we saw in chapter 9, the debate over U.S. healthcare policy is far
from evidence-based, and is largely controlled by corporate media
interests as well as conservative legislators and lobby groups. Examples of distortion are everywhere, with subtle variations in kind.

Despite all of the evidence presented in the last chapter belying
the claimed efficiencies and value of privatized health care and private health insurance, there is widespread and continuing denial,
fueled by stakeholders in the present system, that markets are the
best foundation upon which to base our system. We are led to believe
that the U.S. has the best health care system in the world, despite
strong evidence to the contrary (Starfield, 1998, 2000; World Health
Organization, 2000), while the fact that more than one in seven Americans lacks access to basic health care is played down. We deny that
we ration care by income and class. Supporters of the present system
raise the specter of "class warfare" when challenged on this point,
with denial that class interests are already playing a powerful role in
health care politics. Conservative groups and legislators at the federal level, joined by many moderates, propose shifting responsibility
for Medicaid to the states in the belief that states can do a better job
of assuring health care for the poor. This is a nonstarter policy initiative at a time of dire fiscal deficits in most states, and cutbacks in

funding and eligibility are not mentioned (Aaron & Butler, 2003; Kaiser, 2003; Pear, 2003a; Toner & Stolberg, 2002). Meanwhile corporate insiders rotate back and forth between government and corporate management, thereby perpetuating corporate dominance over government and its regulatory agencies. A classic example of the extent to which Social Darwinism has permeated government today are the suggestions in 2001 by Paul O'Neil, then Secretary of the Treasury and previously a top executive at two large multinational corporations, that corporations should be tax-exempt, like churches, and that Social Security, Medicare, and Medicaid should be eliminated since "able-bodied adults should save enough on a regular basis so that they can provide for their own retirement, and for that matter, health and medical needs" (Hartmann, 2002, p. 177).

Misinformation, based upon political ideology, also plays a large role in the media's coverage of health care. In recent years, misinformation has driven the concept of consumer choice, personal responsibility, and privatized health care. The public is told that we have become a highly taxed nation, and that continued tax cuts are necessary, despite a massive deficit, to stimulate economic growth. This is simply not true—as a share of GDP, federal taxes are at their lowest level since the Eisenhower administration, state and local taxes have been quite stable since the early 1970s, all U.S. taxes combined account for 26.3% of GDP, and the effective tax rate on corporate profits has been cut by one-half since the 1960s (Krugman, 2003). Meanwhile, special interest groups spread misinformation about health issues while posing as reliable sources. A recent example is Fact Checkers, a coalition of such front-group organizations as the Pacific Research Institute, the United Seniors Association, and the Council for Affordable Health Insurance, which promotes itself as "checking the facts so you don't have to". In response to the Proposal of the Physicians' Working Group for single-payer National Health Insurance (Woolhandler, Himmelstein, Angell, Young and Physicians Working Group for Single-Payer National Health Insurance, 2003), the coalition's biased response (Matthews & Jarvis, 2003) raised the issues of rationing (we already ration care), inadequate funding of "government-run systems" (often true, especially as private interests lobby for underfunding of public systems and seek a larger role for themselves) (Sullivan & Baranek, 2002), decreased choice under NHI (although full choice is available to our traditional Medicare system, and constrained in privatized Medicare plans) (Armstrong, 2003; Wolfe, 2003), and waiting lists (disregarding existing waiting times in our present system) (see Figure 13.2) (CSHSC, 2002). This response,

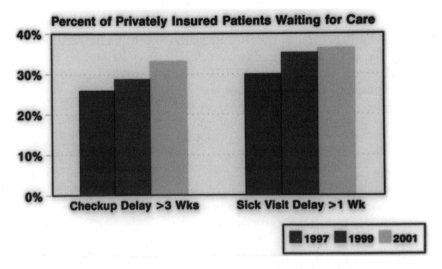

FIGURE 13.2 Waiting lists in the U.S.—even for the privately insured.

Source: Physicians for a National Health Program (2002). Retrieved from *www.pnhp.org* Reprinted with permission.

of course, serves the interests of the for-profit private health insurance industry and other corporate health care interests while not admitting their contributions to the growing unaffordability of U.S. health care.

The extent to which basic health policy issues are obfuscated in everyday coverage by the media is illustrated by these two examples:

- As we saw in the last chapter, privatizing Medicare is being promoted by conservatives, many moderates, and stakeholders in the market-based system despite the mounting evidence of its inefficiencies and problems. Embedded within the debate over a prescription drug benefit for Medicare beneficiaries is a premium-support plan whereby private HMO/PPOs would be subsidized. Traditional Medicare will be expected to "compete" against these more expensive subsidized plans after 2010. As we have already seen, however (chapter 7, p. 131 and chapter 12, p. 230), the traditional Medicare program has already proven itself superior to privatized plans in terms of reliability, continuity, choice, efficiency, value, and patient satisfaction. The implication is that the private market offers seniors more choice and value. More critical reporting would have uncovered this striking similarity. Dean Baker, an economist and co-director of the Center for Economic and Policy Research, recently analyzed the lack of accurate coverage of current Medicare policy issues by major U.S. newspapers (Baker, 2003). And we could easily learn from experience beyond our borders. Australia enacted a publicly-financed system of national health insurance in 1975. Under pressure from conservatives and private interests, duplicative private coverage was permitted in the late 1970s. By the late 1990s, private coverage was unpopular and sought by less than one-third of the population, so a series of rebates were passed by conservatives for the purchase of private plans. A 30% rebate was enacted in 1999, private insurers were allowed to end community rating in 2000, and a later study showed that most of the rebate went to the affluent with only small new enrollment in private plans (Wilcox, 2001).

- IMS Health, which tracks drug prescriptions, estimates that Americans are spending $350 to $650 million each year for prescription drugs from Canada, whether by Internet, mail order, or driving across the border. Health Canada, the Canadian equivalent of our FDA, has not found any counterfeit or other problems in that supply. The pharmaceutical industry engaged a large public relations firm, Edelman, which conducted focus groups around the country on public perceptions. Finding that illegality was not perceived as a barrier to such purchases, Edelman recommended that the drug industry use ads spreading fear over safety concerns of drugs imported from Canada. Despite the lobbying and advertising against Canadian imports, the House passed the Gutknect-Emerson bill in 2003 by a vote of 243 to 186 calling for legalization of imports of drugs from Canada and some other industrialized countries (Hensley, 2003). The drug industry has recently countered by raising the prices of their drugs and reducing sales to Canadian pharmacies. Fearing potential shortages of drugs for Canadians, pharmacy regulators in Canada have recently called on the government to ban exports to the U.S. (Simon, 2003).

WHAT DOES THE PUBLIC WANT?

National polls have shown high levels of support for a national health insurance program on many occasions over the last 60 years. During the 1940s, 74% of the public supported a proposal for national health insurance (Steinmo & Watts, 1995), while Medicare, the country's first universal coverage plan for the elderly, was supported by 61% of respondents in 1965 (Blendon & Benson, 2001). Over the last 25 years, support for national health insurance in national polls has ranged from about 50 to 66%. As shown in Table 13.3, however, when the question is asked in terms of a plan "financed by taxpayers" and a "single government plan," support drops to about 40% (Blendon & Benson, 2001). That wording suggests that taxes may be higher than

TABLE 13.3. Americans' Attitudes About National Health Insurance, 1980–2000

National health Insurance, financed by tax money, and paying for most forms of health care[a]	Favor	Oppose	No Opinion
1980 (February)	50%	41%	9%
1980 (March)	46	43	11
1981	52	37	11
1990 (March–April)	56	34	10
1990 (October)	64	27	8
1991 (June)	60	30	10
1991 (August)	54	33	12
1992 (January)	65	26	9
1992 (July)	66	25	9
1993 (January)	63	26	11
1993 (March)	59	29	12
1995	53	39	8
2000 (August)			
General public	56	32	12
Registered voters	54	34	12

A national health plan, financed by taxpayers, in which all Americans would get their insurance from a single government plan[b]			
1998 (November)	42%	53%	5%
1999 (October)	41	47	11
1999 (December)	39	51	10
2000 (July)			
Registered voters	38	58	3

Sources: Blendon, R. J., & Benson, J. M. (2001). Americans' views on health policy: A fifty-year historical perspective. *Health Affairs (Millwood)*, 20(2), 35. Reprinted with permission.

[a]CBS News/New York Times polls (1980–95); Harvard School of Public Health/ ICR poll (2000).

[b]Kaiser Family Foundation/Harvard School of Public Health polls (1998–99); Washington Post/Kaiser Family Foundation/ Harvard University poll (2000).

people are already paying for health care, that freedom of choice may be limited in a single, publicly-financed plan, and that a private delivery system will not be retained. If the American public were to understand that national health insurance NHI is achievable within current health care expenditures, that free choice of physicians and hospitals will be preserved in a private delivery system, and that a single-payer system will be more efficient than the market-based system, public support for it would likely be overwhelming.

There is growing evidence in recent years that the public is becoming increasingly dissatisfied with the health care system, and more supportive of an expanded role of government in assuring access to care. In a 1997 national survey by the National Coalition on Health Care, four out of five respondents agreed that "medical care has become a big business that puts profits ahead of people," while three of four believed that the federal government should play a more active role in assuring access to care (National Coalition on Health Care, 1997). A 1998 national survey found that one-half of respondents believed that the federal government should guarantee access to health care for all Americans, even if that meant paying an additional annual tax of $2,000 (Hunt, 1998). A 2002 national poll by Harris Interactive surveyed five different groups—public citizens, physicians, employers, hospital managers, and health plan managers. One-half of those polled in all of those groups now favor radical reform of the health care system, not just incremental change. Only 19% of physicians and a smaller proportion of the other four groups believe that only minor changes are needed (Harris Interactive, 2002). Even more recently, an October 2003 national poll by ABC News and the The Washington Post showed that 62% of Americans support national health insurance (Lester, 2003).

Public concern over rising health care costs and the difficulty in affording health care has risen to the top of some current national polls. Just before the 2003 Iraq war, amid terror warnings, a faltering stock market, and a sluggish economy, a survey by USA Today, found that health care costs were the nation's top worry (USA Today, 2003). At the same time, the Kaiser Health Poll report found that 86% of respondents feel that "making health care more affordable" is "very important" (Kaiser, 2003).

Support among health professionals for single-payer national health insurance is strong in many quarters. Two out of three members of the American Medical Women's Association support single-payer national health insurance (PNHP, 2001), while the American Medical Student Association has taken a vigorous activist role toward that goal (Frieden, 2000). A 1999 study of more than 2,100 medical students, residents, faculty, and deans in U.S. medical schools, with an 80% response rate, found that 57% support single-payer national health insurance (Simon, et al., 1999). After a 9-year study of 12 major U.S. health care markets, including almost 2,700 interviews with local health system leaders, the landmark Community Tracking Study (CTS) found deep skepticism that markets can improve the efficiency and quality of our health care system (Nichols, Ginsberg, Berenson, Christianson, Hurley, 2004). Today, 62% of physicians in Massachusetts favor national health insurance (McCormick, Himmelstein, Woolhandler, Bor, 2002). Meanwhile, the AMA continues to oppose any form of national health insurance (AMA, 2003), as it has since the 1930s, but its membership is dropping and now includes only about one-third of U.S. physicians (Page, 2003).

WHERE ARE WE HEADED?

Given the failures of incremental change to reform the U.S. health care system over the last 30 years, what stands in the way of reform? Robert Kuttner's short answer: "Only the insurance industry, the drug companies, the Fortune 500, half the American Medical Association, and the Republican Party, that's all" (Kuttner, 2003).

We are at a political impasse whereby only incremental changes are being considered by legislators, who continue to be pressured by powerful stakeholders in the market-based system to avoid fundamental system reform. The sick elephant, which is our system, has fallen over and cannot get up on its own. It requires more feeding in terms of dollars, but that won't help. Yet the cost of inaction, or of ineffective, incremental "reforms," is too high. A 2003 projection by the National Coalition on Health Care, which includes members from business, labor, purchasers, providers, consumers, and others, concluded that without reform the average annual premium for employer-sponsored family health coverage will reach $14,545 in 2006, when there will be over 53 million uninsured Americans (Pension and Benefits Daily, 2003). We are tracking along, right on schedule, toward the Institute of the Future's worst case scenario for 2010, stormy weather, as shown in Figure 13.3 (Institute for the Future, 2000). Unfortunately, however, Oberlander calls attention to the ultimate paradox of U.S. health care politics: "Rising health costs put health care reform on the agenda, but the more likely a reform proposal is to control costs, the less likely it is to be politically viable" (Oberlander, 2003).

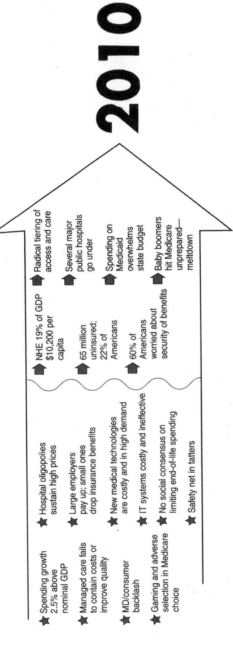

FIGURE 13.3 Scenario for 2010: stormy weather.

Source: Institute for the Future (2000). *Health and health care 2010: The forecast, the challenges.* San Francisco: Jossey-Bass. Adapted with permission.

Concerning the likelihood of structural health care reform, these observations by Victor Fuchs and Bruce Vladeck, two well-known health analysts, are on target:

> National health insurance will probably come to the United States after a major change in the political climate— the kind of change that often accompanies a war, depression, or large-scale civil unrest. Until then, the chief effect of the new plans will be to make young and healthy workers better off at the expense of their older, sicker, colleagues. (Fuchs, 2002, p. 1824)

> This is an old political debate but whatever the advocates of universal health insurance have been doing for the last 30 or 35 years, it obviously hasn't worked very well. There is very little to lose from trying something different. One of the different things that might be tried is to determine in very broad terms what the goals and principles of universal health insurance are by deciding on a set of defining ethical and moral principles and insisting that those goals and objectives be part of every conversation until they are achieved. Perhaps the "Rekindling Reform" initiative will help shape such goals and principles for universal health insurance. (Vladeck, 2003, p. 19)

REFERENCES

Aaron, H. J., & Butler, S. M. (2003). Four steps to better health care. *The Washington Post*.

American Medical Association (AMA). (2003, Aug. 12). Press release. Chicago, Illinois: AMA opposes single-payer health system.

Angell, M. (2001, Sept. 10). Insufficient credits: Why tax breaks won't help the uninsured. *The American Prospect, 23*. Appleby, J. (2002). Health care costs force benefit changes. *USA Today* July 9.

Armstrong, J. (2003). Washington Watch. Medicare + Choice not an option for rural seniors. *Physicians' Financial News, 21*(1) 13.

Baker, D. (2003, Sept./Oct.) Don't follow the money: Misleading Medicare coverage from leading newspapers. *Extra! 16*(5), 6.

Blendon, R. J., & Benson, J. M. (2001). Americans' views on health policy: A fifty-year historical perspective. *Health Affairs (Millwood), 20*(2), 33.

Brand, R., Ford, D., Sager, A., Socolar, D. (1998). Universal Comprehensive Coverage: A Report to the Massachusetts Medical Society, Waltham, Massachusetts.

Bureau of Labor Statistics. (2003, Sept. 17). *Employee benefits in private industry*. Washington, DC: U.S. Department of Labor.

Congressional Budget Office (CBO). (1993, April). Single-payer and all-payer health insurance systems using Medicare's payment rates. Washington, DC: Author.

Commonwealth Fund. (2002, Aug. 29). Only one-fourth of workers would keep health coverage through COBRA if they lost their jobs. Press release.

Center for Studying Health System Change (CSHSC). (2002, Sept. 5). Washington, D.C.

DiPiero, A., & Kilo, C. M. (2000). Will payment innovations benefit your practice? *Hippocrates, 14*(12), 32.

Editorial/Opinion. (2003, Mar. 6). Affordable remedies ignored as nation's health woes soar. *USA Today.*

Enthoven, A. C. (2003). Employment-based health insurance is failing: Now what? *Health Affairs (Millwood), W3,* 237.

Evans, R. G. (1997). Going for the gold: The redistributive agenda behind market-based health care reform. *Journal of Health Politics, Policy and Law, 22*(2), 427.

Freudenheim, M. (2003, Sept. 27). Many California employers face health care mandate. *The New York Times,* p. A13.

Frieden, J. (2000, Apr. 15). Policy and practice: Medical students want national health. *Family Practice News,* 58.

Friedman, E. (2003, Spring). Rocket science. *Health Forum Journal.* Available at *http://www.hospitalconnect.com/healthforumjournal/jsp/voices.jsp?voicepic=emily_pic*

Fuchs, V. (2002). What's ahead for health insurance in the United States? *The New England Journal of Medicine, 346*(23), 13.

Gabel, J. R., Pickreign, J. D., Whitmore, H. H., Schoen, C. (2001).Embraceable you: how employers influence health plan enrollments. *Health Affairs (Millwood), 20*(4), 205.

Gabel, J. R., Lo Sasso, A. T., Rice, T. (2002). Consumer-driven plans: Are they more than talk now? *Health Affairs* Web exclusive, W395.

Government Accounting Office (GAO). (1991). Canadian Health Insurance: Lessons for the United States. Document GAO/HRD-91–90. Washington, DC: Author.

Gruber, J., & Levitt, L. (2000). Tax subsidies for health insurance: Costs and benefits. *Health Affairs (Millwood), 19*(1), 72.

Harris Interactive (2002, Aug. 21). Attitudes toward the United States health care system: Long-term trends—views of the public, employers, physicians, health plan managers are closer now than at any time in the past. Public Opinion Survey. *Harris Interactive, 2*(17).

Hartmann, T. (2002). *Unequal protection: The rise of corporate dominance and the theft of human rights* (pp. 177–8). Emmaus, PA: Rodale Press.

Health costs report says broad reform needed for system ailing from rising costs. (2003, May 20). *Pension and Benefits Daily, 3*(96).

Hensley, S. (2003, Sept. 22). Drug makers cry "danger" over imports. *The Wall Street Journal,* p. B1.

Hibbard, J. H., Jewett, J. J., Engelmann, S., Tusler, M. (1998). Can Medicare beneficiaries make informed choices? *Health Affairs (Millwood), 17*(6), 181.

Himmelstein, D. U., Woolhandler, S., Wolfe, S. M. (2004). Administrative waste in the U.S. health care system in 2003. The cost to the Nation, the States and the District of Columbia, with state-specific estimates of potential savings. *International Journal of Health Services, 34*(1), 79.

Hunt, A. R. (1998, June 25). Public is split on how to pay for access. *The Wall Street Journal,* p. A10.

Institute for the Future. (2000). *Health and health Care 2010: The forecast, the challenges* (p. 123). San Francisco: Jossey-Bass.

Institute of Medicine. (2003). *Hidden costs, value lost: Uninsurance in America.* Washington, DC: National Academy Press.

Joyce, G. F., Escarce, J. J., Solomon, G. D., Goldman, D. P. (2002).Employer drug benefit plans and spending on prescription drugs. *Journal of the American Medical Association, 288*(14), 1733.

Kahn, J., Bodenheimer, T. S., Grumbach, K., Lingpappa, Farey, K., McCann, D. R. (2002). Single-payer proposal for California as analyzed by the Lewin Group. Available at *www.healthcareoptions.ca.gov*

Kaiser Family Foundation (2003, Jan./Feb.). . Health care priorities, health poll report.

Kaiser Commission on Medicaid and the Uninsured (KCMU) (2002, Sept. 22). Kaiser. News release on Medicaid reductions.

Kleinke, J. D. (2001). *Oxymorons: The myth of a U.S. health care system (p. 85).* San Francisco: Jossey-Bass.

Kronick, R., Goodman, D. C., Weinberg, J., Wagner, E. (1993). The marketplace in health care reform: The demographic limitations of managed competition. *The New England Journal of Medicine, 328,* 148.

Krugman, P. (2003). The tax-cut con. *The New York Times,* September 14.

Kuttner, R. (2003, June 11). Face it: We're rationing health. *Boston Globe Online.*

Kuttner, R. (1997). *Everything for sale: The virtues and limits of markets (p. 114).* Chicago: University of Chicago Press.

Lee, C. (2003). Health plan costs up 10.6%. *The Washington Post,* September 17.

Lester, W. (2003, Oct. 19). Poll: Public supports health care for all. *The Washington Post.*

Lu, J. R., & Hsiao, W. C. (2003). Does universal health insurance make health care unaffordable? Lessons from Taiwan. *Health Affairs (Millwood), 22*(3), 77.

Matthews, M., & Jarvis, C. W. (2003). Reality check critique of Physicians' Proposal for National Health Program for the United States. Retrieved September 22, 2003 from Fact Checkers.org

McCormick, D., Himmelstein, D. U. Woolhandler, S., Bor, D. H. (2003). View of single payer national health insurance: A survey of Massachusetts's physicians. *Journal of General Internal Medicine, 17* (suppl), 204.

National Coalition on Healthcare. (1997). A report of a national survey. *Journal of Health Care Finance, 23,* 12.

Navarro, V. (1989). Why some countries have national health insurance, others have national health services, and the United States has neither. *International Journal of Health Services, 19*(3), 383.

Navarro, V. (2003). Policy without politics: The limits of social engineering. *American Journal of Public Health, 93*(1), 64.

Nichols, L. M., Ginsburg, P. B., Berenson, R. A., Christianson, J., Harley, R. E. Are market forces strong enough to deliver efficient health care systems? Confidence is waning. *Health Affairs (Millwood), 23*(2): 8–21, 2004.

Oberlander J. (2003, Aug. 27). The politics of health care reform: why do bad things happen to good plans? *Health Affairs* Web exclusive.

Page, L. (2003, July) Sliding fees, with restructuring dead, the AMA faces membership loss. *Modern Physician, 5.*

Pear, R. (2003a, July). Report criticizes federal oversight of state Medicaid. *The New York Times,* p. A1.

Pear, R. (2003b, Sept. 17). federal workers' insurance premiums to rise less than others. *The New York Times,* p. A14.

Physicians for a National Health Program (PNHP)(2002). Available at *www.pnhp.org*.2002a

Physicians for a National Health Program (PNHP)(2001, May). Data Update. PNHP Newsletter, May, p. 1.

Physicians for a National Health Program (PNHP) (2002, Fall). Data Update. PNHP Newsletter, 10.

Preker, A. S. (1998). The Introduction of Universal Access to Health Care in the OECD: Lessons for Developing Countries. In E. S. Nitagyarumphong & A. Mills, *Achieving Universal Coverage of Health Care,* Bangkok: Ministry of Public Health.

Rasell, M. E. (1995). Cost sharing in health insurance—a re-examination. *The New England Journal of Medicine, 332,* 1164.

Sheils, J. F., & Haught, R. A. (2000). *Analysis of the costs and impact of universal health care models for the state of Maryland: The single-payer and multi-payer models.* Fairfax, VA: The Lewin Group.

Simon, S. R., Pan, R. I., Sullivan, A. M., Clark-Ciarelli, N., Connelly, M. T., Peters, A. S. (1999). Views of managed care—a survey of students, residents, faculty and deans at medical schools in the United States. *The New England Journal of Medicine, 340,* 928.

Simon, B. (2003, Nov. 15). Canadian pharmacy regulators seek to stop exports. *The New York Times,* p. B4.

Smith, R. F. (2001, Nov. 2). Universal health insurance makes business sense. *Rutland Herald.*

Snider, K. (2002, June 23). Unions fight cuts in health benefits. *Seattle Times.*

Starfield, B. (2000). *Primary care, Balancing health needs, services, and technology.* New York: University Press.

Starfield B. (2000). Is U.S. health really the best in the world? *Journal of the American Medical Association, 284,* 483.

Starr, P. (1982). *The social transformation of American medicine.* New York: Basic Books.

Steinmo, S., & Watts, J. (1995). It's the institutions, stupid! Why comprehensive national health insurance always fails in America. *Journal of Health Politics, Policy and Law, 20,* 329.

Sullivan, T., & Baranek, P. M. ((2002). *First do no harm: Making sense of Canadian health reform.* Vancouver, BC: UBC Press.

Synthesis Project (2003, May). Tax subsidies for private health insurance: Who currently benefits and what are the implications for new policies? Princeton, NJ: The Robert Wood Johnson Foundation.

Tamblyn, R., Laprise, R., Hanley, J. A., Abrahamowicz, M., Scott, S., & Mayor, N. et al. (2001). Adverse events associated with prescription drug cost-sharing among poor and elderly persons. *Journal of the American Medical Association, 285,* 421.

Taylor, H. (2002). How and why the health insurance system will collapse. *Health Affairs (Millwood), 21*(6), 195.

Tejada, C. (2002, Sept. 25). A special news report about life on the job—and trends taking shape there. *The Wall Street Journal,* p. B5.

Toner, R., & Stolberg, S. G. (2002, Aug. 11). Decade after health care crisis, soaring costs bring new strains. *The New York Times.*

Vladeck, B. (2003). Universal health insurance in the United States: Reflections on the past, the present, and the future. *American Journal of Public Health, 93*(1), 16.

Wilcox, S. (2001). Promoting private health insurance in Australia. *Health Affairs (Millwood), 20*(3), 152.

Wolfe, S. M. (2003). Bush Administration plan to privatize Medicare would limit seniors' choice of doctors. *Health Letter, 19*(7), 1.

Woolhandler, S., & Himmelstein, D. U. (2002a). Paying for national health insurance—and not getting it. *Health Affairs (Millwood), 21*(4), 88.

Woolhandler, S., & Himmelstein, D. U. (2002b, Jan.). Vouchers by another name: Defined contribution and premium support plans. *PNHP Newsletter, 19.*

Woolhandler, S., Himmelstein, D. U. Angell, M., Young, Q. D., and Physicians Working Group for Single-Payer National Health Insurance (2003a). Proposal of the Physicians' Working Group for Single-Payer National Health Insurance. *Journal of the American Medical Association, 290,* 798.

Woolhandler, S., Campbell, T., Himmelstein, D. U. (2003b). Costs of health care administration in the United States and Canada. *The New England Journal of Medicine, 349,* 768.

World Health Organization (WHO) (2000). Report Available at *http:// www.who.int/whr/2000en.report.htm*

Chapter 14

AN APPROACH TO REFORM

This report and the work of the Committee on the Consequences of Uninsurance not only provide information about the costs resulting from the lack of coverage and some of the costs and benefits of expanding it to everyone, it also presents us with an ethical dilemma. In light of the information and analyses that the Committee has developed about choices we have not made as a society, as well as those we have made to invest heavily in health care, we cannot excuse the unfairness and insufficient compassion with which our society deploys its considerable health care resources and expertise. Providing all members of American society with health insurance coverage would contribute to the realization of democratic ideals of equality of opportunity and mutual concern and respect. By tolerating a society in which a significant minority lacks the health care and coverage that most Americans enjoy, we are missing opportunities to become more fully the nation we claim to be.

—*Committee on the Consequences of Uninsurance*
Institute of Medicine

The last two chapters exposed the current realities of our failing health care system as well as the political clout of stakeholders resisting serious system reform. The urgent question remains as to whether, and how, this political impasse can be broken and the social, moral, and ethical dilemma described above (Institute of Medicine, 2003) resolved. As Vladeck urged at the conclusion of the last chapter, and as other industrialized nations learned as they took on the challenge of adopting one or another form of social health insurance, national consensus around its supporting principles is the *sine qua non* for success.

This chapter has five goals: (1) to compare and note the commonalities of principles for reform which have been proposed by various professional groups in this country and elsewhere; (2) to discuss briefly how reform issues can best be framed, with examples of negative framing; (3) to show how reform proposals can be compared and graded against principles; (4) to present some useful approaches to building political momentum for reform; and (5) to summarize our conclusions and offer an answer to the subtitle of this book: *Can the public interest still be served?*

PRINCIPLES FOR HEALTH CARE REFORM

The last attempt (1993–1994) by the U.S. to establish a national plan for universal health care coverage provides an excellent case study of how *not* to do it. The attempt failed for many reasons, but the failure to start with any broad principles or goals contributed in large part to its later demise. The Task Force was carefully selected to represent the key groups and interests involved in the medical-industrial complex. The goal was to enlist their support for whatever improvements in coverage they deemed acceptable. However, these vested interests were divided, even within groups. For example, the interests of large employers differed sharply from those of small employers, while large insurers had few objectives in common with small insurers. After a long series of political compromises among diverse vested interests, a bill of 1,342 pages died in committee in Congress. The Clinton Health Plan was widely criticized, even by early supporters, for its complexity, expense, and lack of coherence. It attempted to combine an employer mandate with some cost controls, and ended up confusing the public and alienating all of the stakeholders (Andrews, 1995; Gordon, 1995).

Fortunately, many fine minds have been focused for some years on value-driven principles which can best underpin a rational and humane health care system. We have a rich treasury of useful principles from which to draw in adapting to the needs of our system in a new century. Several examples warrant our attention:

- An international work group from four countries (the United States, the United Kingdom, Mexico, and South Africa) convened several years ago in London to draft ethical principles which could and (should) underlie any health care system. The Tavistock Group, as it came to be known, included physicians, nurses, academicians, ethicists, health care executives, an economist, a philosopher, and a jurist. These were their recommendations:

"1. Health care is a human right.
2. The care of individuals is at the center of health care delivery, but must be viewed and practiced within the overall context of continuing to generate the greatest possible health gains for groups and populations.
3. The responsibilities of the health care delivery system include the prevention of illness and the alleviation of disability.
4. Cooperation with each other, and with those served, is imperative for those working within the health care delivery system.
5. All individuals and groups involved in health care, whether they provide access or services, have the continuing responsibility to help improve its quality."

- A series of lectures and workshops was held in New York City in 2002 bringing together a broad cross-section of health-professional and health-worker groups, advocacy organizations, unions, university departments and associations, and faith-based organizations. A special issue of the *American Journal of Public Health* was devoted to their proceedings in January 2003, including lessons from four other countries—Canada, the U.K, France, and Germany (Birn & Fein, 2003). As part of these discussions, the following principles, each addressing more than one of five intertwined goals, was proposed as a vision for a restructured health care system in the U.S.:

"1. Everyone should have access to the care they need when they need it, and without financial hardship (access, equality).
2. The cost of the entire system should not be excessive because everyone pays more when costs increase; costs should be controlled by eliminating waste, not by restricting effective services. Cost and access are related because when costs go up, access often goes down (cost, access).
3. Everyone should receive all the care that is effective in preventing illness and improving health, and no one should receive care that is ineffective or harmful (quality, equality).
4. Caregivers' work should be organized so that caregivers can serve the public to the best of their abilities under conditions that do not create undue job stress or burnout (caregiver friendliness, quality).
5. Health care should be delivered and paid for in an equitable way. People with more money should pay the same propor-

tion of their wealth for health care (or a higher proportion) as people with less money, and everyone should be afforded equal access and quality (equality, access, quality)." (Bodenheimer, 2003)

- Still another formulation of useful principles has been offered by the Ad Hoc Committee to Defend Health Care, a group of Massachusetts physicians and nurses, and endorsed in its *Call to Action* by some 2,500 of their colleagues across the state (The Ad Hoc Committee to Defend Health Care, 1997).

"1. Medicine and nursing must not be diverted from their primary tasks: the relief of suffering, the prevention and treatment of illness, and the promotion of health. The efficient deployment of resources is critical, but must not detract from these goals.

2. Pursuit of corporate profit and personal fortune have no place in caregiving.

3. Potent financial incentives that reward overcare or undercare weaken patient-physician and patient-nurse bonds and should be prohibited. Similarly, business arrangements that allow corporations and employers to control the care of patients should be proscribed.

4. A patient's right to choose a physician must not be curtailed.

5. Access to health care must be the right of all."

Many of these principles overlap, but they coalesce into a smaller group of principles, such as universal access, affordability, comprehensiveness and continuity of care, quality assurance, public accountability, and a population perspective. In stark contrast, the Clinton Health Plan, with its 1,342 pages and lack of overarching principles, was 1,329 pages longer than the Canada Health Act of 1984, which embodied five basic principles: *public administration, comprehensiveness, universality, portability,* and *accessibility* in successfully establishing the Canadian system of social health insurance (Armstrong & Armstrong, 1998). In 2003, as part of the Romanow Report, Canada adopted a sixth basic principle, *accountability* (Romanow, 2002).

FRAMING THE ISSUES FOR REFORM

As G. K. Chesterton observed many years ago, "it isn't that we can't see the solution, it's that we can't see the problem" (Goldsmith, 2003). It makes all the difference in the world how an issue is framed, and by whom. Consider this example: The current debate still raging over how a prescription drug benefit can be provided to Medicare beneficiaries has been diverted from the real problem—the soaring costs of pharmaceutical products—to such far removed issues as privatizing and dismantling Medicare itself. Based upon what we saw in chapters 9 and 10, it is readily apparent why this is occurring—it best serves the interests of the drug industry and private health plans and fits into the political agenda of conservative legislators who want to eliminate entitlement programs and downsize government. The drug industry fiercely opposes price controls, and lobbies against any increased expansion of public programs which would result in more effective discounting of their prices through bulk purchasing.

As is well documented in earlier chapters, these are some of the real problems which need to be addressed by health care reform:

- increasing unaffordability of health care and insurance coverage, with decreasing access to that care
- a tattered safety net at a time of fiscal deficits at all levels of government
- poor, and often preventable, outcomes of care for many millions of Americans due to access and cost problems
- failure of the public and the body politic to perceive that the market-based system cannot deliver an equitable system of care
- increasing cost shifting from insurers and employers to patients under the guise of increased choice and personal responsibility
- continued opposition by stakeholders who want to maintain the status quo, which has blocked reform at every turn
- lack of transparency and accountability of the corporate health care sector as it pursues profits at the expense of patients
- the inherent problem of voluntary, competitive health insurance—the *inverse coverage law*—which holds that those that need coverage most are least likely to get it (Keen, Light, Mays, 2001).

Although these problems may seem diverse at first, for the purposes of reform they can be readily grouped under a small number of principles such as affordability and accessibility of care, comprehensiveness of necessary services, freedom of choice, quality of care, and accountability to the public. Here again, it will be dialogue over the principles—without diversion to technical details—which will enable the political process to go forward toward health care reform.

Many frame the debate over health care policy according to the ideologies of the major political parties, but this also distorts the issues and supports the interests of stakeholders in the existing system. National health insurance is but one of many examples; it has often been portrayed by its opponents over the years as some sort of socialist, or far-left radical scheme inconsistent with American political values. One needs to question, however, whether it is a radical idea to favor an affordable health care system accessible to the whole population instead of what we have.

Indeed, there is a strong conservative case to be made in favor of national health insurance, from the standpoints of eliminating waste, improving efficiency of the system, and making U.S. industries more competitive in global markets. U.S. employers now spend more than $6,600 per family each year for health insurance premiums and these costs have grown by almost 40% in the last three years. (Wessel, 2004). The National Association of Manufacturers, representing hundreds of small employers across the country, believes that U.S. companies are at a competitive disadvantage abroad because of their high health care costs. (Andrews, 2004). The Vice Chairman of Ford Motor Company recently had this to say on the subject: "Right now the country is on an unsustainable track and it won't get any better until we begin—business, labor and government in partnership—to make a pact for reform. A lot of people think a single-payer system is better." (Downey, 2004).

As Don McCanne, former President of Physicians for a National Health Program, observes:

> Why is this a partisan issue? Democrats are interested in ensuring access to affordable, comprehensive health care for everyone, or at least they should be. Republicans are interested in sound business principles which reduce administrative waste and contain costs, or at least they should be. (McCanne, 2003).

COMPARING ALTERNATIVE REFORM PROPOSALS BASED ON PRINCIPLES

As we have seen, incremental attempts to reform the U.S. health care system have been put forward into the political process and lobbied heavily for or against by supporters and critics, without much consideration of guiding principles or goals. The challenge, therefore, is twofold: first, to develop some degree of national consensus around the basic principles of the health care system, and second, to compare reform alternatives based on these principles before adopting changes of health policy.

If we take two basic principles for health care reform—universal coverage and affordability through effective cost controls—reform alternatives at the state or national level should be compared based on these principles. In California, for example, nine different reform proposals were recently studied by the Lewin Group as that state grapples with the problem of no insurance for 21% of its population. These proposals included six different combinations of employer or individual mandates, as well as three kinds of single-payer plans. With regard to universal coverage and costs, none of the employer/individual mandate proposals would achieve universal coverage, and all would increase costs. Only the single-payer proposals would provide universal coverage, while at the same time lowering costs (by up to $7 billion a year) (California Health Care Options project, 2002).

An important 1996 book by Daniels, Light, and Caplan, *Benchmarks of Fairness for Health Care Reform*, injects an essential element—fairness—into the debate over health care reform. This collaboration between a philosopher, a sociologist, and an economist, puts together a system of 10 benchmarks against which to evaluate and grade different reform proposals, including four major alternative bills debated in Congress in 1993–1994:

- The Michel Bill ("Affordable Health Care Now"), a minimally regulated, free-market proposal without any mandates and with government subsidies for low-income people
- The Cooper Bill ("Managed Competition Act"), another market-based proposal with moderate regulation of the private insurance market as well as proposals for state and regional purchasing pools and a required standard benefits package
- The Clinton Bill ("Health Security Act"), which guaranteed universal coverage through a heavily managed approach without effective cost controls
- The McDermott/Wellstone Bill ("American Health Security Act"), a public, tax-financed, single-payer plan for universal coverage with budgetary cost containment.

Table 14.1 shows how Daniels and his colleagues scored these four proposals against these 10 benchmarks. Each of the benchmarks is self-explanatory except for Benchmark 9, which refers to the extent to which the total budget for health care spending can be calculated and compared with the cost of all other goods and services in society (Daniels, Light, & Caplan, 1996).

The Institute of Medicine's Committee on the Consequences of Uninsurance has recently completed a comprehensive multi-year study of this problem. In its 2004 report *Insuring America's Health: Principles and Recommendations,* it called for a national effort to achieve universal coverage by 2010. Without taking a position on which of four prototype approaches could best meet that goal, each of the prototypes were compared against the Committee's five principles, as shown in Table 14.2 (Committee on the Consequences of Uninsurance (2004).

SOME USEFUL APPROACHES TOWARD REFORM

Based on the foregoing, I suggest below five targeted approaches as practical steps toward structural health care reform. The implementation of each is challenging in itself, given the powerful resistance to reform of stakeholders in the present system. But together they could lead to a political movement which can lead to reform when the failures of the market-based system become too intolerable for society to bear.

1. *Focus on national health insurance with universal coverage.* This book is filled with evidence that all incremental market-based reforms stack up poorly against the kinds of principles we should be basing them upon. The health care system, as one-seventh of the nation's economy, is admittedly enormous and difficult to reform. But, if and when a national system of social health insurance is achieved, many other system problems will be effectively addressed. As universal access to medically necessary care is assured, the fairness and outcomes of care will improve for the whole population. Global budgets can facilitate more effective cost containment while redirecting more of our already adequate health care spending from bureaucratic waste and profiteering to direct patient care. Monitoring of quality of care can be improved through simplified administrative and electronic information systems.

2. *Add cost effectiveness to regulatory reviews and the health policy debate.* Although cost-effectiveness of health care treatments and services should be uncontroversial, this criterion is often not applied in everyday clinical practice. Many treatments provided are of marginal benefit, are sometimes more harmful than beneficial, and are often provided without regard to cost. (Schuster, McGlynn, Brook, 1998;

TABLE 14.1. Benchmarks of Fairness for United States Health Care Reform Proposals

	Public Financing/ Private Practice (McDermont (Wellstone)	Heavily Regulated Market Approach (Clinton)	Moderately Regulated Market Approach (Cooper)	Least Regulated Free Market Approach (Michel)
Benchmark 1:				
Universal Access—Coverage and Participation				
Mandatory Coverage and Participation	4.5	4.0	1.5	0.5
Prompt Phase-in	4.5	4.0	2.0	1.5
Portability	5.0	4.0	2.0	1.5
Average Score for Benchmark 1	4.7	4.0	1.8	1.2
Benchmark 2:				
Minimizing Nonfinancial Barriers				
Minimizing Maldistributions	5.0	4.5	0.5	0.5
Reform of Health Professional Education	4.0	4.0	4.0	0.0
Minimizing Language, Culture, Class Barriers	2.0	3.0	0.0	0.0
Minimizing Educational and Informational Barriers	2.0	4.5	3.5	3.0
Average Score for Benchmark 2	3.3	4.0	2.0	0.9
Benchmark 3:				
Comprehensive and Uniform Benefits				
Comprehensiveness	4.5	15	1.5	0.0
Reduced Tiering and Uniform Quality	3.0	2.5	1.5	0.0
Benefits Not Dependent on Savings	5.0	4.0	0.0	0.0
Average Score for Benchmark 3	4.2	3.3	1.0	0.0
Benchmark 4:				
Equitable Financing—Community-rated Contributions				
True Community-rated Premiums	5.0	3.5	2.0	1.5
Minimum Discrimination via Cash Payments	5.0	1.5	0.5	0.0
Average Score for Benchmark 4	5.0	2.5	1.3	0.8
Benchmark 5:				
Equitable Financing—By Ability to Pay	5.0	2.0	1.0	0.0

Benchmark 6:				
Value For Money—Clinical Efficacy				
Emphasis on Primary Care	2.0	4.5	4.0	1.0
Emphasis on Public Health and Prevention	1.5	2.5	2.0	1.0
Systematic Assessment of Outcomes	4.5	3.5	2.5	2.0
Minimizing Overmilization and Underutilization	4.0	4.0	3.5	2.0
Average Score for Benchmark 6	3.0	3.6	3.0	1.5
Benchmark 7:				
Value For Money—Financial Efficacy				
Minimizing Administrative Overhead	5.0	3.0	2.5	2.0
Tough Contractual Bargaining	5.0	3.5	0.0	0.0
Minimizing Cost Shifting	5.0	3.0	2.0	0.0
Anti-Fraud and Abuse Measures	3.0	3.5	2.0	3.5
Average Score for Benchmark 7	4.5	3.3	1.6	1.4
Benchmark 8:				
Public Accountability				
Explicit Public Procedures for Evaluation	4.0	4.5	3.0	2.5
Explicit Democratic Procedures for Resource Allocation	2.0	2.0	0.5	0.0
Fair Grievance Procedures	1.0	5.0	4.0	2.0
Adequate Privacy Protection	-1.0	1.0	-1.0	1.0
Average Score for Benchmark 8	1.5	3.1	1.6	1.4
Benchmark 9:				
Comparability	5.0	3.0	0.0	0.0
Benchmark 10:				
Degree of Consumer Choice				
Choice of Primary-Care Provider	5.0	3.5	1.0	0.5
Choice of Specialists	5.0	-1.5	-3.5	-1.0
Choice of Other Health Care Providers	5.0	-2.0	-2.0	-1.0
Choice of Procedure	5.0	-3.0	-3.0	0.0
Average Score for Benchmark 10	5.0	-0.8	-1.9	-0.4
TOTAL: Average Score Across All Benchmarks	4.1	2.8	1.1	0.7

Explanation of Scores: Reform proposals were judged according to how much they would increase, or decrease the fairness of the U.S. Health Care System. A score of zero represents no change from the status quo of 1994. Santa, range from–5.0 to +5.0.

Source: Daniels, N., et al. (1996). *Benchmarks of fairness for health care reform.* New York: Oxford University Press. Reprinted with permission.

TABLE 14.2. Summary Assessment of Prototypes Based on Committee Principles

Principles	Status Quo	Prototype 1 Major Public Program Extension and New Tax Credit
Coverage should be universal	Not universal; 43 million uninsured	*Would not achieve universality because voluntary,* but would reduce uninsured population
Coverage should be continuous	*Not continuous;* income, age, family, job, and health-related *gaps in coverage*	Family- and job-related *gaps in coverage*
Coverage should be affordable for individuals and families	*Private coverage unaffordable* to many moderate- and low-income persons	*More affordable than current system* for those with low or moderate income
Strategy should be affordable and sustainable for society	*Not affordable or sustainable for society;* uninsurance is growing; cost of poorer health and shorter lives is $65–$130 billion; some participants contribute; no limit on aggregate health expenditures or on tax expenditures-spending is higher than other countries, sustainability of current public programs depends on economy and political support	All participants contribute; *aggregate expenditures not controlled; new public expenditures for only the public program expansion and tax credit;* sustainability of public program depends on revenue sources and political support; size of credit depends on political support
Coverage should enhance health through high-quality care	*Quality of care* for the population *limited* because one in seven is uninsured	Opportunities to promote quality improvements *similar to current system*

continued

Fisher & Welch, 1999; Leape, 1992). Although other countries integrate cost-effectiveness into their regulatory review of drugs (e.g., Australia), our FDA has been unwilling to add cost-effectiveness to its regulatory review process, knowing that it would create a firestorm of protest from industry (Abboud & McGinley, 2003). Archie Cochrane, a well known international leader in health services research, has emphasized the primacy of cost-effectiveness for attaining efficiency in any health care system. Table 14.3 presents the Cochrane Test for health care systems, which if taken seriously by

TABLE 14.2. *(continued)*

Prototype 2	Prototype 3	Prototype 4
Employer Mandate, Premium Subsidy, and Individual Mandate	Individual Mandate and Tax Credit	Single Payer
Coverage likely to be high; depends on enforcement of mandates	Depends on size of tax credit, *enforcement*, and cost of individual insurance	Likely to achieve universal *coverage*
Brief gaps related to life and job transitions	*Minimal gaps*	*Continuous* until death or age 65
Yes for workers, assuming adequate employer premium assistance; *public program designed to be affordable* for all enrollees	Subsidy based only on income and family size leaves *older, less healthy, and those in expensive areas with less affordable coverage*	*Minimal cost sharing*, but could be problem for lowest income
All participants contribute; *basic package less costly than current employment coverage;* revenue from patients in public program; sustainability depends on revenue sources for employers' premium assistance and public program	No limit on aggregate health expenditures or on tax expenditure, though federal costs relatively predictable and controllable through size of credit; *sustainable through federal income tax base;* size of credit depends on political support	Nearly all participants contribute; *aggregate expenditures controllable,* utilization not directly or centrally controlled; *high cost to federal budget;* administrative savings; sustainability depends on revenue source and political support
Could design quality incentives in expanded public program and basic benefit package; current employer incentives for quality remain	*Similar incentives to current private insurance* system, consumer could choose quality plans	*Potentially yes;* depends on proper design

U.S. health policy, would move our system toward greater efficiency, improved quality, and substantial cost savings (Cochrane, 1972; Light, 1991).

3. *Build new coalitions toward a political movement.* Meaningful health care reform has been blocked at every turn for many years by the politics of divisiveness and blame. The insured have been pitted against the uninsured, patients against providers, and employers against employees. As we have also seen, each major group is often

TABLE 14.3. The Cochrane Test

(1) Consider anything that works
(2) Make effective treatments available to all
(3) Minimize ill-timed interventions
(4) Treat patients in the most cost-effective place
(5) Prevent only what is preventable
(6) Diagnose only if treatable

Source: Light, D. W. (1991). Effectiveness and efficiency under competition: The Cochrane test. *British Medical Journal, 303,* 1254. Reprinted with permission.

divided within itself, as is the case with large insurers and employers versus their smaller counterparts. As observed by Jamie Court, well-known consumer advocate and co-author of *Making a Killing: HMOs and the Threat to your Health,* "The hope for a new political dynamic arises because the system is so broken that only radical change can save any one group" (Court, 2002). Reform will become most likely and politically feasible when both the benefits and costs of proposed reforms are distributed widely (Thai, Qiao, & McManus, 1998). When the interests of the major segments of society for fundamental health care reform coincide with the public interest, the longstanding political logjam can be broken. The most important groups for coalition building would appear to be business, employees (including organized labor), health professionals, faith-based groups (especially the Catholic church), and consumers.

4. *Leadership by health professionals.* Physicians, nurses, and other health professionals see up close the problems being experienced every day by their patients in a collapsing health care system, as well as the often preventable adverse clinical outcomes resulting from delayed care. They also encounter the mindless bureaucracy that handicaps our complex and fragmented system, and which increasingly diverts their energies from direct patient care. They are in an excellent position to call attention within their communities and professional organizations to ways in which our system is failing their patients, and to advocate for system reform.

Organized medicine has a poor track record in this regard, having opposed any system of universal coverage throughout the last century. The widespread inequities of our present system, however, present new opportunities for medicine to take a more active leadership role in reform. Recent years have seen calls for renewed professionalism in medicine (Pellegrino, 2000; Bulger, 2000; Mechanic, 2000) which would provide obvious opportunities for active involvement:

- Recommit to service as the raison d'etre of medicine.
- Embrace evidence-based and population-based medicine, while preserving a personal partnership with patients.
- Re-examine professional roles in an effort to avoid conflicts of interest that work against the needs of patients or populations being served.
- Take a leadership role in determining necessary care and delivering appropriate care of the best possible quality within available resources.
- Redesign practice systems based on evidence-based guidelines, with the goal of increasing efficiencies and cost-effectiveness of health care services.
- Join with other health professionals in advocating for major structural reform of the health care system to serve the public interest exclusively, not the interests of special groups.

5. *Better educate the public about health policy issues.* As we saw in chapter 9, much of the information being presented by the media about the health care system is biased by the self-interest of stakeholders in the present market-based system. More responsible coverage of health care issues by the media will be required to educate the public about needed reforms in the public interest. More disclosure about conflicts of interest and transparency concerning funding sources for public education reports and programs are urgently needed. Health professionals have both an opportunity and a responsibility to expose disinformation and clarify misconceptions through their research, associations, and publications.

CONCLUDING COMMENTS

Our journey through many parts of the enormous and complicated U.S. health care system has revealed extensive evidence that it has been transformed over the last 30 years by a for-profit corporate business ethic. This sea change has been detrimental to the health of individual citizens and the population as a whole. Based on their track record, we are forced to conclude that market-based policies favoring corporate interests do not serve the public interest well, and that corporations are not sufficiently self-regulating. The health care system needs to be rebuilt based on principles of fairness that will assure access, affordability, and quality of care for everyone.

A case has been made for the conversion to a publicly-financed system of social health insurance, whether on a state-by-state basis or, preferably, as a national system. A case has also been made to convert much of health care from a for-profit business to a public utility model.

As the nation becomes immersed in political campaigns for the 2004 election, widespread concerns over soaring health care costs, and the growing numbers of uninsured and insecurely insured Americans have risen to the top of the domestic agenda according to many national polls. Rising health care costs are now recognized as one cause of the country's "jobless recovery" (Pollack, 2003) It is becoming more obvious every day that the health care system is not sustainable on its present course. Meanwhile, "incremental reforms" which neither control costs nor assure universal coverage are being proposed nationally and in statehouses across the country.

Fortunately, there is a solution to the travails of the U.S. health care system. In his recent editorial commenting upon the 2003 Proposal of the Physicians' Working Group for Single-Payer National Health Insurance, endorsed by over 12,000 U.S. physicians (Woolhandler, et al., 2003), Rashi Fein, a well-known economist, had this to say:

> The American health care system and American society face a real problem and are compelled to search for an answer . . . The members of the Physicians' Working Group have done their job by raising the issue of national health insurance once again. Those who like their proposal should join with them. Those who do not should develop and propose something better, more effective, and with fewer untoward side effects. No one should sit back and bemoan the existing state of affairs. The "health care mess" is too real for anyone to ignore it. (Fein, 2003).

So what will happen? We cannot yet know, but this observation by Marcia Angell, former editor-in-chief of *The New England Journal of Medicine,* is on target:

> Either the United States can join every other advanced nation and develop a national single-payer health care system, or we can keep going the way we are and eventually have a three-tier system in which the wealthy get whatever health care they want, the middle-class gets some kind of stripped-down managed care, and the rest get nothing. In that respect, we would be just like a Third World country. (Angell, 2003)

The health care crisis is real. The stakes are high and how we approach the problems as a society and nation will test our democracy to its core.

REFERENCES

Abboud, L., & McGinley, L. (2003, April 16). FDA chief embarks on novel mission: cut drug costs. *Wall Street Journal*, pA4.

Andrews, C. (1995). *Profit fever: The drive to corporatize health care and how to stop it.* Monroe, ME: Common Courage Press.

Andrews, E. L. (2004, Feb. 24). Small business. Health care heights. *New York Times*, E1.

Angell, M. (2003, Jan. 5). Outlook. They can see it coming. *The Washington Post*.

Armstrong, P., & Armstrong, H. (1998). *Universal health care: What the United States can learn from the Canadian experience.* New York: The New Press.

Birn, A. E., & Fein, O. (2003). Why "rekindling reform?" *American Journal of Public Health, 93*, 15.

Bodenheimer, T. (2003). The movement for universal health insurance: Finding common ground. *American Journal of Public Health, 93*, 112.

Bulger, R. J. (2000). The quest for a therapeutic organization. *Journal of the American Medical Association 283*, 2431.

California Health Care Options Project (2002). Draft proposals. Available at *http://www.healthcareoptions.ca.gov/doclib.asp*

Cochrane, A. (1972). Effectiveness and efficiency: Random refections on health services. London: Nuffield Provincial Hospitals Trust.

Committee on the Consequences of Uninsurance. Institute of Medicine (2004). *Insuring America's Health: Principles and recommendations.* National Academy Press, Washington, DC,: 150–151.

Court, J. (2002, Dec. 9). Universal coverage will take universal sacrifice. Available at *www.consumerwatchdog.org/ftcr/co/co0029.php3*

Daniels, N., Light, D. W., Caplan, R. L. (1996). *Benchmarks of fairness for health care reform.* New York: Oxford University Press.

Downey, K. (2004, March 6). A heftier dose to swallow. *The Washington Post*.

Fein, R. (2003). Universal health insurance—let the debate resume. *Journal of the American Medical Association, 290*, 817.

Fisher, E. S., & Welch, H. G. (1999). Avoiding the unintended consequences of growth in medical care: How might more be worse? *Journal of the American Medical Association 281*, 446.

Geyman, J. P. (2002). *Health care in America: Can our ailing system be healed?* (p. 418). Woburn, MA: Butterworth-Heinemann.

Goldsmith, J. (2003). The road to meaningful reform: A conversation with Oregon's John Kitzhaber. *Health Affairs (Millwood), 22*(1), 124.

Gordon, C. (1995). *The Clinton Health Care Plan: Dead on arrival.* Westfield, NJ: Open Magazine Pamphlet Series.

Institute of Medicine (2003). Committee on the Consequences of Uninsurance. *Hidden costs, value lost: Uninsurance in America (p. 179)*. Washington, DC: National Academy Press.

Keen, J., Light, D., Mayo, N. (2001). *Public-private relations in health care*. London: King's Fund.

Leape, L. L. (1992). Unnecessary surgery. *Annual Review Public Health 13*, 363.

Light, D. W. (1991). Effectiveness and efficiency under competition: The Cochrane Test. *British Medical Journal, 303,* 1254.

McCanne, D. (2003). Quote of the Day. Accessed May 21, 2003. from mccanne.org

Mechanic, D. (2000). Managed care and the imperative for a new professional ethic. *Health Affairs (Millwood), 19*(5), 100.

Pellegrino, E.D. (2000). Medical professionalism: Can it, should it survive? *Journal of the American Board of Family Practice, 13,* 147.

Pollack, R. (2003, Sept. 30). Executive Director, *Families USA:* 43.6 million uninsured Americans. Fox News.

Romanow, R. (2002, Nov. 28). Commission on the Future of Health Care in Canada. Final Report, Ottawa, Ontario.

Schuster, M., McGlynn, E. A. Brook, R. H. (1998). How good is the quality of health care in the United States? *Milbank Quarterly, 76*(4), 517.

The Tavistock Group. (1999). A shared statement of ethical principles for those who shape and give health care: A working draft. *Effective Clinical Practice, 2,* 143.

Thai, K. V., Qiao, Y., McManus, S. M. (1998). National health care reform failure: The political economy perspective. *Journal of Health and Human Services Administration, 21*(2), 236.

The Ad Hoc Committee to Defend Health Care (1997). For our patients, not for profits: A call for action. *JAMA, 278*(21): 1733–1738.

Wessel, D. Health care costs blamed for hiring gap. *Wall Street Journal* March 11, 2004: A2.

Woolhandler, S., Himmelstein, D. U. Angell, M., Young, Q. D., and the Physicians Working Group for Single-Payer National Health Insurance (2003). Proposal of the Physicians' Working Group for Single-Payer National Health Insurance. *Journal of the American Medical Association, 290,* 798.

APPENDIX 1

THE "UNITED STATES NATIONAL HEALTH INSURANCE ACT," H.R. 676

("Expanded & Improved Medicare For All Bill")
*Introduced by Cong. John Conyers, Jim McDermott, Dennis Kucinich, and Donna Christensen

BRIEF SUMMARY OF LEGISLATION

- The **United States National Health Insurance Act** establishes a new American program by creating a single payer health care system. The bill would create a publically financed, privately delivered health care program that uses the already existing Medicare program by expanding and improving it to all U.S. residents, and all residents living in U.S. territories. The goal of the legislation is to ensure that all Americans, guaranteed by law, will have access to the highest quality and cost effective health care services regardless of one's employment, income, or health care status.
- With over **75 million** uninsured Americans, and another **50 million** who are under insured, the time has come to change our inefficient and costly fragmented health care system.
- The USNHI would reduce health spending in **2005** from **$1,918 billion to 1,861.3 billion.** Over-all government spending would be reduced by **56 billion** while covering all of the uninsured. In **2005**, without reform, the average employer that offers coverage will contribute **$2,600** to health care per employee (for much skimpier benefits). Under this proposal, the average costs to employers for an employee making **$30,000** per year will be reduced to **$1,155** per month, less than **$100** per month. Previous Medicare For All studies concluded that an average family of three would pay a total of **$739.00** annually in total health care costs.

WHO IS ELIGIBLE?

- Every person living in the United States and the U.S. Territories would receive a **United States National Health Insurance Card**

and i.d. number once they enroll at the appropriate location. Social Security numbers may not be used when assigning i.d. cards. No co-pays or deductibles are permissible under this act.

BENEFITS/PORTABILITY

- This program will cover **all medically necessary services,** including primary care, inpatient care, outpatient care, emergency care, prescription drugs, durable medical equipment, long term care, mental health services, dentistry, eye care, chiropractic, and substance abuse treatment. Patients have their **choice of physicians, providers, hospitals, clinics, and practices.**

Conversion to a Non-Profit Health Care System

- Private health insurers shall be **prohibited under this act from selling coverage that duplicates the benefits of the USNHI program.** They shall not be prohibited from selling coverage for any additional benefits not covered by this Act; examples include cosmetic surgery, and other medically unnecessary treatments.

Cost Containment Provisions/Reimbursement

- The National USNHI program will annually set reimbursement rates for physicians, health care providers, and negotiate prescription drug prices The national office will provide an annual lump sum allotment to each existing Medicare region, which will then administer the program. Payment to health care providers include fee for service, and global budgets.
- The conversion to a not-for-profit health care system will take place over a 15 year period, through the sale of U.S. treasury bonds; payment will not be made for loss of business profits, but only for real estate, buildings, and equipment.

FUNDING & ADMINISTRATION

- The United States Congress will establish annual funding outlays for the USNHI program through an annual entitlement. The USNHI program will operate under the auspices of the **Dept of Health & Human Services,** and be administered in the former Medicare offices. All current expenditures for public health insurance programs such as S-CHIP, Medicaid, and Medicare will be placed into the USNHI program.

- **A National USNHI Advisory Board** will be established, comprised primarily of health care professionals and representatives of health advocacy groups.

PROPOSED FUNDING FOR USNHI PROGRAM

- Maintaining current federal and state funding of existing health care programs. A modest payroll tax on all employers of **3.3%**. A **5%** health tax on the top **5%** of income earners. A small tax on stock and bond transfers. Closing corporate tax shelters. Charitable contributions. For more details, see Physicians For A National Health Program *Financing National Health Insurance.*

*For more information, contact Joel Segal, legislative assistant, Rep. John Conyers, at 202-225-5126, or e-mail at Joel.Segal@mail.house.gov.

APPENDIX 2

Potential administrative savings by state, 2003, achievable with a single-payer national health insurance program

	Projected 2003 health expenditures ($ millions annually)	Admininistrative expenses in 2003 ($ millions annually)	Potential administrative savings in 2003 ($ millions annually)	Uninsured Residents in 2001 (thousands)	Administrative savings per uninsured resident ($)
United States	1,660,500	399,356	285,961	41,206	6,940
Alabama	22,541	6,205	4,459	573	7,781
Alaska	3,011	787	565	100	5,650
Arizona	21,673	5,848	4,296	950	4,522
Arkansas	12,319	3,341	2,360	428	5,515
California	162,943	45,041	33,699	6,718	5,016
Colorado	19,568	5,231	3,802	687	5,534
Connecticut	22,144	5,967	4,225	346	12,212
Delaware	4,433	1,186	837	73	11,468
District of Columbia	6,226	1,816	1,244	70	17,771
Florida	87,077	23,578	17,071	2,856	5,977
Georgia	39,293	10,765	7,805	1,376	5,672
Hawaii	6,612	1,798	1,325	117	11,321
Idaho	4,937	1,289	919	210	4,378
Illinois	63,778	17,389	12,339	1,676	7,362
Indiana	30,641	8,367	5,902	714	8,266
Iowa	14,716	3,987	2,777	216	12,857
Kansas	13,441	3,610	2,562	301	8,511
Kentucky	20,895	5,718	4,042	492	8,216
Louisiana	23,729	6,622	4,680	845	5,538
Maine	7,068	1,884	1,325	132	10,037
Maryland	28,166	7,647	5,509	653	8,437
Massachusetts	43,603	12,090	8,556	520	16,453
Michigan	50,907	13,591	9,638	1,028	9,375
Minnesota	28,862	7,885	5,793	392	14,777
Mississippi	13,044	3,609	2,537	459	5,527
Missouri	30,539	8,440	5,931	565	10,498
Montana	4,122	1,115	784	121	6,477
Nebraska	47,320	12,625	1,637	160	10,233
Nevada	8,821	2,362	1,577	344	4,585
New Hampshire	8,058	2,134	1,277	119	10,733
New Jersey	6,656	1,773	9,030	1,109	8,143
New Mexico	7,745	2,108	1,500	373	4,022
New York	122,958	33,664	23,437	2,916	8,037
North Carolina	38,733	10,552	7,472	1,167	6,403
North Dakota	3,854	1,073	745	60	12,415
Ohio	60,353	16,530	11,644	1,248	9,330
Oklahoma	15,734	4,273	3,038	620	4,899
Oregon	15,811	4,069	2,938	443	6,631
Pennsylvania	73,293	19,932	14,053	1,119	12,559
Rhode Island	6,353	1,672	1,174	80	14,677
South Carolina	18,780	5,057	3,569	493	7,240
South Dakota	4,005	1,104	780	69	11,305
Tennessee	31,474	8,690	6,256	640	9,775
Texas	98,742	27,082	19,469	4,960	3,925
Utah	8,567	2,241	1,607	335	4,798
Vermont	2,963	774	552	58	9,513
Virginia	31,994	8,566	6,130	774	7,920
Washington	27,912	7,265	5,254	780	6,735
West Virginia	10,129	2,743	1,939	234	8,286
Wisconsin	28,598	7,727	5,527	409	13,513
Wyoming	2,019	534	376	78	4,814

Source: Woolhandler S, Campbell T, and Himmelstein DU. "Administrative Waste in the U.S. Health Care System in 2003: The Cost to the Nation, the States, and the District of Columbia, with State-Specific Estimates of Potential Savings"; *International Journal of Health Services*, 34:1, 79-86, 2004.

INDEX

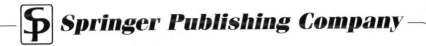

Springer Publishing Company

Linking Medical Care and Community Services

Practical Models for Bridging the Gap

Walter Leutz, PhD, Merwyn R. Greenlick, PhD, and Lucy Nonnenkamp, MA

How can a medical care system structure itself best to serve the total needs of the frail and disabled members of its population? Kaiser Permanente set out to answer this question. Its extraordinary 32-site demonstration program investigated the issues linking two systems (medical and long-term care) to improve how helping professionals and organizations can cooperate to assist people in their struggles to cope with chronic illness and disability.

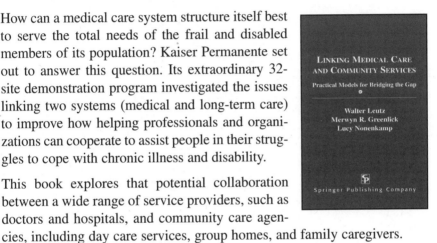

This book explores that potential collaboration between a wide range of service providers, such as doctors and hospitals, and community care agencies, including day care services, group homes, and family caregivers.

Contents:
* Introduction
* Coping with Aging and Disability, *W. Leutz*
* Manifesto 2005, *W. Leutz, M. Greenlick, and K. Brody*
* Reaching Out and Linking Up, *W. Leutz, M. Hillier, E. Hunkeler, et al.*
* Individuals with Disabilities and Their Families, *W. Leutz, A. Au, K. Brody, et al.*
* Looking Inward: Making Changes in Complex Organizations,
  W. Leutz, J. Bath, L. Johns, et al.
* Infants, Children, and Non-Elderly Adults with Disabilities, *C. Green,*
  N. Vuckovic, P. Bourgeois, et al.
* Challenges and Opportunities -- Strengths and Weaknesses,
  W. Leutz, M. Greenlick, and L. Nonnenkamp
* A Prototype for 2005, *W. Leutz, M. Greenlick, R. DellaPenna, et al.*

2003 256pp 0-8261-1754-6 hard

11 West 42nd Street, New York, NY 10036-8002 • Fax: 212-941-7842
Order Toll-Free: 877-687-7476 • Order On-line: www.springerpub.com

Springer Publishing Company

The Business of Medical Practice
Advanced Profit Maximization
Techniques for Savvy Doctors
2nd Edition

David Edward Marcinko, MBA, CFP, CMP, Editor

"Dr. Marcinko has once again...produced what is arguably the essential medical management work for physicians in today's dynamically changing and increasingly business oriented practice environment."
  —**Robert James Cimasi,** ASA, CBA, AVA, FCBI
President, Health Capital Consultants, LLC
St. Louis, Missouri

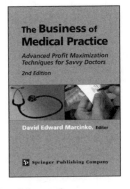

An interdisciplinary team of experts teaches newcomers how to open, staff, and equip an insurance-friendly office for patients, and how to raise the capital necessary for it. New coverage in the second edition includes how to write a medical office business plan; compliance methods, risks and programs, and the insurance CPT coding issues; six-sigma initiatives; futuristic information technology to track clinical outcomes, treatment results and medical care; physician recruitment, and more!

Partial Contents:
Section I: Qualitative Aspects of Medical Practice • Healthcare Economics in Medical Practice • Medical Practice Strategic Operating Plan • Establishing Healthy Medical Partner Relationships

Section II: Quantitative Aspects of Medical Practice • Cash Flow Analysis and Management • Medical Office Expense Modeling • Accounting for Mixed Practice Costs • Medical Activity Based Cost Management

Section III: Contemporary Aspects of Medical Practice • Medical Information Systems and Office Business Equipment • Human Resource Outsourcing for the Physician Executive • Medical Practice Non Compete Agreements • Physician Recruitment

2004   520pp   0-8261-2375-9   hard

11 West 42nd Street, New York, NY 10036-8002 • **Fax: 212-941-7842**
Order Toll-Free: 877-687-7476 • **Order On-line: www.springerpub.com**